TWENTY ONE DAY LOAN

This item is to be returned on
or before the date stamped below

UNIVERSITY OF PLYMOUTH

PLYMOUTH LIBRARY

Tel: (01752) 232323

This item is available for the student loan period of 21 days
It is subject to recall if required by another reader
CHARGES WILL BE MADE FOR OVERDUE BOOKS

DERMATOLOGY
AND THE
NEW GENETICS

DERMATOLOGY AND THE NEW GENETICS

CELIA MOSS

MA, DM(Oxford), MRCP(London)

Consultant Dermatologist
The Children's Hospital
Ladywood, Birmingham, UK

JOHN SAVIN

MA, MD(Cantab),
FRCP(London and Edinburgh), DIH

Consultant Dermatologist
Royal Infirmary
Edinburgh, UK

b

Blackwell
Science

For our families

©1995 by
Blackwell Science Ltd
Editorial Offices:
Osney Mead, Oxford OX2 0EL
25 John Street, London WC1N 2BL
23 Ainslie Place, Edinburgh EH3 6AJ
238 Main Street, Cambridge
  Massachusetts 02142, USA
54 University Street, Carlton
  Victoria 3053, Australia

Other Editorial Offices:
Arnette Blackwell SA
  1, rue de Lille, 75007 Paris
  France

Blackwell Wissenschafts-Verlag GmbH
  Kurfürstendamm 57
  10707 Berlin, Germany

  Feldgasse 13, A-1238 Wien
  Austria

First published 1995

Set by
EXPO Holdings, Malaysia
Printed and bound in Italy
by Vincenzo Bona srl, Turin

DISTRIBUTORS

Marston Book Services Ltd
PO Box 87
Oxford OX2 0DT
(*Orders*: Tel: 01865 791155
    Fax: 01865 791927
    Telex: 837515)

North America
Blackwell Science, Inc.
238 Main Street
Cambridge, MA 02142
(*Orders*: Tel: 800 215-1000
    617 876-7000
    Fax: 617 492-5263)

Australia
Blackwell Science Pty Ltd
54 University Street
Carlton, Victoria 3053
(*Orders*: Tel: 03 347-0300
    Fax: 03 349-3016)

A catalogue record for this title
is available from the British Library

ISBN 0–632–03582–X

Library of Congress
Cataloging-in-Publication Data

Moss, Celia.
    Dermatology and the new genetics/
    Celia Moss, John Savin.
        p.   cm.
    Includes bibliographical references
    and index.
    ISBN 0–632–03582–X
    1. Skin—Diseases—Genetic aspects.
    I. Savin, John.   II. Title.
    [DNLM: 1. Skin Diseases—genetics.
    WR 218 M913d 1995]
    RL72.M67 .1995
    616.5′042—dc20
DNLM/DLC
for Library of Congress   94–33892
                                             CIP

CONTENTS

PREFACE

Dermatology needed the new genetics. It had fallen into a rut. Its clinical rarities had long since been collected and stuck in textbooks in neat rows, like stamps. Many associations between uncommon disorders had been ferreted out and recorded, but this had become an end in itself. Some smugness may have crept in, but, surprisingly, this limited and apparently sterile approach allowed the new genetics, when it came, to sweep quickly through a highly ordered subject.

At that point a fog lifted and much of dermatology could be seen clearly, for the first time. Many clinical mysteries now make sense and the topics illuminated range right from the somatic mosaicism of birth marks to the oncogenes of the tumours of old age. This massive expansion of knowledge has been the main impact of the new genetics.

It continues apace. The total number of genes mapped to specific chromosomes has doubled since 1988 and the whole human genome will surely be mapped over the next few years. No aspect of dermatology will be left untouched. But it is all happening so fast that many busy dermatologists are in danger of being left behind.

They have little time to read about molecular biology or animal genetics, yet they need to know about recent advances in their field to practice to a high standard. They dislike the way the subject seems to be accelerating out of their grasp. As clinical dermatologists we have shared their difficulties, and it is for them we have written this book.

The task has not been easy. We have had to struggle to clarify matters which are inherently complicated, and apologize for any oversimplifications we have preferred to obscurities. We have also tried to be both comprehensive and focused at the same time. To achieve the first aim we have mentioned all of the conditions listed in McKusick's *Mendelian Inheritance in Man*, which we thought would be of interest to dermatologists, accepting that others might have selected differently. To achieve the second aim we have spent more time on advancing subjects than on static ones. We have also broken away from the custom of most books on genodermatology by including common skin diseases.

Our theme has not been how to recognize skin disorders, or how to manage them, but how to bridge the gap between clinical dermatology and the new genetics. We have included a number of clinical photographs and there are many excellent atlases already in existence that can, of course, be used in conjunction with our book. For those who are not familiar with the jargon of genetics there is a glossary of terms at the back of the book.

INTRODUCTION:
GENES AND THE SKIN

Genetics has advanced over the past 50 years not in a steady stream but in waves, as each new technological floodgate has opened. The study of genes and their function began with Mendel, whose principles were well established by the beginning of the 20th century. Although Garrod wrote about the inheritance of alkaptonuria in 1902, it was nearly 50 years before genetics became biochemical with the recognition of protein products of genes. Techniques for banding chromosomes developed in the 1960s and opened up the science of cytogenetics; and in the 1980s methods of analysing DNA ushered in the era of molecular genetics.

Many more technological barriers have been washed away by this latest wave. The structure of DNA was established by Watson and Crick in 1953, but its repetitive simplicity evaded further analysis until restriction enzymes were discovered. Fragments of DNA, cleaved by restriction enzymes and separated by electrophoresis, were difficult to manipulate until a method was developed to 'blot' them on to a more robust substrate. Identification of DNA sequences became possible with recombinant technology, which utilizes the ability of single-stranded DNA to anneal only to an exactly complementary strand of DNA or RNA. These three principles are used sequentially in Southern blotting. The scantiness of the available material has been another obstacle, as each gene occurs only once in each cell. This has been overcome by ingenious methods of amplification including gene cloning and the polymerase chain reaction (PCR).

Molecular genetics looks not only at the structure of genes but also at how they are arranged on chromosomes, what they do, how they are controlled and how mistakes may occur.

The process of gene mapping began with Mendel and with the X chromosome: a condition that was sex-linked was X-linked. The X-linked disorders were at first mapped roughly, according to whether they were linked to colour blindness, now known to lie towards the end of the long arm. Autosomal mapping awaited the development of cytogenetics. The first genes mapped were those associated with a chromosomal abnormality: a chromosomal break may indicate the position of the abnormal gene. The banded pattern of chromosomes still provides the essential backbone for gene mapping, but molecular techniques have added greatly to the power of cytogenetics. DNA probes have largely replaced phenotypic and biochemical traits as markers in family linkage studies. They are also used to locate genes more directly in chromosomes that have been physically separated; for example, in a mitotic spread (*in situ*), or by somatic cell hybridization, or in a fluorescence activated chromosome sorter.

Gene function can be elucidated in a variety of ways. Once the DNA sequence has been established it can be used to deduce the nature of the protein product. Even if the complete sequence is unknown, the gene may be amplified by cloning or PCR for further functional study; for example, in hybrid cells or transgenic animals. Deducing the pathogenesis of a disorder by mapping and cloning the gene, rather than by studying the pathophysiology of the condition is called reverse genetics. More often genetics is bidirectional, for example, knowledge of the biochemistry of a disorder may suggest a candidate gene, the role of which can be tested by linkage studies or by looking for mutations in that gene in affected individuals.

Genetic errors are frequent. Genes may be duplicated or contain additional material, or they may be deleted in part or completely, sometimes along with a contiguous gene. Point mutations, described as missense, nonsense, stop-codon or frameshift, distort gene transcription in different ways. Splice mutations disturb the removal of introns. Mutations may affect not the gene itself but its promoters or other regulatory sequences. New types of mutation discovered in one situation are looked for in other situations, and often found —an application of the law stating that if something can go wrong it will.

Recent genetic discoveries seem almost to wash away Mendel's tenets altogether. We are bombarded with novel ideas such as genomic imprinting, uniparental disomy, variable number repeats, compound heterozygosity and gonadal mosaicism. But the fact that Mendel was able to distil a set of simple and timeless principles from such a complex system is reassuring: these newer concepts are fascinating and important but essentially simple variations on the classical theme.

What has all this to do with dermatology? The skin, as every medical student knows, is the largest organ in the body. It is also the most accessible. Disorders that differ only subtly, perhaps in their shade of pink or the arrangement of their spots, can be identified accurately in the skin but would be indistinguishable in the brain, lungs or liver. Genetic mosaicism is dramatically visible in the skin. The skin can be tested *in situ*, physically or chemically, and the results measured accurately. It can be biopsied and grafted. The component cells can be cultured *in vitro*, genetically engineered, and restored to the host, making it ideal for gene therapy. The superb research opportunities afforded by dermatology were a well-kept secret, until the advent of molecular genetics. Now, rare dermatoses feature in the mainstream scientific literature and skin cells have colonized every major molecular laboratory. Dermatologists are learning to swim with the tide.

Further reading

Archives of Dermatology. Molecular medicine issues. 1993; 129 (11 and 12).

Brock DJH. *Molecular Genetics for the Clinician*. Cambridge: Cambridge University Press, 1993.

Journal of Investigative Dermatology. The genetics of skin disease. 1994; 103 (5) (suppl.): 1S–154S.

Moss C. Dermatology and the human gene map. *Br. J. Dermatol.* 1991; 124: 3–9.

Priestley GC (ed) *Molecular Aspects of Dermatology*. Chichester: John Wiley and Sons, 1993.

Savin JA. The impact of the new genetics on dermatology. *Br. J. Hosp. Med.* 1994; 52: 264–268.

Weatherall DJ. *The New Genetics and Clinical Practice*, 3rd edn. Oxford: Oxford University Press, 1991.

A NOTE ON MIM NUMBERS

A few dermatologists glancing through this book may be puzzled by MIM numbers. These have nothing to do with the *Monthly Index of Medical Specialties*, but refer to the most influential textbook on genetics, Victor McKusick's *Mendelian Inheritance in Man* [1].

McKusick catalogues every genetic trait known, giving a brief description of the phenotype and the nature of the basic defect, with a summary of genetic information including mapping, molecular genetic details and key references. In the 10th edition there are nearly 6000 entries with 43387 references. Dermatological journals lie sixth in the order of specialty journals most often cited, after genetics itself, paediatrics, neurology, haematology and ophthalmology, and ahead of many other major specialties such as orthopaedics, cardiology, endocrinology, metabolism and chest medicine.

Each entry is assigned a six-digit number. The first digit indicates the mode of inheritance: 1 is autosomal dominant, 2 is autosomal recessive, and 3 is X linked. Within these three categories, entries are numbered in alphabetical order. There are spaces between the numbers (most end in 0) to allow for new entries. Like all genetic textbooks, each edition of *Mendelian Inheritance in Man* is out of date as soon as it is published, but it is constantly updated: new editions come out every 2 years, and an on-line version is also available (OMIM) [2]. There were 869 new entries between the ninth and tenth editions, while 96 entries were deleted or reassigned, usually because the gene responsible for a particular condition had been established. For example, some patients with Dowling–Meara epidermolysis bullosa simplex (MIM 131760) have a mutation in a keratin 14 gene (MIM 1480066).

McKusick is a mine of information. The casual reader will be intrigued by ACHOO syndrome (MIM 100820), dysmelodia (MIM 191200) and inability to smell freesias (MIM 229250), and may succumb to hyperlexia (MIM 238350). More important, geneticists around the world all turn to McKusick for an unambiguous designation. For example, the International Human Gene Mapping Workshops are based on McKusick numbers.

In this book, for the first time, dermatological terms are given alongside McKusick numbers, in the hope of making the vast genetic literature accessible to dermatologists, and vice versa.

References

1 McKusick VA. *Mendelian Inheritance in Man*. 11th edn. Catalogues of autosomal dominant, autosomal recessive and X-linked phenotypes. Baltimore: Johns Hopkins University Press, 1994.
2 OMIM™ (on-line *Mendelian Inheritance in Man*) available via SprintNet from the Welch Medical Library, Johns Hopkins University, 1830 East Monument Street, Third Floor, Baltimore, Md. 21205; Tel: 410-955-7058; Fax: 410-614-0434; e-mail: omimhelp@welch.jhu.edu.

1
SKIN DEVELOPMENT AND ITS DISORDERS

Embryogenesis

Embryology ought to help us understand congenital skin diseases, which must be due to antenatal errors, but most embryological events remain obscure. Studies of human fetuses give only snapshot pictures of this complex dynamic process, and experimental work on human embryos is still, as it were, in its infancy. However, information flows in both directions. Elucidating the genetic basis of developmental disorders such as ectodermal dysplasias, aplasia cutis and naevi will advance our knowledge of normal development.

The mechanics of skin development

Keratinocytes

At first the fetus is covered by periderm, a temporary protective monolayer derived from embryonic ectoderm. At about 4 weeks a basal layer appears in patches beneath the periderm, and by 11 weeks there are intermediate layers. Hemidesmosomes can be seen by 10 weeks; and by 14 weeks the epidermal keratins are all expressed, as is filaggrin by 15 weeks. The granular layer is present at 21 weeks and at 24 weeks the periderm separates.

In an adult, the cells produced by the basal layer move towards the surface in columns, but in the rapidly growing fetus they must also move sideways. The direction of proliferation is presumably dictated by the predominant direction of growth of the embryo. These aspects are considered in the section on Blaschko's lines (p. 8).

Hair follicles

The first sign of a developing hair follicle appears at 9 weeks as a focal aggregation of mesenchymal cells, precursors of the dermal papilla, just below the basal layer. Transient expression of mRNA for bone morphogenetic protein 4 coincides with this event and may constitute a message to the epidermis. A message from the epidermis then initiates the formation of a dermal papilla [1], towards which basal cells grow forming a follicle that is complete by 16 weeks. Hair follicles arise *in vitro* from single-cell suspensions of embryonic rat skin biopsied at 15 days (before the appearance of follicles), demonstrating that a dermal influence on the epidermis has already occurred [2].

In animals, several cell adhesion molecules (L-CAM, N-CAM, integrin, tenascin) are involved and various patterns of abortive hair growth can be produced experimentally using monoclonal antibodies to these proteins [3].

The arrector pili muscles develop from adjacent collections of mesenchymal cells. Sebaceous glands form in the side of the hair follicle and are functional after 15 weeks: they are highly active in the fetus, contributing to the vernix caseosa, but involute rapidly after birth.

Factors controlling the regional distribution and slope of hair are discussed in the section on hair patterns (p. 32).

Sweat glands

These begin as undulations in the basal layer and grow down into the dermis, reaching their maximum depth at 15 weeks. Cadherin cell adhesion molecules (uvomorulin) may be involved in sweat duct development [4].

Nails

The nail first appears as a thickened plaque at the tip of the digit, and migrates to the back of the terminal phalanx. It keratinizes, forming a 'false nail', under which the true nail grows forwards from the depths of the proximal nail fold. Nails are usually absent in syndromes with missing terminal phalanges, such as the Adams–Oliver syndrome.

Melanocytes

These originate in the neural crest. They are present in the epidermis by 8 weeks, and contain melanosomes by 10 weeks. The routes they take and the forces that carry them remain unknown. Cell-to-cell and cell-to-matrix adhesion must be important: certainly melanocytes attach to and migrate on fibronectin, an interaction that is probably mediated by integrins [5]. Melanocytes are probably transported initially by the streaming mesodermal cells. Once they reach the epidermis they must be carried with the movement of the surrounding keratinocytes, but may also move through the epidermis by migration or directional proliferation. In fetal skin, melanocytes lie in groups both basally and suprabasally, whereas after birth they are distributed singly among the basal keratinocytes. These arrangements are reproduced *in vitro* in fetal and neonatal skin equivalent models [6].

Waardenburg syndrome and piebaldism, in which there are mutations of the *Pax-3* and *C-kit* genes respectively, may be disorders of melanocyte migration. The ash-leaf macule of tuberous sclerosis usually parallels Blaschko's lines (and hair lines) and may represent an area populated by a clone of melanocytes produced intraepidermally from an individual abnormal melanocyte that has migrated from the neural crest.

Langerhans cells

These are derived from haemopoietic tissue, and enter the epidermis at 12 weeks. Studies using monoclonal antibodies to epidermal Langerhans cells in rats suggest that they enter the epidermis as macrophages, which then differentiate into dendritic cells and post-natally into Langerhans cells [7].

The control of skin development

The complex processes described above require even more complex mechanisms to ensure that they happen at the right time, in the right place and to the right degree. Many factors have been implicated in epidermal morphogenesis in animals, including activins [8], epimorphin [9], fibroblast growth factors [10] and electrical fields

[11]. In human epidermopoiesis there are sequential changes in expression of integrins (cell-surface proteins important for intercellular adherence) [12]. However, the most important genes masterminding skin development are probably the homeobox (*HOX*) genes [13].

HOX genes have been studied intensively in the fruit fly. Mutations cause major disruptions, such as appearance of an antenna where a leg should be. Thirty-eight human homeobox genes are known, arranged in four clusters on separate chromosomes. These genes are highly conserved, all containing a common 183-base-pair homeodomain.

HOX genes are expressed particularly in early fetal development. The protein product functions by binding to other genes (including other homeobox genes), regulating transcription. Minor differences in amino-acid sequence confer specificity with regard to DNA binding. The target sequences are usually 10–12 base pairs around a TAAT motif. *HOX* gene products interact with other regulatory factors and with each other to induce or repress gene function.

HOX genes themselves are regulated by growth factors and cytokines as well as by their own and other *HOX* gene products. Retinoic acid, a major morphogen, controls several *HOX* genes, hence the teratogenicity of retinoids.

Mutations have been found in several human *HOX* genes; for example, Wolf–Hirschhorn syndrome in which there is midline scalp aplasia with other developmental defects, and Waardenburg syndrome in which defective melanocyte migration produces a white forelock. The mutant gene in the latter is in fact a member of a subclass of *HOX* genes called *PAX* (paired-box) genes.

Aplasia cutis congenita

Strictly speaking this is due to a failure of skin development, but a similar appearance can follow antenatal skin loss due to epidermolysis bullosa (Bart syndrome), or congenital varicella. For these cases the term congenital absence of skin is more accurate.

In aplasia cutis congenita (ACC), both the dermis and epidermis are defective (the focal dermal hypoplasias are discussed elsewhere). Underlying structures are covered initially by a thin glistening membrane containing easily visible blood vessels. Later the area develops scarring, sometimes keloidal. There may also be an underlying bony defect.

Congenital absence of skin may be localized to the scalp or widespread, alone or associated with other malformations. These two variables are the basis for the classification used here (Table 1.1), although others have assigned ACC disorders to nine categories [14].

Simple aplasia cutis of the scalp (Fig. 1.1)

This is usually a round defect at the crown. Its situation suggests that the forces involved in the migration of skin to the cranial end of the embryo are the same as those determining hair slope. Both dominant and recessive modes of inheritance have been reported (MIM 107600, 207700). A similar lesion has followed the treatment of hyperthyroidism in pregnancy with methimazole [15]. Sometimes symmetrical parietal defects lie on either side of the sagittal suture, as seen in five generations of the Catlin family (MIM 168500) and probably due to incomplete closure of the fontanelle between frontal and parietal bones [16].

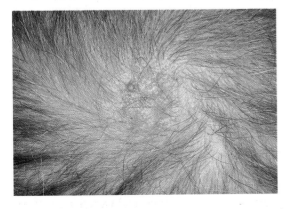

Fig. 1.1 Simple aplasia cutis of the scalp situated at the crown.

Aplasia cutis of the scalp with associated abnormalities

The scalp defect in these conditions is usually over the posterior fontanelle. An exception is when it accompanies a naevus sebaceus, which can occur anywhere on the scalp and may be part of the epidermal naevus syndrome. Only the best recognized syndromes are described here.

Adams–Oliver syndrome (MIM 100300)

Distal limb reduction anomalies, particularly absence of toes, cutis marmorata and large parietal scalp defects with normal intellect are the hallmarks of this condition. Lethal haemorrhage or meningitis may complicate the scalp defect. The manifestations are highly variable within families. Inheritance is autosomal dominant. The pathogenesis is unknown, but the association with cutis marmorata suggests that the abnormalities may be due to vascular disruption [17].

Johanson–Blizzard syndrome (MIM 243800)

This condition is also included elsewhere as an ectodermal dysplasia–deafness syndrome. The other features are hypoplasia of the alae nasi, hypothyroidism, growth and mental retardation, absent permanent teeth and imperforate anus, as well as scalp aplasia cutis [18]. The scalp defect may overly the anterior as well as the posterior fontanelle. The predominance of this syndrome in females initially suggested an X-linked dominant inheritance with male lethality, but autosomal recessive transmission has now been established. Pathogenesis is unknown.

Trisomy 13 (Bartholin–Patau syndrome)

This is found in 1 in 5000 births but only 18% of babies survive their first year. Features include severe mental defect due to incomplete development of the forebrain, polydactyly, cardiac anomalies (usually septal defects), clefting, portwine stain on the forehead and other abnormalities, in addition to scalp aplasia cutis [19]. As

Table 1.1 Classification of aplasia cutis congenita (ACC)

MIM*	Characteristic features
1 *Isolated ACC of scalp*	
107600 and 207700	ACC of vertex of scalp
168500	Catlin marks (ACC lesions on either side of sagittal sinus)
—	ACC associated with methimazole in pregnancy
2 *Scalp ACC with associated abnormalities*	
100300	Adams–Oliver syndrome (ACC of scalp, limb reductions, cutis marmorata)
243800	Johanson–Blizzard (ectodermal dysplasia, hypothyroidism, deafness)
—	Trisomy 13 (holoprosencephaly, polydactyly, cardiac anomalies, clefting)
194190	Wolf–Hirschhorn syndrome (4p- syndrome) (closure defects including cleft lip/palate, coloboma of eye, cardiac septal defects)
101120[1]	Sakati–Nyhan syndrome (craniosynostosis, polysyndactyly, cardiac defects)
129550[2]	Ectodermal dysplasia with adrenal cyst
134100[3]	ACC with unilateral facial palsy and lop-ear
181250	Scalp defects with postaxial polydactyly
181270[4]	Scalp–ear–nipple syndrome
233430[5]	XY gonadal dysgenesis (feminization, with meso- and ectodermal defects)
207731[6]	ACC and intestinal lymphangiectasia
—	ACC adjacent to organoid naevus, sometimes in epidermal naevus syndrome[7]
—	ACC with meningeal angiomatosis[8]
3 *Isolated aplasia cutis congenita of trunk/limbs*	
—	ACC with fetus papyraceus and limb constriction bands
	Congenital erosions and vesicles healing with reticulate scarring
4 *ACC of trunk or limbs with associated abnormalities*	
207730	Carmi syndrome (gastrointestinal atresia)
164180	Delleman–Orthuys syndrome (cerebral and ocular defects, skin tags)
—	ACC overlying developmental malformations, e.g. omphalocoele
—	Amnion rupture malformation sequence

* First digit of MIM number indicates inheritance: 1 = autosomal dominant; 2 = autosomal recessive; 3 = X-linked.

1 Sakati N, Nyhan WL, Tisdale WK. A new syndrome with acrocephalosyndactyly, cardiac disease and distinctive defects of the ear, skin and lower limbs. *J. Pediatr.* 1971; 79: 104–109.

2 Tuffli GA, Laxova R. New autosomal dominant form of ectodermal dysplasia. *Am. J. Med. Genet.* 1983; 14: 381–384.

3 Anderson CE, Hollister D, Szalay GC. Autosomal dominantly inherited cutis aplasia congenita, ear malformations, right-sided facial paresis and dermal sinuses. *Birth Defects* 1979; 15: 265–270.

4 Finlay AY, Marks R. An hereditary syndrome of lumpy scalp, odd ears and rudimentary nipples. *Br. J. Dermatol.* 1978; 99: 423–430.

5 Brosnan PG, Lewandowski RC, Toguri AG *et al.* A new familial syndrome of 46XY gonadal dysgenesis with anomalies of ectodermal and mesodermal structures. *J. Pediatr.* 1980; 97: 586–590.

6 Bronspiegel N, Zelnick N, Rabinowitz H *et al.* Aplasia cutis congenita and intestinal lymphangiectasia: an unusual association. *Am. J. Dis. Child.* 1985; 139: 509–513.

7 Frieden I, Golabi M. Aplasia cutis congenita and the epidermal naevus syndrome: a previously unrecognised association. *Clin. Res.* 1985; 33: 130.

8 Pozzati E, Podovani R, Franco F *et al.* Leptomeningeal angiomatosis and aplasia congenita of the scalp. *J. Neurosurg.* 1983; 58: 937–940.

in Down's syndrome, mean maternal age is increased, and cytogenetic studies are indicated in young mothers, to look for the rare balanced translocation.

Wolf–Hirschhorn syndrome (4p- syndrome) (MIM 194190)

This is characterized by retardation of both physical growth and mental development, facial anomalies including hyperteleorism and clefting, talipes, cryptorchidism and cardiac defects, as well as posterior midline scalp aplasia cutis.

This is the only aplasia cutis syndrome in which there is a clue to its molecular basis. Wolf–Hirschhorn syndrome is associated with deletion of the short arm of chromosome 4 (4p). The critical zone on chromosome 4 for the development of this syndrome is distal to the Huntington disease locus D4S10, at 4p16.3 [20,21], the deletion being usually on the paternal chromosome [22]. The deletion includes the human homeobox gene *HOX7* (MIM 142983). The mouse homologue of *HOX7* is expressed during development in heart valves, mandibular and hyoid arches and limb buds. It seems likely that deletion of *HOX7* is responsible for this particular malformation sequence with failure of midline fusion [23]. This is the first *HOX* gene to be implicated in a developmental anomaly.

Isolated aplasia cutis congenita of trunk or limbs

Multiple, symmetrical linear and stellate areas of ACC are sometimes found in the survivor of a twin (or triplet) pregnancy in which the other fetus died during the second trimester, leaving a fetus papyraceus [24]. Fibrous constriction bands may also be present. The skin defect has been attributed to placental transfer of thromboplastin from the dead fetus.

A similar appearance is found in congenital erosive and vesicular dermatosis healing with reticulate scarring, a sporadic condition of unknown aetiology [25].

Extensive ACC of this type involving the trunk and distal extremities occurred in a baby with an unbalanced translocation between chromosomes 1 and 12 resulting in trisomy for the distal portion of 1q and monosomy for the end of 12q. The baby died, apparently from skin sepsis, and no other abnormalities were found [26].

Aplasia cutis congenita of trunk or limbs with associated abnormalities

The Carmi syndrome, with widespread ACC and gastrointestinal atresia, may be a form of epidermolysis bullosa [27]. Delleman–Orthuys (oculo-cerebrocutaneous) syndrome [28], characterized by asymmetrical eye, skull and brain defects with periorbital skin tags and widespread aplastic skin lesions, may be due to mosaicism for a lethal gene [29]. Midline fusion defects are presumably responsible for aplasia cutis overlying both large congenital herniations of brain, spine or viscera, and occult spinal and vertebral malformations [30]. Early amnion rupture leads to a variety of malformations including aplasia cutis congenita attributed to adhesion between the fetus and the chorion [31].

References

1   Holbrook KA, Smith LT, Kaplan ED *et al.* Expression of morphogens during human follicle development *in vivo* and a model for studying follicle morphogenesis *in vitro. J. Invest. Dermatol.* 1993; 101: 39–49S.
2   Ihara S, Watanabe M, Nagao E, Shioya N. Formation of hair follicles from a single cell suspension of embryonic rat skin by a two step procedure *in vitro. Cell Tissue Res.* 1991; 266: 65–73.
3   Chuong CM, Chen HM, Jiang TX, Chia J. Adhesion molecules in skin development: morphogenesis of feather and hair. *Ann. N.Y. Acad. Sci.* 1991; 642: 263–280.
4   Fujita M, Furukawa F, Horiguchi Y *et al.* Expression of cadherin cell adhesion molecules during human skin development: morphogenesis of epidermis, hair follicles and eccrine sweat ducts. *Arch. Derm. Res.* 1992; 284: 159–166.
5   Scott G, Ryan DH, McCarthy JB. Molecular mechanisms of human melanocyte attachment to fibronectin. *J. Invest. Dermatol.* 1992; 99: 787–794.

6   Haake AR, Scott GA. Physiologic distribution and differentiation of melanocytes in human fetal and neonatal skin equivalents. *J. Invest. Dermatol.* 1991; 96: 71–77.

7   Mizoguchi S, Takahashi K, Takeya M *et al.* Development, differentiation and proliferation of epidermal Langerhans cells in rat ontogeny studied by a novel monoclonal antibody against epidermal Langerhans cells, RED-1. *J. Leukoc. Biol.* 1992; 52: 52–61.

8   Ohuchi H, Noji S, Koyama E *et al.* Expression pattern of the activin receptor type IIA gene during differentiation of chick neural tissues, muscle and skin. *FEBS Lett.* 1992; 303: 185–189.

9   Hirai Y, Takebe K, Takashina M *et al.* Epimorphin: a mesenchymal protein essential for epithelial morphogenesis. *Cell* 1992; 69: 471–481.

10 Peters KG, Werner S, Chen G *et al.* Two FGF receptor genes are differentially expressed in epithelial and mesenchymal tissues during limb formation and organogenesis in the mouse. *Development* 1992; 114: 233–243.

11 Hotary KB, Robinson KR. Evidence for a role for endogenous electrical fields in chick embryo development. *Development* 1992; 114: 985–996.

12 Hertle MD, Adams JC, Watt FM. Integrin expression during human epidermal development *in vivo* and *in vitro. Development* 1991; 112: 193–206.

13 Scott GA, Goldsmith LA. Homeobox genes and skin development: a review. *J. Invest. Dermatol.* 1993; 101: 3–8.

14 Frieden IJ. Aplasia cutis congenita: a clinical review and proposal for classification. *J. Am. Acad. Dermatol.* 1986; 14: 646–660.

15 Ferner RE, Smith JM. Disorders of the fetus and infant. In *Textbook of Adverse Drug Reactions*, 4th edn. (Davies DM ed). Oxford: Oxford Medical Publications, 1991: 73.

16 Little BB, Knoll KA, Klein VR, Heller KB. Hereditary cranium bifidum and symmetrical parietal foramina are the same entity. *Am. J. Med. Genet.* 1990; 35: 453–458.

17 Der Kaloustian VM, Hoyme HE, Hogg H *et al.* Possible common pathogenetic mechanisms for Poland sequence and Adams–Oliver syndrome. *Am. J. Med. Genet.* 1991; 38: 69–73.

18 Hurst JA, Baraitser M. Johanson–Blizzard syndrome. *J. Med. Genet.* 1989; 26: 45–48.

19 Abuelo D, Feingold M. Scalp defects in trisomy 13. *Clin. Paediatr.* 1969; 8: 416–417.

20 Anvret M, Nordenskjold M, Stolpe L *et al.* Molecular analysis of 4p deletion associated with Wolf–Hirschhorn syndrome moving the 'critical segment' towards the telomere. *Hum. Genet.* 1991; 86: 481–483.

21 McKeown C, Read AP, Dodge A *et al.* Wolf–Hirschhorn locus is distal to D4S10 on short arm of chromosome 4. *J. Med.. Genet.* 1987; 24: 410–412.

22 Quarrel OWJ, Snell RG, Curtis MA *et al.* Paternal origin of the chromosomal deletion resulting in Wolf–Hirschhorn syndrome. *J. Med. Genet.* 1991; 28: 256–259.

23 Ivens A, Flavin N, Williamson R *et al.* The human homeobox gene HOX7 maps to chromosome 4p16.1 and may be implicated in Wolf–Hirschhorn syndrome. *Hum. Genet.* 1990; 84: 473–476.

24 McCrossin DB, Robertson NRC. Congenital skin defects: twins and toxoplasmosis. *J. Roy. Soc. Med.* 1989; 82: 108–109.

25 Gupta AK, Rasmussen JE, Headington JT. Extensive congenital erosions and vesicles healing with reticulate scarring. *J. Am. Acad. Dermatol.* 1987; 17: 369–376.

26 Khan JY, Roper HP, Moss C. Extensive aplasia cutis congenita in association with chromosome 12q abnormality (in preparation).

27 Vivona G, Frontali M, Di Nunzio ML, Vendemiati A. Aplasia cutis congenita and/or epidermolysis bullosa. *Am. J. Hum. Genet.* 1987; 26: 497–502.

28 Al-Gazali LI, Donnai D, Berry SA *et al.* The oculocerebrocutaneous (Delleman) syndrome. *J. Med. Genet.* 1988; 25: 773–778.

29 Happle R. Lethal genes surviving by mosaicism: a possible explanation for sporadic birth defects involving the skin. *J. Am. Acad. Dermatol.* 1987; 16: 899–906.

30 Higginbottom MC, Jones KL, James HE *et al.* Aplasia cutis congenita: a cutaneous marker of occult spinal dysraphism. *J. Pediatr.* 1980; 96: 687–689.

31 Higginbottom MC, Jones KL, Hall BD *et al.* The amniotic band disruption complex: timing of amniotic rupture and variable spectra of consequent defects. *J. Pediatr.* 1979; 95: 544–549.

Mosaicism and Blaschko's lines

Blaschko's lines, well known to dermatologists, are at last attracting the wider audience they deserve. Geneticists and molecular biologists are waking up to the fact that these curious skin markings are probably cutaneous signs of genetic mosaicism.

Blaschko, a 19th century dermatologist, was intrigued by the bizarre linear and whorled patterns of epidermal naevi and by their constancy from one individual to the next. He documented the lesions in over a hundred patients, transferred them to a wax doll, and so constructed the system known as Blaschko's lines [1] (Fig. 1.2). We recognize them in many dermatoses, but the cause of the pattern is still speculative. Its constancy in so many different disorders suggests that is a function of normal skin biology rather than being due to any particular pathological process.

Montgomery in 1901 [2] dismissed various anatomical candidates: Blaschko's lines do not correspond to vascular or lymphatic territories, to Voigt's lines, which demarcate areas supplied by the major cutaneous nerve branches, to Langer's lines of skin tension or to embryological body segments. Although on the limbs they roughly correspond to dermatomes, on the trunk they differ in several respects: on the back, dermatomes lie at right angles to the midline while Blaschko's lines form a central V shape; unlike dermatomes, Blaschko's lines form an S-shaped or whorled pattern on the flanks; they are also closer together than dermatomes. Montgomery concluded that Blaschko's lines reflect the streams or trends of growth of embryonic tissues, and this view, although unproven, is still held.

This hypothesis may account for the orientation of the lines but two further questions remain. First, why do some dermatoses characteristically follow this pattern while others never do? Second, in patients showing Blaschko's lines, why does most of the skin remain unaffected by the dermatosis? The answers seem to be that only genetically determined skin disorders follow Blaschko's lines, and that the patchy distribution represents genetic mosaicism, with clones of normal skin cells separated by clones of affected ones.

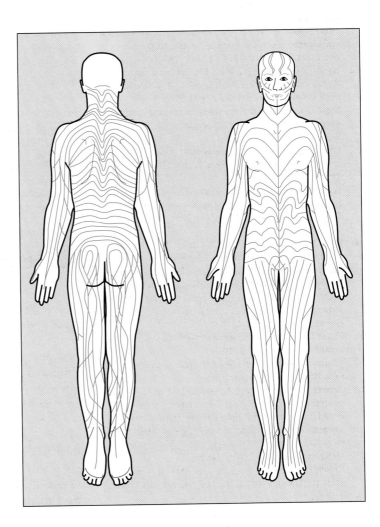

Fig. 1.2 Blaschko's lines, originally charted by Blaschko in 1901.

These ideas were first expressed in 1978 when Shuster suggested that the whorled appearance of many naevi is 'best related to the developmental movement of a clone of cells' and that 'susceptibility even to a common disease such as eczema may be focal with a bizarre linear and whorled appearance in a "clonal" pattern' [3]. Happle has developed the hypothesis that disorders following Blaschko's lines are due to genetic mosaicism or chimaerism [4–6]. Before considering the evidence for this, the various mechanisms by which mosaicism can arise will be discussed.

Mechanisms of mosaicism and chimaerism

Lyonization

A female has two X chromosomes, and therefore twice as many X-linked genes as males, who have one X chromosome and a very small Y chromosome. Perhaps to compensate for this overprovision, females express only one X chromosome in each cell, the other remaining as the inactive Barr body. The process of X inactivation is called lyonization after Mary Lyon who discovered it [7]. The inactivation process takes place early in embryogenesis and is random: some cells inactivate the paternal X and some the maternal X chromosome. All daughter cells express the same X chromosome as their parent cell, therefore two different clones grow up. Adult females are therefore mosaic with regard to expression of their maternal and paternal X chromosome.

If only one X chromosome is expressed per cell why are females who lack one X chromosome abnormal? Presumably, before lyonization, expression of both is essential for prevention of Turner syndrome.

Chimaerism

Geneticists use the words chimaera and mosaic rather precisely. Mosaic describes an organism with two or more cell lines that differ in one or a few genes or chromosomes, but are for the most part genetically identical. The two cell lines are rather like identical twins, one of whom has developed a mutation. By contrast, the different cell lines in a chimaera are like fraternal twins: their genetic constitution is quite different. They may even be of different sex (hermaphroditism). In fact, chimaerism may arise in the same way as dizygotic twinning, but the two zygotes fail to separate; for example, when two sperm fertilize a single ovum. It is exceedingly rare.

Somatic mutation

A mutation occurring in a single cell in a developing fetus will result in a clone of abnormal cells within an otherwise normal individual. The size of the abnormal clone depends on the timing of the mutation: if it occurs very early, before tissue differentiation, many organs will be mosaic; the later it occurs the more the mosaicism will be confined to a single region or organ. The size of the abnormality can range from a single-point mutation to a large chromosomal rearrangement arising from a mistake during cell division (somatic non-dysjunction) which may be detectable cytogenetically.

Mutation of a gene for a recessive disorder will have no effect, unless by chance the individual is already heterozygous for that disorder. Mosaicism for a dominant mutation will produce a mild or patchy form of the condition: affected individuals will have no antecedent family history of that disorder, but might pass the condition on to their offspring if some of their gametes carry the mutation (gonadal mosaicism) [8].

There is some evidence that a tendency to nondysjunction may be inherited, giving rise to familial mosaicism (MIM 158250, 257300).

Half-chromatid mutation

If an error occurs in a gene during the last stage of meiosis (gametogenesis), one chromatid in the affected gamete will contain two strands of DNA that are not exactly complementary at the locus. After fertilization, at the first mitotic division in the zygote, those two strands separate to act as templates for two daughter cells. Because the templates are different, two populations of daughter cells arise, one normal and the other carrying the mutation, so the individual is mosaic.

Mosaic conditions in which Blaschko's lines are seen

X-linked disorders

The skin abnormalities in females that are heterozygous for several X-linked dominant skin disorders (incontinentia pigmenti, focal dermal hypoplasia and X-linked chondrodysplasia punctata) follow Blaschko's lines. This probably reflects lyonization: cells expressing the normal paternal X chromosome make up the normal skin, while cells in which the abnormal maternal X chromosome is active produce the lesions [9]. The same argument applies to female carriers of recessive X-linked hypohidrotic ectodermal dysplasia, who show patches of sweating and non-sweating skin along Blaschko's lines.

A pattern equivalent to Blaschko's lines is seen in female animals heterozygous for certain X-linked skin genes. The Lyon hypothesis in fact arose from the observation of variegated fur in female mice heterozygous for sex-linked genes for coat colour. Often the pattern is mottled, but there is a basic arrangement of transverse bands around the body lacking the dorsal V shape seen in humans. The same pattern is seen in animal versions of human X-linked skin disorders, including murine hypohidrotic ectodermal dysplasia [10], 'bare patches' in mice that may be analogous to chondrodysplasia punctata [11], and streaked hairlessness in Holstein–Friesian cattle, which is probably equivalent to incontinentia pigmenti [12]. These observations, combined with findings in chimaeric animals with the same stripy pattern (see below) provide strong evidence for the clonal hypothesis of Blaschko's lines.

In some X-linked skin disorders in humans, the lesions so characteristic of affected males are minimal or absent in female carriers and do not follow Blaschko's lines. This may appear to be contrary to the hypothesis. Examples include α-galactosidase deficiency (Fabry's disease),

Wiskott–Aldrich syndrome, steroid sulphatase-deficient ichthyosis, chronic granulomatous disease, Menkes syndrome and dyskeratosis congenita. However, in most of these the biochemical or immunological disorder is generalized and the skin manifestations are secondary. For an X-linked disorder to be confined to Blaschko's lines, it seems that the defective gene has to be expressed in epidermal cells. Steroid sulphatase deficiency appears to be an exception to this rule, but although the enzyme is produced in epidermal cells its function is extracellular, affecting the lipid matrix of the stratum corneum, so the lipid production by enzyme from normal cells of the heterozygous females may compensate for the deficiency. Steroid sulphatase deficiency is also complicated by incomplete inactivation of the gene, so females are not as deficient as if they were totally heterozygous. Female carriers of Menkes kinky hair syndrome show a mixture of normal and anomalous hair, but no particular pattern has been reported [13]; however, in one carrier a pigmentary pattern following Blaschko's lines was seen on the trunk [14], perhaps because tyrosinase is a copper-dependent enzyme.

Chimaerism

Animal chimaeras can be produced by fusing zygotes taken from two different animals, and implanting the product into the uterus of a pseudopregnant female. If the zygotes differ genetically with regard to coat colour, the chimaeric animals have stripes in the pattern described above [15]. If they differ with regard to certain epidermal antigens, this again can be detected in a linear pattern [16]. Thus, the pattern in animals corresponding to Blaschko's lines is clearly due to migrating clones of genetically different epidermal cells.

Human chimaerism is extremely rare, and may be detected by the presence of two types of blood group or by hermaphroditism. Findlay and Moores traced the donors of the only two samples in more than a million routine blood tests that showed evidence of chimaerism [17]. Both were women with an XX/XX genotype, and both were racially pigmented with odd patches of darker skin. In one woman, the darker areas followed Blaschko's lines; in the other there was a large block of darker pigment on one side of the trunk that did not cross the midline and that extended down the posterior aspect of the arm but had rather more horizontal upper and lower borders than Blaschko's lines. Reports of three other chimaeras were reviewed: although the pigmentary changes often followed Blaschko's lines, some showed rounded areas like cafe-au-lait macules, while others had rectangular blocks with a ventral midline demarcation. The three earlier cases were XX/XY chimaeras, so it was possible to differentiate two cell lines in culture on the basis of the sex chromosomes. Fibroblasts were grown from light and dark areas of skin, to see whether the skin type corresponded to the karyotype. In fact, a mixture of XX and XY cells was seen in one or both biopsies from all three patients, perhaps because the cells studied were fibroblasts rather than epidermal cells.

Chromosomal mosaicism

This results from somatic non-dysjunction. Thomas *et al.* [18] described eight patients with mosaicism for a variety of chromosomal defects, and patchy pigmentation. Their literature review revealed 36 similar cases, most of which were unclassified, but 14 had been diagnosed as Pallister syndrome (retardation, linear pigmentation and additional material on the short arm of chromosome 12), and some had been labelled hypomelanosis of Ito. There are now many reports of chromosomal mosaicism in patients with linear dyspigmentation [18–22]. In chromosomal mosaics, as in chimaeras, the pigmentary pattern does not always follow Blaschko's lines but there is always midline demarcation.

The hypothesis that Blaschko's lines reflect clonality has been tested in patients with chromosomal mosaicism and linear dyspigmentation. There have been many cytogenetic studies on fibroblasts cultured from light and dark skin, but the findings are similar to those in human chimaeras: hardly any show pure cultures of the two different cell lines in the two different biopsies; there is usually a mixture in one or both biopsies [18–22].

The most likely explanation for this, as for the corresponding result in chimaeras, is that fibroblasts do not conform to Blaschko's lines. Most dermatoses following Blaschko's lines affect ectodermal derivatives, namely melanocytes, keratinocytes or epidermal appendages. Similarly, all the chimaeric animal studies involve epidermal cells. One of the authors has therefore investigated chromosomes in cultured keratinocytes from light and dark skin from patients with linear dyspigmentation [23]. It would have been more logical to look for the abnormality in melanocytes, but it is more difficult to grow them. Two girls with hypomelanosis of Ito who had no clear cytogenetic abnormality in lymphocytes or fibroblasts, showed definite chromosomal mosaicism in keratinocytes; in both girls the cells from normal skin had a normal karyotype and the light skin cells showed a chromosomal abnormality. This provides firm evidence that Blaschko's lines represent epidermal clones.

It is curious that the skin change common to such diverse chromosomal defects is dyspigmentation, rather than dyskeratosis or a difference in any other property of the skin. Perhaps melanocyte migration is non-specifically affected by the presence of different cell lines, regardless of the abnormality [24]. This would explain the findings in chimaeras, where neither cell line is abnormal. Alternatively, perhaps the difference between the light and dark areas in the chimaeras is no greater than may be found between normal siblings. Most patients with chromosomal mosaicism do not have pigmentary dysplasia: Thomas *et al.* [18] found 36 cases of chromosomal mosaicism with dyspigmentation but 200 cases without. The control of pigmentation is complex and polygenic, and it is just possible that in 36 out of 236 cases the rearrangement involved a pigment-related gene. In support of this, the experiments described above on keratinocytes showed the chromosomal abnormality to lie in the abnormal (pale) epidermis, and not in the normal epidermis [23].

Autosomal dominant disorders

Autosomal dominant disorders may occur in a mosaic form, as a result of half-chromatid or somatic mutation. If the condition is due to a gene expressed in the skin, the abnormality should follow Blaschko's lines. One such condition is autosomal dominant bullous ichthyosiform erythroderma (BIE). Certain linear epidermal naevi, called ichthyosis hystrix, show the characteristic histology of BIE, namely epidermolytic hyperkeratosis. Sometimes a parent has the linear form and a child has the generalized form of BIE, as one would expect if the parent had gonadal as well as cutaneous mosaicism for the gene [25]. Epidermal mosaicism for the BIE mutation has now been demonstrated in three such parents [26].

Another dominant disorder in which this phenomenon has been observed is von Recklinghausen's neurofibromatosis (NF-1) [27]. Families have been reported in which a parent has a limited cutaneous distribution of neurofibromas or cafe-au-lait macules (segmental NF), and a child has generalized NF-1.

Some other dominant skin disorders may occur in a linear distribution with no antecedent family history: these include Darier's disease [28], linear porokeratosis, alopecia mucinosa [29], primary cutaneous amyloidosis [30], eczema [31] (lichen striatus), psoriasis [32,33], and lichen planus. The latter is not usually thought of as heritable, but there are well-documented families with many affected members (MIM 151620). The last three are probably polygenic disorders in which expression depends on immunity, and the linear pattern could be explained by a clonal susceptibility defect. Affected offspring have not yet been reported.

There are some conditions that occur in Blaschko's lines but are never seen in a generalized form, such as epidermal naevus, Proteus syndrome, McCune–Albright syndrome [34], CHILD syndrome (congenital *h*emidysplasia with *i*chthyosiform erythroderma and *l*imb *d*efects), and ILVEN (Inflammatory *l*inear *v*errucous *e*pidermal *n*aevus). The last two of these may be extreme forms of the same disorder [35]. Happle has suggested that these are all due to lethal dominant genes 'rescued' by mosaicism [36]; in other words, if all cells were affected the individual would die. The prediction, that parents with such naevi should have a higher than average rate of fetal loss, has not been tested. Other possibly mosaic syndromes are Parry–Romberg hemifacial atrophy (MIM 141300) and Goldenhaar syndrome of hemifacial microsomia with ipsilateral radial defect (MIM 141400).

Dermal disorders in Blaschko's lines

If it is true that any dermatosis occurring in Blaschko's lines is determined by a gene expressed in keratinocytes or melanocytes, how can we explain linear disorders that do not primarily affect the epidermis?

Happle has regarded port-wine stains, in particular Sturge–Weber syndrome, as examples of cutaneous mosaicism [36]. We feel that capillary haemangiomas follow a dermatomal distribution rather than Blaschko's lines, in keeping with the idea that they are caused by a failure of innervation. They may still represent a mutation, but their distribution is determined by migration of nerves rather than epidermis.

Patients with segmental neurofibromatosis tend to have either localized freckling or localized neurofibromas, but rarely both. If the individual lesions are widely separated it may be difficult to see whether the distribution is dermatomal or in Blaschko's lines. Depending on whether the mutation affects mainly nerves or melanocytes, the distribution might be determined by either neural or cutaneous migration, or both.

The linear lesions of focal dermal hypoplasia are difficult to reconcile with the idea that fibroblast clones are not constrained by Blaschko's lines. Perhaps fibroblasts do initially migrate in a linear manner but subsequently move randomly, so a defect in the dermis might take up a linear shape if it were expressed and became fixed at an early stage of development. It should be noted, however, that the epidermis overlying focal dermal hypoplasia is profoundly defective, and the primary defect might be absence of some epidermal factor necessary for normal dermal development.

The expression of psoriasis is determined by many factors, both cutaneous and systemic. The Koebner phenomenon (development of a psoriatic lesion at the site of trauma) indicates local as well as general susceptibility. Some cases of linear psoriasis are associated with an inflammatory linear verrucous epidermal naevus (ILVEN): presumably this epidermal abnormality provides the local susceptibility allowing expression of psori-asis. Linear psoriasis arising on apparently normal skin might be due to a mutation in one of the genes for psoriasis [33], or in one causing a more subtle epidermal alteration which again 'koebnerizes'. The same explanation may apply to linear lichen planus, and lichen striatus, a transient linear inflammatory dermatosis clinically and histologically resembling eczema. As in the case of psoriasis, it could represent either a clone of eczema cells in an otherwise non-eczematous person, or a clone of particu-larly susceptible cells in a mildly eczematous individual.

Variations on Blaschko's lines

Not all mosaic skin disorders follow exactly the pattern described by Blaschko, although all show midline demarcation. Several of the human chimaeras showed large blocks of pigment with rather horizontal borders on the trunk. This pattern is also seen in McCune–Albright syndrome, now known to be a mosaic disorder. Epidermal naevi can run the whole length of a limb in a narrow continuous line, while the lesions of incontinentia pigmenti tend to be more reticulate and irregular. These differences may reflect the migratory behaviour of the particular cell line expressing the abnormality; for example, keratinocytes move outwards by directional proliferation and are therefore more likely to form a continuous line, while melanocytes move out separately. Finally, there seem to be anatomical sites particularly prone to manifest Blaschko's lines, in

Table 1.2 Linear dermatoses explained on the basis of mosaicism

Skin condition	Characteristics of abnormal clone of epidermal cells	Cause of mosaicism
Incontinentia pigmenti Goltz syndrome Chondrodysplasia punctata	Lethal X-linked dominant gene	Lyonization
Epidermal naevus McCune–Albright syndrome CHILD syndrome ILVEN Proteus syndrome	Lethal autosomal dominant gene	Half chromatid or somatic mutation
Epidermolytic hyperkeratosis Linear Darier's disease Segmental neurofibromatosis Linear amyloid Linear porokeratosis Linear psoriasis Linear lichen planus Linear eczema (lichen striatus)	Non-lethal autosomal dominant gene	Half chromatid or somatic mutation
Hypomelanosis of Ito	Chromosomal abnormality	Somatic non-dysjunction
Linear dyspigmentation	Normal	Chimaerism

particular the axial lines at the back of the thigh and on the upper arm (see p.31).

Incontinentia pigmenti (MIM 308300)

Clinical features [37]

Incontinentia pigmenti (IP) is characterized by skin lesions that follow Blaschko's lines, and by a spectrum of other ectodermal, ophthalmic and neurological manifestations (Figs 1.3–1.5; Table 1.3). Despite these, IP is usually not as serious a disease as was once believed, since most adult patients have only minor abnormalities of their skin and teeth.

The skin lesions usually start in the neonate as lines and whorls of blisters that evolve into verrucous lesions. These usually disappear within a year leaving the classical 'marble cake' pigmented whorls and streaks, which themselves fade and may have disappeared by the age of 20. In adults the only remaining skin lesions may be pale, hairless, anhidrotic streaks on the backs of the legs and radiating from the vertex of the scalp [38]. In general, the most severe blistering is on the legs and culminates in these linear scars, while the less marked truncal blisters become the pigmented lesions.

Some patients show only the late lesions, with no preceding blisters. In these cases the blistering has presumably occurred *in utero*.

Table 1.3 Non-cutaneous manifestations of incontinentia pigmenti

Other ectodermal	Lack of hair and sweat glands in affected skin
	Partial anodontia
	Conical and peg-shaped teeth
	Nail tumours
	Nail dystrophy
Ophthalmic	Retinal vascular anomalies
	Pseudoglioma
	Cataract
	Optic atrophy
Neurological	Retardation
	Epilepsy
	Spastic diplegia/tetraplegia
Skeletal	Skull anomalies
	Scoliosis

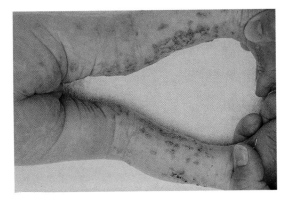

Fig. 1.3 Incontinentia pigmenti: linear blisters in a newborn girl.

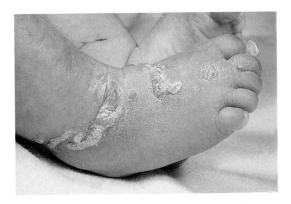

Fig. 1.4 Incontinentia pigmenti: the verrucous stage.

Genetic aspects

IP is an X-linked dominant disorder, usually lethal before birth in males. Occasional males with otherwise typical IP have been reported: some have had Klinefelter syndrome and are presumably protected by the extra X chromosome [39]; most were sporadic cases and the defect may have arisen during early embryogenesis as a somatic mutation. Another possibility is a half-chromatid mutation [40] during gametogenesis: if a mutation occurs in half of a base pair during the final reduction division, the chromosome passed on to the fetus comprises two strands of DNA that are not exactly complementary; thus, from these two different templates, two populations of daughter

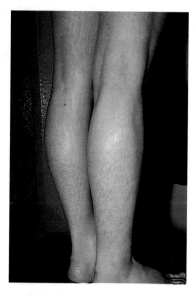

Fig. 1.5 Incontinentia pigmenti: linear scars at the sites of earlier blisters on the legs may be the only remaining signs in an adult.

cells are produced, one normal and the other carrying the mutation. However, some males with inherited IP and a normal karyotype have been reported, and cannot be accounted for by these arguments [41].

The gene was mapped to Xp11 on the basis of several patients with X-autosome translocations at this locus, but linkage studies failed to confirm this localization in affected families [42]. It now seems likely that there are two IP mutations: one at Xq28, which causes familial IP, and another at Xp11, which causes the more severe sporadic disease. However, some families show recombination at both loci [43].

Pathogenesis

The pattern of skin involvement in females is attributable to lyonization (random X inactivation). Lines of affected and unaffected skin then represent clones of cells in which the abnormal or normal (respectively) X chromosome is active. However, attempts to test this hypothesis gave unexpected results. Females were studied who had IP and were also heterozygous for another

X-linked polymorphism (either glucose-6-phosphate dehydrogenase (G6PD) or a DNA polymorphism), so that the two X chromosomes could be differentiated. Fibroblasts cultured from the affected and unaffected areas of IP patients heterozygous for G6PD all expressed the same G6PD type, demonstrating that the same X chromosome was active in all cells. This was confirmed using a DNA probe and a methylation-sensitive restriction endonuclease, which picks out the inactive X chromosome: it was the paternal X that was active in all tissues studied, including blood and skin [44]. In some cases the maternal X was expressed, but the proportion was heavily skewed towards the paternal X.

A likely explanation for this finding is that lyonization is initially random, with equal numbers of cells expressing each X chromosome, but the IP mutation is so serious that cells in which the abnormal X is active cannot survive. In males this results in early fetal death, while in females the affected cells die out and the cells expressing the normal X take over. The fact that much less than half of the skin surface is affected by IP can be explained by the proliferative advantage of the cells expressing the normal X chromosome. The final result is indistinguishable from non-random lyonization.

This phenomenon was responsible for the manifestation of haemophilia (inherited from the father) in a girl with IP inherited from her mother [45]. The same principle can be used as a diagnostic blood test in girls with the IP phenotype, but with a normal 46XX karyotype and no family history of IP [46]. If X-inactivation studies show that all cells express the X chromosome derived from one parent, this implies that the X chromosome from the other parent carried a lethal mutation, which in the clinical context must be IP. Whereas in familial cases the maternal X chromosome is preferentially inactivated, in sporadic cases the X chromosome derived from either parent may carry the mutation. This test is not always reliable, however, because the degree of skewing may be quite small in IP patients, comparable to levels occasionally found in normal females [47].

Although IP is usually thought of as a pigmentary disorder, the intense eosinophilic infiltration of the vesicular phase is directed at the whole of the epidermis, not particularly at melanocytes, and the pigmentary incontinence is simply postinflammatory hyperpigmentation. The pathogenesis of the inflammation is unknown. In some ways IP is like a severe form of ectodermal dysplasia: the dental abnormalities are indistinguishable, and in females with IP a linear arrangement of sweating and non-sweating skin can be demonstrated [38], just as in female carriers of X-linked hypohidrotic ectodermal dysplasia [5]. However, the gene for X-linked hypohidrotic ectodermal dysplasia at Xq12 is distinct from the IP genes.

Focal dermal hypoplasia (Goltz syndrome: MIM 305600)

Clinical features (Fig. 1.6) [48]

Focal dermal hypoplasia (FDH) is a rare but genetically important condition. Less than 200 cases have been published; however, mild examples may well escape detection. The main skin changes are:

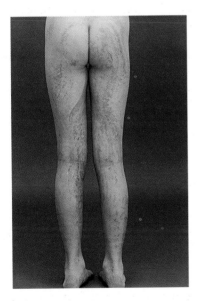

Fig. 1.6 Areas of focal dermal hypoplasia in Goltz syndrome: these also follow Blaschko's lines.

1 Linear areas of pinkish atrophy, which may look pale on a dark skin, lying along Blaschko's lines;
2 Soft, raised, yellowish areas of fat herniation;
3 Multiple raspberry-like papillomas around orifices and in the flexures.

Various skeletal abnormalities include syndactyly and the presence of fine parallel lines seen on X-ray at the metaphyses of long bones. Dental hypoplasia and ocular abnormalities (coloboma or microphthalmia) may also occur.

Genetic aspects

Over 90% of cases are female: most occur sporadically but in some families affected females have been seen in four generations [49]. These families have a high proportion of miscarriages. The best explanation is that FDH is inherited as an X-linked dominant trait with male hemizygote lethality. Manifestation in a male may be due to mosaicism for a somatic mutation on the X chromosome, or to lyonization in a male with Klinefelter syndrome. The few recorded instances of father-to-daughter transmission [50] can be explained by paternal mosaicism. Some patients have had deletions on the short arm of the X chromosome, placing the FDH gene tentatively on Xp22.31 [51,52].

Pathogenesis

The linear skin lesions, and presumably the bone striations also, fit with the Lyon hypothesis and are due to functional X-chromosome mosaicism. Cells expressing the abnormal allele may experience a selective disadvantage [53] as in incontinentia pigmenti. In affected areas the dermis is greatly thinned and subcutaneous fat lies close to the epidermis. Fibroblasts from an affected patient have been shown to have a reduced proliferative capacity. Although the obvious cutaneous change is dermal hypoplasia, the overlying epidermis is also thin and lacking appendages. Given that disorders following Blaschko's lines are usually epidermal, the dermal defect may be secondary to a focal abnormality in the epidermis. The precise defect has not yet been identified, although deletion of the gene on chromosome 9q34.3 for the pro-α1 (V) chain of collagen has been found in one patient with features both of the Goltz and the nail–patella syndromes [54].

Hypomelanosis of Ito
(mosaic dyspigmentation) (MIM 146150)

In 1952 Ito described a healthy 22-year-old female with a cutaneous pattern of hypopigmented lines resembling a negative image of incontinentia pigmenti. He called this incontinentia pigmenti achromians [55]. The name hypomelanosis of Ito is now used in order to distinguish this from incontinentia pigmenti. Ironically, the original patient may actually have had incontinentia pigmenti, as Ito himself believed, rather than the disorder that now bears his name. The depressed, atrophic, anhidrotic white lesions in Ito's patient sound remarkably like the late lesions of incontinentia pigmenti [38], which were not recognized until 1955 [56]. The label of hypomelanosis of Ito is now used for patients with linear hypopigmentation and neurological deficit (although Ito's patient was neurologically normal). It now seems that hypomelanosis of Ito is not a single condition, but rather a non-specific manifestation of chromosomal mosaicism [21,22]. For all these reasons, the term hypomelanosis of Ito should probably now be dropped. The term pigmentary dysplasia has been used [21,22], but a more suitable alternative would be mosaic dyspigmentation, which recalls the cutaneous pattern as well as its probable cause.

Clinical features (Fig. 1.7)

The essential feature is a pattern of pale whorls and streaks, often markedly asymmetrical, following Blaschko's lines. This is easily seen at birth in racially pigmented skin, but in white skin may not become apparent until the adjacent skin becomes tanned: it is much more readily seen under ultraviolet light. In most patients the only abnormality in these lines is hypopigmentation, but sometimes there may also be lack of hair and

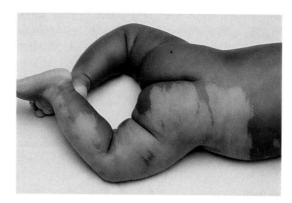

Fig. 1.7 Hypomelanosis of Ito: segmental hypopigmentation in a child with mental retardation and mosaicism for a chromosome 15 anomaly.

of sweating [57], atrophy and a difference in vascular responsiveness so that, for example, the lesions are more obvious after a hot bath when the patient is generally vasodilated. Some individuals have hyper- as well as hypopigmentation.

It is important to note these variable features, because they may reflect the heterogeneity of the disorder. Because this is not a single disorder, many different associated extracutaneous features have been reported [58], and it is impossible to define precise diagnostic criteria. Most would diagnose hypomelanosis of Ito in a patient with linear hypopigmentation and neurological deficit. In the light of current knowledge, all patients with linear dyspigmentation and chromosomal mosaicism, whatever their associated features, should probably be included in the same category.

Linear hypopigmentation may also be seen in vitiligo, tuberous sclerosis and epidermal naevi, and may follow lichen striatus. It may occur alone as naevus depigmentosus: whether this has the same basis as hypomelanosis of Ito is not yet known.

Genetic aspects

Cases of hypomelanosis of Ito are usually sporadic. The few reports claiming to show autosomal dominant inheritance are not well documented. There is a 2.5-fold excess of females with this condition but some of these actually have had incontinentia pigmenti misdiagnosed as hypomelanosis of Ito, and this must always be considered when counselling females [57].

Many patients diagnosed clinically as having hypomelanosis of Ito show chromosomal mosaicism, that is karyotypic abnormalities in some cells but not in others [21,22]. Such mosaicism is generally not transmissible from one generation to the next, and this is consistent with the sporadic occurrence of the disorder. Mosaicism, moreover is not excluded by a routine report stating normal karyotype. Up to a hundred cells must be examined to detect it, and this is not done unless specifically requested. In addition, the karyotype may be normal in lymphocytes but abnormal in cultured fibroblasts or keratinocytes [57], therefore a skin biopsy may be required. In fact, all patients with hypomelanosis of Ito are likely to have some form of genetic mosaicism, but this may be too subtle to be detected by current techniques.

The cytogenetic abnormalities in hypomelanosis of Ito can be anywhere, on any chromosome, and the clinical picture may be complicated or dominated by the phenotype attributable to the particular chromosomal abnormality, especially if a large proportion of cells has the abnormal karyotype [59]. One group has been recognized (Killian–Pallister mosaic syndrome) in which there is a linear dyspigmentation, retardation and a distinctive facies associated with mosaic 12p tetrasomy. A disproportionate number of karyotypic abnormalities reported in hypomelanosis of Ito involve the X chromosome, particularly Xp11, the incontinentia pigmenti locus: it is possible that hypomelanosis of Ito can not only mimic incontinentia pigmenti, but can also arise as an allelic variant [23,60].

The finding of chromosomal mosaicism has resulted in the lumping together of patients, previously thought to have different conditions, on the basis of this common feature. However, in future the group will probably be split up again, as phenotypes associated with particular cytogenetic defects emerge. At present only the Killian–Pallister syndrome can be separated on this basis, but the patients with ectodermal defects within the lesions may well represent another subgroup.

Pathogenesis

The patches of different skin colour probably represent clones of cells with a different genetic constitution. However, this has been remarkably difficult to demonstrate: fibroblasts cultured from any area show a mixture of cell types rather than a single clone. This is probably because Blaschko's lines are epidermal not dermal and cytogenetic studies should be directed at keratinocytes rather than fibroblasts [23].

We do not yet know why such a wide variety of different karyotypes should result in a similar linear dyspigmentation. The control of pigmentation is certainly complex and polygenic, but pigment genes are not likely to be at all these loci. Furthermore, a similar phenomenon of patchy pigmentation, sometimes in Blaschko's lines, is seen in chimaeras, individuals composed of two different but genetically intact cell lines [17]. Possibly the pigmentary disturbance is due to some as yet unexplained incompatibility between different cell lines migrating contiguously [24]. The common and rather non-specific feature of mental retardation may arise in the same way.

References

1 Blaschko A. Die Nevenverteilung in der Haut in ihrer Beziehung zu den Ekrankungen der Haut. *Beilage zu den Verhandlungen der Deutschen Dermatologischen Gesellschaft VII Congress, Breslau.* Wien: Braumuller, 1901.

2 Montgomery DW. The cause of the streaks in naevus linearis. *J. Cutan. Genitourin. Dis.* 1901; 19: 455–464.

3 Shuster S. *Dermatology in Internal Medicine.* Oxford: Oxford Medical Publications, 1978: 21.

4 Happle R. Genetische Interpretation streifenformiger Hautanomalien. *Hautarzt* 1978; 29: 357–363.

5 Happle R. Lyonization and the lines of Blaschko. *Hum. Genet.* 1985; 70: 200–206.

6 Happle R. Cutaneous manifestation of lethal genes. *Hum. Genet.* 1986; 72: 280.

7 Lyon MF. Gene action in the X-chromosome of the mouse (*Mus musculus* L.). *Nature* 1961; 190: 372–373.

8 Bernards A, Gusella JF. The importance of genetic mosaicism in human disease. *New Engl. J. Med.* 1994; 331: 1447–1449.

9 Curth HO, Warburton D. The genetics of incontinentia pigmenti. *Arch. Dermatol.* 1965; 92: 229–235.

10 Blecher SR. Anhidrosis and absence of sweat glands in mice hemizygous for the Tabby gene: supportive evidence for the hypothesis of homology between Tabby and human anhidrotic (hypohidrotic) ectodermal dysplasia (Christ–Siemens–Touraine syndrome). *J. Invest. Dermatol.* 1986; 87: 720–722.

11 Happle R, Phillips RJS, Roessner A, Junemann G. Homologous genes for X-linked chondrodysplasia punctata in man and mouse. *Hum. Genet.* 1983; 63: 24–27.

12 Eldridge FE, Atkeson FW. Streaked hairlessness in Holstein–Friesian cattle: a sex-linked, lethal character. *J. Hered.* 1953; 44: 265–271.

13 Collie WR, Moore CM, Goka TJ, Howell RR. Pili torti as marker for carriers of Menkes disease. *Lancet* 1978; i: 607–608.

14 Volpintesta EJ. Menkes kinky hair syndrome in a black infant. *Am. J. Dis. Child.* 1974; 128: 244–246.

15 Mintz B. Gene control of mammalian pigmentary differentiation. I. Clonal origin of melanocytes. *Proc. Natl. Acad. Sci. USA* 1967; 58: 344–351.

16 Schmidt GH, Blount MA, Ponder BAJ. Immuno chemical demonstration of the clonal organisation of chimaeric mouse epidermis. *Development* 1987; 100: 534–541.

17 Findlay GH, Moores PP. Pigment anomalies of the skin in human chimaera: their relation to systematised naevi. *Br. J. Dermatol.* 1980; 103: 489–498.

18 Thomas IT, Frias JL, Cantu ES *et al.* Association of pigmentary anomalies with chromosomal and genetic mosaicism and chimaerism. *Am. J. Hum. Genet.* 1989; 45: 193–205.

19 Donnai D, Read AP, McKeown C, Andrews T. Hypomelanosis of Ito: a manifestation of mosaicism or chimaerism. *J. Med. Genet.* 1988; 25: 809–818.

20 Flannery DB, Byrd JR, Freeman WE, Perlman SA. Hypomelanosis of Ito: a cutaneous marker of chromosomal mosaicism. *Am. J. Hum. Genet.* 1985; 37: A93.

21 Flannery DB. Pigmentary dysplasias, hypomelanosis of Ito and genetic mosaicism. Editorial. *Am. J. Med. Genet.* 1990; 35: 18–21.

22 Ohashi H, Tsukahara M, Murano I *et al.* Pigmentary dysplasias and chromosomal mosaicism: report of nine cases. *Am. J. Med. Genet.* 1992; 43: 716–721.

23 Moss C, Larkins S, Stacey M *et al.* Epidermal mosaicism and Blaschko's lines. *J. Med. Genet.* 1993; 30: 752–755.

24 Read AP, Donnai D. Association of pigmentary anomalies with chromosomal and genetic mosaicism and chimaerism. *Am. J. Hum. Genet.* 1990; 47: 166–167.

25 Nazzaro V, Ermacora E, Santucci B, Caputo R. Epidermolytic hyperkeratosis: generalised form in children from parents with systematised linear form. *Br. J. Dermatol.* 1990; 122: 417–422.

26 Paller A, Syder AJ, Chan Y-M *et al.* Genetic and clinical mosaicism in a type of epidermal nevus. *New Engl. J. Med.* 1994; 331: 1408–1415.

27 Moss C, Green SH. What is segmental neurofibromatosis? *Br. J. Dermatol.* 1994; 130: 106–110.

28 Munro CS, Cox NH. An acantholytic dyskeratotic epidermal naevus with other features of Darier's disease on the same side of the body. *Br. J. Dermatol.* 1992; 127: 168–171.

29 Tosti A, Fanti PA, Peserico A, Variotti C. Linear alopecia mucinosa along Blaschko's lines. *Acta Derm. (Stockh)* 1992; 72: 155–156.

30 Bourke JF, Berth-Jones J, Burns DA. Diffuse primary cutaneous amyloidosis. *Br. J. Dermatol.* 1992; 127: 641–644.

31 Taieb A, el Youbi A, Grosshans E, Maleville J. Lichen striatus: a Blaschko linear acquired inflammatory skin eruption. *J. Am. Acad. Dermatol.* 1991; 25: 637–642.

32 Atherton DJ, Kahana M, Russell-Jones R. Naevoid psoriasis. *Br. J. Dermatol.* 1989; 120: 837–841.

33 Happle R. Hypothesis: somatic recombination may explain linear psoriasis. *J. Med. Genet.* 1991; 28: 337.

34 Schwindinger WF, Francomano CA, Levine MA. Identification of a mutation in the gene encoding the alpha subunit of the stimulatory G-protein of adenylyl cyclase in McCune–Albright syndrome. *Proc. Natl. Acad. Sci. USA* 1992; 89: 5152–5156.

35 Moss C, Burn J. CHILD + ILVEN = PEN OR PENCIL. *J. Med. Genet.* 1990; 27: 390–391.

36 Happle R. Lethal genes surviving by mosaicism: a possible explanation for sporadic birth defects involving the skin. *J. Am. Acad. Dermatol.* 1987; 16: 899–906.

37 Landy SJ, Donnai D. Incontinentia pigmenti (Bloch–Sulzberger syndrome). *J. Med. Genet.* 1993; 30: 53–59.

38 Moss C, Ince P. Anhidrotic and achromians lesions in incontinentia pigmenti. *Br. J. Dermatol.* 1987; 116: 839–849.

39 Garcia-Dorado J, Unamuno P, Fernandez-Lopez P *et al.* Incontinentia pigmenti: XXY male with a family history. *Clin. Genet.* 1990; 38: 128–138.

40 Lenz W. Half chromatid mutations may explain incontinentia pigmenti in males. *Am. J. Hum. Genet.* 1975; 27: 690–691.

41 Hecht F, Hecht BK, Austin WJ. Incontinentia pigmenti in Arizona Indians including transmission from mother to son inconsistent with the half chromatid mutation model. *Clin. Genet.* 1982; 21: 293–296.

42 Sefiani A, Sinnett D, Abel L *et al.* Linkage studies do not confirm the cytogenetic location of incontinentia pigmenti on Xp11. *Hum. Genet.* 1988; 80: 282–286.

43 Hyden-Granskog C, Salonen R, von Koskull H *et al.* Three Finnish incontinentia pigmenti families with recombinations with the incontinentia pigmenti loci at Xq28 and Xp11. *Hum. Genet.* 1993; 91: 185–189.

44 Migeon BR, Axelman J, Beur SJ *et al.* Selection against lethal alleles in females heterozygous for incontinentia pigmenti. *Am. J. Hum. Genet.* 1989; 44: 100–106.

45 Coleman R, Genet SA, Harper JI. Interaction of incontinentia pigmenti and factor VIII mutations in a female with biassed X-inactivation resulting in haemophilia. *J. Med. Genet.* 1993; 30: 497–500.

46 Moss C, Goodship J. A novel diagnostic test for incontinentia pigmenti. *Br. J. Dermatol.* 1991; 125 (Suppl. 38): 87.

47 Harris A, Collins J, Vetrie D *et al.* X inactivation as a method of selection against lethal alleles: further investigation of incontinentia pigmenti and X-linked lymphoproliferative disease. *J. Med. Genet.* 1992; 29: 608–614.

48 Temple IK, MacDowall P, Baraitser M, Atherton DJ. Focal dermal hypoplasia (Goltz syndrome). *J. Med. Genet.* 1990; 27: 180–187.

49 Goltz RW, Henderson RR, Hitch JM, Ott JE. Focal dermal hypoplasia: a review of the literature and report of two cases. *Arch. Dermatol.* 1970; 101: 1–11.

50 Mahe A, Couturier J, Mathe C *et al.* Minimal focal dermal hypoplasia in a man: a case of father-to-daughter transmission. *J. Am. Acad. Derm.* 1991; 25: 879–881.

51 Friedman PA, Rao KW, Teplin SW, Aylsworth AS. Provisional deletion mapping of the focal dermal hypoplasia (FDH) gene to Xp22.31. *Am. J. Hum. Genet.* 1988; 43: A50.

52 Naritomi K, Izumikawa Y, Nagataki S. *et al.* Combined Goltz and Aicardi syndromes in a terminal Xp deletion: are they a contiguous gene syndrome? *Am. J. Med. Genet.* 1992; 43: 839–843.

53 Gorski JL. Father-to-daughter transmission of focal dermal hypoplasia associated with nonrandom X-inactivation: support for X-linked inheritance and paternal X chromosome mosaicism. *Am. J. Med. Genet.* 1991; 40: 332–337.

54 Ghiggeri GM, Caridi G, Altieri P. *et al.* Are the nail–patella syndrome and the autosomal Goltz-like syndrome the phenotypic expressions of different alleles of the COL5A1 locus? *Hum. Genet.* 1993; 91: 175–177.

55 Ito M. Incontinentia pigmenti achromians: a singular case of naevus depigmentosus systematicus bilateralis. *Tohoku J. Exp. Med.* 1952; 55: 57–59.

56 Cramer JA, Schmidt WJ. Incontinentia pigmenti: report of six cases. *Arch. Dermatol.* 1955; 71: 699.

57 Moss C, Burn J. Genetic counselling in Hypomelanosis of Ito: case report and review. *Clin. Genet.* 1988; 34: 109–115.

58 Takematsu H, Sato S, Igarashi M, Seiji M. Incontinentia pigmenti achromians (Ito). *Arch. Dermatol.* 1983; 119–395.

59 Sybert VP. Hypomelanosis of Ito: a description not a diagnosis. *J. Invest. Dermatol.* 1994; 103 (Suppl.): 141–143S.

60 Koiffman., de Souza DH, Diament A *et al.* Incontinentia pigmenti achromians (hypomelanosis of Ito, MIM 146150): further evidence of localisation at Xp11. *Am. J. Med. Genet.* 1993; 46: 529–533.

Naevi

Definition

A naevus is a skin hamartoma consisting of normal skin components in an abnormal distribution. Usually naevi are congenital (birth marks) but some, for example melanocytic naevi, can arise later in life. Some dermatologists complicate this further by using naevus cell to mean immature melanocyte, hence the confusing terms naevocytic naevus and naevoid basal-cell carcinoma.

Naevi presenting at or soon after birth are included in this chapter, while acquired naevi are discussed under benign tumours (pp. 127–138). This division is artificial but convenient.

Cause

Isolated naevi are probably due to somatic mutations in genes responsible for normal development, the normal skin carrying the normal genotype, and the abnormal patches being composed of the mutant clone. In some cases the mutation is one which, if generalized, causes a characteristic autosomal dominant disorder; for example, Darier's disease, psoriasis or bullous ichthyosiform erythroderma (see p. 13). In others, the naevus has no generalized counterpart. Happle [1,2] has suggested that these are due to lethal genes rescued by mosaicism: if all cells carried the mutation the fetus would be aborted. If the patient is indeed genetically mosaic, he or she may also have gonadal mosaicism, and could in theory pass on either a normal or a mutant chromosome, with a risk of transmitting the disease in a generalized, lethal form resulting in an increased fetal loss.

Sometimes a tendency to develop naevi is generalized or familial, in which case presumably all cells carry a premutation, and naevi develop only when the full mutation occurs.

There are innumerable types of naevi all of which must embody clues to normal development, but in most cases the pathogenesis is unknown. We include only those that are multiple, familial or associated with other features in characteristic syndromes.

Shape

In general, naevi that follow Blaschko's lines are epidermal. Their arrangement probably reflects the lines of migration of embryonic ectodermal clones (see pp. 8–10).

Non-linear naevi may also arise in the epidermis. Oval sebaceous naevi may be found on the scalp, and have a propensity to develop secondary tumours within themselves, particularly basal-cell carcinoma and syringocystadenoma papilliferum. It seems likely that these naevi are also clonal defects, but the mutations occur later than the linear epidermal migrations that determine Blaschko's lines. The same argument presumably applies to congenital pigmented naevi: giant hairy naevi affect large areas of the trunk or a limb with no respect for Blaschko's lines; cafe-au-lait macules are generally oval and may cross the midline; and Becker's naevus is quite irregular in outline. However, linearity may be imposed on these lesions (presumably by an earlier epidermal mutation), as in zosteriform lentiginous naevus and segmental neurofibromatosis (see pp. 136–137).

Port-wine stains conform to dermatomes rather than Blaschko's lines. This may reflect a neurological basis, the primary abnormality being the neural control of vascular tone.

Naevi in the epidermis

Verrucous, sebaceous and inflammatory epidermal naevi

These may be small or extensive, single or multiple, isolated or associated with numerous other abnormalities. Histologically, a brown, warty, 'verrucous epidermal naevus' simply shows epidermal thickening, while the smooth, yellowish, papular 'sebaceous naevus' shows sebaceous differentiation, sometimes with comedone formation (a comedone naevus) (Figs 1.8 and 1.9). Indeed, an individual patient may show different histology in different areas and at different times [3], sebaceous differentiation being more common on the head and neck and after puberty. It is not surprising, therefore, that a confusing variety of names is used (including verrucous naevus, organoid naevus, naevus unius lateris, naevus sebaceus of Jadassohn, etc.).

Epidermal naevi are occasionally familial [4], inherited in an autosomal dominant manner. The explanation for inheritance of an apparently mosaic disorder, as discussed above, may be inheritance of an unstable premutation.

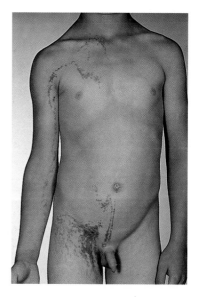

Fig. 1.8 Verrucous epidermal naevi corresponding to Blaschko's lines.

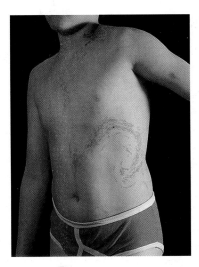

Fig. 1.9 Verrucous epidermal naevi: the characteristically whorled pattern is seen on the flank.

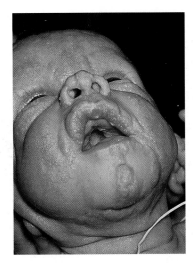

Fig. 1.10 Extensive naevus sebaceous in a child with the epidermal naevus syndrome.

Linear epidermal naevi occur in the epidermal naevus syndrome and Proteus syndrome.

Epidermal naevus syndrome (Schimmelpenning–Feuerstein–Mims syndrome) (MIM 163200, 165630)

Clinical features [5]

The essential feature is one or more linear epidermal naevi, which may show verrucous, sebaceous or comedone differentiation [6]. The naevus may be a single, small, linear group of papules, or extensive and bilateral (systematized) [7] (Fig. 1.10). Its extent does not correlate with the severity of associated defects, but the site is relevant in that neurological abnormalities are much more common in people with an epidermal naevus on the head, and usually occur on the same side.

The associated features are very variable, the most constant being mental retardation, epilepsy and ocular abnormalities, particularly colobomas (fusion defects). In practice, any combination of an epidermal naevus and a significant skeletal, neurological or ocular abnormality is included in the epidermal naevus syndrome [5]. It has been estimated that one-third of patients with a linear epidermal naevus have other abnormalities, but these include common defects such as genu valgum and inguinal hernia [5].

Genetic aspects

Epidermal naevus syndrome is usually sporadic, and is thought to be due to a dominant mutation incompatible with survival except when rescued by mosaicism [1].

Pathogenesis

If the epidermal naevus syndrome is a mosaic disorder due to a somatic mutation, the question arises as to what sort of mutation could give rise to such protean manifestations. Hamartomas can arise in many different tissues, suggesting that the mutation occurs very early, before any tissue differentiation, and that the defect involves a generally expressed gene controlling cell proliferation.

ILVEN

ILVEN (inflammatory *l*inear *v*errucous *e*pidermal *n*aevus) usually develops in the first few years of life as a red, scaly, itchy area following Blaschko's lines anywhere on the body. It has been confused with linear psoriasis, but is distinguishable by its persistence and resistance to antipsoriatic medication, as well as by histology. In some cases an ILVEN on the limb has been associated with a terminal limb defect, which has led to the suggestion of overlap with CHILD syndrome (see below). ILVEN is not seen in epidermal naevus syndrome.

CHILD syndrome (MIM 308050)

The acronym is derived from *c*ongenital *h*emidysplasia with *i*chthyosiform erythroderma and *l*imb *d*efects [8]. The classical appearance is dramatic with a sharp midline demarcation between the two halves of the body, one being normal, and the other having red, scaly skin and limb reductions. Internal organs may be hypoplastic on the affected side. In most cases demarcation is less absolute, with linear spared areas of skin on the affected side and linear red scaly lesions on the other. The appearance and histology of the skin are more like ILVEN than ichthyosiform erythroderma. The limb reductions sometimes associated with ILVEN also suggest an overlap. It has been suggested therefore that ILVEN and CHILD syndrome are manifestations of the same disorder and would be better designated PEN or PENCIL, that is *p*soriasiform *e*pidermal *n*aevus plus or minus *c*ongenital *i*psilateral *l*imb defects [9]. Happle, who devised the acronym CHILD, has disputed this [10].

Genetic aspects

Happle *et al.* [8] reported 18 females and one male, and possible increased antenatal loss of males, suggesting X-linked dominant inheritance with mosaicism due to lyonization.

Pathogenesis

Increased synthesis of prostaglandin E^2 in affected dermal fibroblasts has been reported in one case [11]. Holbrook's group found reduced expression of differentiation markers and increased expression of the basal keratins K5 and K14 in affected epidermis, and abnormal accumulation of intercellular vesicles in cell cultures [12].

Congenital pigmented naevi

Moles, freckles and lentigines usually appear in childhood or early adult life, and syndromes involving these features are included in the chapter on benign tumours. Syndromes with congenital moles include giant, pigmented, hairy naevus [13] (MIM 137550), which may be associated with multiple moles in relatives, and neurocutaneous melanosis [14] (MIM 249400), in which extensive melanocytic naevi involve the meninges as well as the skin.

Naevus spilus, which is essentially a cafe-au-lait macule with small, dark, melanocytic naevi speckled within it, is usually present at birth and may be segmental when it is termed zosteriform lentiginous naevus. The latter may be related to segmental neurofibromatosis [15].

Cafe-au-lait macules are characteristically present at birth, but become more obvious and perhaps more numerous with age. They occur classically in neurofibromatosis but also in Bloom and Fanconi syndromes, and in Russell–Silver dwarfism (MIM 270050).

Large areas of cafe-au-lait-type pigmentation sometimes occur in a segmental distribution in an otherwise normal child: in some cases this might be the sole manifestation of McCune–Albright syndrome, a mosaic disorder with patchy pigmentation in which there is a mutation causing activation of a gene that stimulates cAMP in endocrine glands and presumably in the melanocyte.

Hypopigmented naevi

Hypopigmented naevi resemble segmental vitiligo but are fixed at birth. They are usually unassociated, but the same lesions accompany neurological deficit in hypomelanosis of Ito. In the latter there is chromosome mosaicism in the skin: this has not been studied in isolated hypopigmented naevi.

Naevi in the dermis

Non-vascular naevi

Most dermal hamartomas appear in late childhood or adult life, and are discussed in the chapter on benign tumours. Table 1.4 lists some syndromes in which dermal naevi are found early in childhood.

Vascular naevi

There are several distinct types, which usually occur singly but may be multiple. Different types may coexist in multiple naevus syndromes such as Proteus and Klippel–Trenaunay syndromes.

Raised capillary haemangiomas (strawberry naevi) (Fig. 1.11)

A strawberry naevus develops as a mass of proliferating endothelial cells, which becomes canalized and subsequently involutes. These changes correspond to the clinical signs of postnatal enlargement and subsequent regression. They are sometimes familial and may be multiple. Complications of large strawberry naevi include

consumption coagulopathy (Kasabach–Merritt syndrome, MIM 141000, a non-genetic syndrome).

Strawberry naevi are found in the syndromes listed in Table 1.5.

Flat capillary naevi (port-wine stains)

The port-wine stain and salmon patch are not angiomas, but naevoid areas of reduced capillary tone with vascular dilatation and increased blood flow.

Unna's naevus or 'stork mark' is a common finding in normal individuals [16]. The nuchal salmon patch is more persistent than the forehead component.

Port-wine stains are frequently segmental in distribution (Fig 1.12. and 1.13). However, their arrangement conforms more to dermatomes than to Blaschko's lines: this is particularly apparent in facial lesions and may indicate a neurological basis.

These lesions occur in many syndromes (Tables 1.6 and 1.7), some of which are sporadic and probably mosaic disorders, the vascular naevi presumably representing somatic mutations. Inherited syndromes with vascular naevi presumably involve susceptibility genes (see Introduction). Expression is variable within

Table 1.4 Syndromes featuring dermal naevi in early childhood

MIM*	Name	Naevi/hamartomas present in infancy
191100	Tuberous sclerosis	Sacral collagenoma (shagreen patch)
166700	Buschke–Ollendorf[1]	Elastomas (with osteopoikilosis)
—	Encephalocraniocutaneous lipomatosis[2]	Multiple lipomas of head, neck and brain
—	Michelin-tyre baby syndrome[3,4]	Diffuse lipomatous hypertrophy
167730	Coloboma–lipoma syndrome[5]	Lipomas around the eyes

* First digit of MIM number indicates inheritance: 1 = autosomal dominant; 2 = autosomal recessive; 3 = X-linked.
1 Verbov J, Graham R. Buschke–Ollendorf syndrome: disseminated dermatofibrosis with osteopoikilosis. *Clin. Exp. Dermatol.* 1986; 11: 17–26.
2 Sanchez NP, Rhodes AR, Mandell F *et al.* Encephalocraniocutaneous lipomatosis: a new neurocutaneous syndrome. *Br. J. Dermatol.* 1981; 104: 89–96.
3 Gardner EW, Miller HM, Lowney ED. Deletion of chromosome 11 in babies with Michelin tyre syndrome. *Arch. Dermatol.* 1980; 116: 622.
4 Niikawa N, Ishikiriyama S, Shikimani T. The 'Michelin tire baby' syndrome—an autosomal dominant trait. *Am. J. Med. Genet.* 1985; 22: 637–638.
5 Akarsu AN, Sayli BS. Nasopalpebral lipoma–coloboma syndrome. *Clin. Genet.* 1991; 40: 342–344.

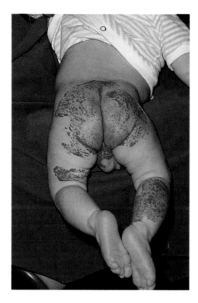

Fig. 1.11 Extensive strawberry naevi.

families; for example, relatives of a patient with Klippel–Trenaunay syndrome may have multiple port-wine stains [17].

There is considerable overlap between syndromes; for example the neurocutaneous disorders Sturge–Weber syndrome and Wyburn–Mason syndrome may coexist [18].

A mid-forehead port-wine stain is a rather non-specific finding in many different disorders (Table

1.7). For several of these there is a clue to the genetic locus, including Beckwith–Wiedemann syndrome on 11p [19], Rubinstein–Taybi syndrome on 16p [20], diastrophic dysplasia on 5q [21] and trisomy 13, but there is no known unifying pathogenetic factor.

Klippel–Trenaunay syndrome (MIM 149000)

Clinical features

The classical triad is cutaneous vascular naevus, varicose veins and limb hypertrophy [17]. When significant arteriovenous anastomoses are present the name of Parkes–Weber is added. Occasionally limb hypotrophy has occurred [22].

Genetic aspects

This is probably a mosaic disorder, caused by somatic mutation for a lethal gene rendered survivable by mosaicism (see above). There is considerable phenotypic overlap between Klippel–Trenaunay, Sturge–Weber, Proteus and epidermal naevus syndromes, all of which are thought to be mosaic conditions. In two Belgian families there was possible dominant inheritance of Klippel–Trenaunay syndrome, with a strong history of vascular naevi in relatives [23]. This is consistent with the idea of a susceptibility gene,

Table 1.5 Syndromes featuring strawberry naevi

MIM*	Name	Associated features
106070	Disseminated haemangiomatosis	Internal and cutaneous haemangiomas
140850[1]	—	Facial haemangiomas + supra-umbilical midline raphe
149000	Klippel–Trenaunay	Mixed vascular anomalies; hemihypertrophy
153480	Bannayan–Zonana[2,3]	Macrocephaly, skin + visceral haemangiomas, lipomas
153480	Riley–Smith[3]	Macrocephaly, pseudopapilloedema
176920	Proteus	Epidermal naevi, localized hypertrophy
234800	—	Cutaneous haemangiomas, joint hyperextensibility

* First digit of MIM number indicates inheritance: 1 = autosomal dominant; 2 = autosomal recessive; 3 = X-linked.

1 Igarashi M, Uchida H, Kajii T. Supraumbilical midabdominal raphe and facial cavernous haemangiomas. *Clin. Genet.* 1985; 27: 196–198.

2 Israel J, Lessick M, Szego K, Wong P. Translocation 19; Y in a child with Bannayan-Zonana phenotype. *J. Med. Genet.* 1991; 28: 427–428.

3 Cohen MM Jr. Bannayan–Riley–Ruvacalba syndrome: renaming three formerly recognized syndromes as one etiologic entity. *Am. J. Med. Genet.* 1990; 35: 291.

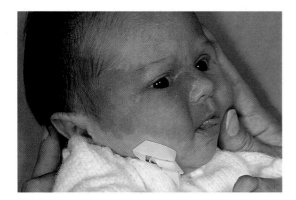

Fig. 1.12 Port-wine stain: maxillary distribution.

which is dominantly inherited, but must be associated with a second mutation for a lesion to occur.

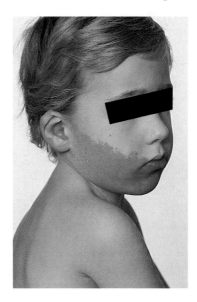

Fig. 1.13 Port-wine stain: mandibular distribution.

Table 1.6 Syndromes featuring flat capillary naevi

MIM*	Name	Associated features
163000	Multiple port-wine stains[1]	Usually no associations
106070	Hereditary neurocutaneous angioma[2]	Widespread cutaneomeningospinal angiomas
185300	Sturge–Weber[3]	Ophthalmic port-wine stain + epilepsy/retardation
—	Wyburn–Mason[3]	Ipsilateral retinal arteriovenous malformation, facial port-wine stain and cerebral arteriovenous malformation
—	Cobb[4]	Spinal port-wine stain + overlying spinal angioma
176920	Proteus[5]	Epidermal and vascular naevi with local overgrowth
149000	Klippel–Trenaunay[6]	Mixed vascular naevi + hemihypertrophy
274000	TAR[7]	Thrombocytopenia, absent radius, unilateral port-wine stain
—	Phakomatosis pigmentovascularis[8]	Port-wine stain, oculocutaneous melanosis, central nervous system defect

* First digit of MIM number indicates inheritance: 1 = autosomal dominant; 2 = autosomal recessive; 3 = X-linked.

1 Pasyk KA. Familial multiple lateral telangiectatic nevi (port wine stains or nevi flammei). *Clin. Genet.* 1992; 41: 197–201.
2 Hurst J, Baraitser M. Hereditary neurocutaneous angiomatous malformations: autosomal dominant inheritance in two families. *Clin. Genet.* 1988; 33: 44–48.
3 Ward KB, Katz NNK. Combined phakomatoses: a case report of Sturge–Weber and Wyburn–Mason syndrome occurring in the same individual. *Ann. Ophthalmol.* 1983; 15: 1112–1116.
4 Kaplan P, Hollenberg RD, Fraser C. A spinal arteriovenous malformation with hereditary cutaneous haemangiomas. *Am. J. Dis. Child.* 1976; 130: 1329–1331.
5 Samlaska CP, Levin SW, James WD *et al.* Proteus syndrome. *Arch. Dermatol.* 1989; 125: 1109–1114.
6 Aelvot GE, Jorens PG, Roelen LM. Genetic aspects of the Klippel–Trenauney syndrome. *Br. J. Dermatol.* 1992; 126: 603–607.
7 Ashinoff R, Geronemus RG. Thrombocytopenia–absent radii syndrome and lack of response to the pulsed-dye laser. *Arch. Dermatol.* 1990; 126: 1520–1521.
8 Ruiz-Maldonado R, Tamayo L, Laterza AM *et al.* Phacomatosis pigmentovascularis: a new syndrome? *Pediatr. Dermatol.* 1987; 4: 189–196.

Table 1.7 Syndromes featuring mid-forehead port-wine stain

MIM*	Name	Associated features
163100	Unna's naevus[1]	Familial naevus of mid-forehead and nape of neck
108110	Arthrogryposis multiplex congenita	Widespread joint contractures
130650	Beckwith–Wiedemann[2]	Exomphalos, macroglossia, gigantism
253290	Lethal multiple pterygium syndrome[3]	Joint contractures, pterygium, stillbirth
146510	Pallister–Hall	Hypopituitarism, abnormal lungs, poly/syndactyly, anal defects
180700	Robinow	Short forearms, flat face, hypoplastic genitalia
268300	Robert[4]	Hypomelia, hypotrichosis, clefting
180849	Rubinstein–Taybi[5]	Broad thumbs/toes, small jaw, low IQ, down-slanting eyes
—	Trisomy 13	Holoprosencephaly, polydactyly, scalp aplasia cutis
222600	Diastrophic dysplasia[6]	Dwarfism with skeletal abnormalities

*   First digit of MIM number indicates inheritance: 1 = autosomal dominant; 2 = autosomal recessive; 3 = X-linked.

1   Merlob P, Reisner SH. Familial nevus flammeus of the forehead and Unna's nevus. *Clin. Genet.* 1985; 27: 165–166.

2   Weksburg R, Glaves M, Teshima I *et al*. Molecular characterization of Beckwith–Wiedmann syndrome (BWS) patients with partial duplication of chromosome 11p excludes the gene MYOD1 from the BWS region. *Genomics* 1990; 8: 693–698.

3   Hall JG, Reed SG, Rosenbaum J *et al*. Limb pterygium syndromes: a review and report of eleven cases. *Am. J. Med. Genet.* 1982; 12: 377–409.

4   Romke C, Froster-Iskenius U, Heyne K *et al*. Roberts' syndrome and SC phocomelia: a single genetic entity. *Clin. Genet.* 1987; 31: 170–177.

5   Trommerup N, van der Hagen CB, Heiberg A. Tentative assignment of a locus for Rubinstein–Taybi syndrome to 16p13.3 by a *de novo* reciprocal translocation t (7; 16) (q 34; p13.3). *Cytogenet. Cell Genet.* 1991; 58: 2002–2003.

6   Hastbacka J, Katila I, Sistonen P, de la Chapelle A. Diastrophic dysplasia gene maps to the distal long arm of chromosome 5. *Proc. Natl. Acad. Sci. USA* 1990; 87: 8056–8059.

Proteus syndrome (MIM 176920)

Clinical features

Characteristically there are vascular naevi, localized hypertrophy particularly of hands and feet, and epidermal naevi [24] (Fig. 1.14). There may be other vascular malformations and hamartomas, particularly lipomas. This highly variable syndrome is named after the Greek god who could change his form [25]. It seems likely that the massive hypertrophy suffered by John Merrick, the 'Elephant Man', was due to Proteus syndrome rather than neurofibromatosis.

Genetic aspects and pathogenesis

The condition is usually sporadic. It is thought to be a mosaic disorder, due to somatic mutation for a lethal gene, like epidermal naevus

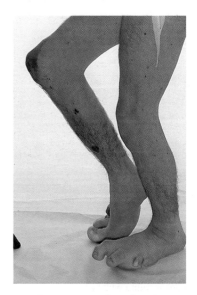

Fig. 1.14 Focal gigantism and capillary haemangiomas in Proteus syndrome. (Courtesy of Dr J. S. Comaish.)

syndrome and Klippel–Trenaunay syndrome. Apparent dominant inheritance in one family may be due to a dominant premutation or susceptibility gene [26].

Naevus anaemicus

This is apparently the reverse of a port-wine stain: a naevus in which capillary tone is increased resulting in reduced blood flow (Fig. 1.15). It probably has a pharmacological basis [27]. Occasionally naevus anaemicus and port-wine stain occur together, and Happle has suggested that this is due to somatic recombination [28]. Naevus anaemicus is more common in patients with neurofibromatosis than in the general population [29] and may be inherited alone [30].

Telangiectatic naevi

Telangiectases (end-vessel dilatations) appear as red dots in the skin. They occur in two segmental naevi, angioma serpiginosum [31] (MIM 106050) and unilateral naevoid telangiectasia [32]. Both are more common in females. Some cases may represent mosaic forms of the dominant disorders hereditary haemorrhagic telangiectasia (MIM 187300) or hereditary benign telangiectasia (MIM 187260).

Fig. 1.15 Naevus anaemicus unmasked by rubbing: the typical confluent round white areas fail to vasodilate, in contrast to the pinkness induced in the surrounding normal skin.

Reticulate vascular naevi

Cutis marmorata telangiectatica congenita (MIM 219250) is usually localized to a limb, which may show hypotrophy. A variety of associated systemic features have been reported, the majority only once [33]. Familial occurrence has been reported [34]. In the Divry–van Bogaert syndrome (MIM 206570) there are central nervous system abnormalities due to diffuse leptomeningeal angiomatosis, and some patients have had recurrent strokes and other evidence of microvascular disease [35].

Angiokeratomatous naevi

Angiokeratoma circumscriptum may occur alone or as part of a mixed vascular malformation such as Klippel–Trenaunay syndrome. The possibility that these naevoid lesions represent mosaicism for a generalized angiokeratomatous disorder has not been explored.

Venous naevi

In Mafucci syndrome (MIM 166000), zosteriform venous haemangiomas are associated with acral enchondromas. Blue rubber bleb naevus syndrome (MIM 112200) is characterized by visceral as well as cutaneous venous angiomas. The two conditions may coexist [36]. In Klippel–Trenaunay syndrome there are venous as well as capillary malformations.

References

1 Happle R. Cutaneous manifestation of lethal genes. *Hum. Genet.* 1986; 72: 280.
2 Happle R. Lethal genes surviving by mosaicism: a possible explanation for sporadic birth defects involving the skin. *J. Am. Acad. Dermotal.* 1987; 16: 899–906.
3 Mehregan AH, Pinkus H. Life history of organoid nevi. *Arch. Dermatol.* 1965; 91: 574–588.
4 Sahl WJ. Familial nevus sebaceous of Jadassohn: occurrence in three generations. *J. Am. Acad. Derm.* 1990; 22: 853–854.
5 Rogers M, McCrossin I, Commens C. Epidermal nevi and the epidermal nevus syndrome. *J. Am. Acad. Dermatol.* 1989; 20: 476–488.

6   Solomon LM, Fretzin DF, Dewald RL. The epidermal nevus syndrome. *Arch. Dermatol.* 1968; 97: 273–285.

7   Moss C, Parkin JM, Comaish JSC. Precocious puberty in a boy with a widespread linear epidermal naevus. *Br. J. Dermatol.* 1991; 125: 178–182.

8   Happle R, Koch H, Lenz W. The CHILD syndrome. Congenital hemidysplasia with ichthyosiform erythroderma and limb defects. *Eur. J. Pediatr.* 1980; 134: 27–33.

9   Moss C, Burn J. Hypothesis: CHILD + ILVEN = PEN or PENCIL. *J. Med. Genet.* 1990; 27: 390–391.

10 Happle R. CHILD naevus is not ILVEN. *J. Med. Genet.* 1991; 28: 214.

11 Goldyne ME, Williams ML. CHILD syndrome: phenotypic dichotomy in eicosanoid metabolism and proliferative rates among cultured dermal fibroblasts. *J. Clin. Invest.* 1989; 84: 357–360.

12 Dale BA, Kimball JR, Fleckman P *et al.* CHILD syndrome: lack of expression of epidermal differentiation markers in lesional ichthyotic skin. *J. Invest. Dermatol.* 1992; 98: 442–449.

13 Goodman RM, Caren J, Ziprkowski M *et al.* Genetic considerations in giant pigmented hairy naevus. *Br. J. Dermatol.* 1971; 85: 150–157.

14 Kaplan AM, Itabashi HH, Hanelin LG, Lu AT. Neurocutaneous melanosis with maligant leptomeningeal melanoma. *Arch. Neurol.* 1975; 32: 669–671.

15 Moss C, Green SH. What is segmental neurofibromatosis? *Br. J. Dermatol* 1993; 130: 106–110.

16 Merlob P, Reisner SH. Familial nevus flammeus of the forehead and Unna's nevus. *Clin. Genet.* 1985; 27: 165–166.

17 Aelvoet GE, Jorens PG, Roelen LM. Genetic aspects of the Klippel–Trenaunay syndrome. *Br. J. Dermatol.* 1992; 126: 603–607.

18 Ward JB, Katz NNK. Combined phakomatoses: a case report of Sturge–Weber and Wyburn–Mason syndrome occurring in the same individual. *Ann. Ophthalmol.* 1983; 15: 1112–1116.

19 Weksberg R, Glaves M, Teshima I *et al.* Molecular characterisation of Beckwith–Wiedemann syndrome (BWS) patients with partial duplication of chromosome 11p excludes the gene MYOD1 from the BWS region. *Genomics* 1990; 8: 693–698.

20 Tommerup N, van der Hagen CB, Heiberg A. Tentative assignment of a locus for Rubinstein–Taybi syndrome to 16p13.3 by a *de novo* reciprocal translocation t(7; 16) (q34; p13.3). *Cytogenet. Cell Genet.* 1991; 58: 2002–2003.

21 Hastbacka J, Kaitila I, Sistonen P, de la Chapelle A. Diastrophic dysplasia gene maps to the distal long arm of chromosome 5. *Proc. Natl. Acad. Sci. USA* 1990; 87: 8056–8059.

22 Moss C, Robson BJ. Haemangiectatic hypotrophy associated with Perthe's disease. *Clin. Exp. Dermatol.* 1988; 13: 237–239.

23 Viljoen DL. Klippel–Trenaunay–Weber syndrome (angio-osteohypertrophy syndrome). *J. Med. Genet.* 1988; 25: 250–252.

24 Samlaska CP, Levin SW, James WD *et al.* Proteus syndrome. *Arch. Dermatol* 1989; 125: 1109–1114.

25 Wiedemann HR, Burgio GR, Aldenhoff P *et al.* The Proteus syndrome: partial gigantism of the hands and/or feet, nevi, hemihypertrophy, subcutaneous tumours, macrocephaly or other skull anomalies and possible accelerated growth and visceral affections. *Eur. J. Pediatr.* 1983; 140: 5–12.

26 Goodship J, Redfearn A, Milligan D *et al.* Transmission of Proteus syndrome from father to son? *J. Med. Genet.* 1991; 28: 781–785.

27 Greaves M, Birkett D, Johnson C. Nevus anemicus: a unique catecholamine dependent nevus. *Arch. Dermatol.* 1970; 102: 172–176.

28 Happle R, Koopman R, Mier OD. Hypothesis: vascular twin naevi and somatic recombination in man. *Lancet* 1990; i: 376–378.

29 Piorkowski PO. Nevus anemicus (Voerner). *Arch. Dermatol.* 1944; 50: 374–377.

30 Cardoso H, Vignale R, Abreu de Sastre H. Familial naevus anaemicus. *Am. J. Hum. Genet.* 1975; 27: 24A.

31 Marriott PJ, Munro DD, Ryan T. Angioma serpiginosum–familial incidence. *Br. J. Dermatol.* 1975; 93: 701–706.

32 Wilkin JK, Graham-Smith J, Collison DA *et al.* Unilateral dermatomal superficial telangiectasia. *J. Am. Acad. Dermatol.* 1983; 8: 468–477.

33 Picascia DD, Esterley NB. Cutis marmorata telangiectasia congenita: report of 22 cases. *J. Am. Acad. Dermatol.* 1989; 20: 1098–1104.

34 Andreev VC, Pramatorov K. Cutis marmorata telangiectatica congenita in two sisters. *Br. J. Dermatol.* 1979; 101: 345–349.

35 Baxter P, Gardner-Medwin D, Green SH, Moss C. Congenital livedo reticularis and recurrent stroke-like episodes. *Dev. Med. Child Neurol.* 1993; 35: 917–926.

36 Sakurane HF, Sugai T, Saito T. The association of blue rubber bleb nevus and Maffucci's syndrome. *Arch. Dermatol.* 1967; 95: 28–36.

Pigmentary demarcation lines

The natural boundaries of pigmentation that occur in racially pigmented skin can easily be misinterpreted as linear pigmentary anomalies.

1 The anterior brachial (Futcher's) line (MIM 13700) [1] runs down the front of the upper arm separating a darker lateral region from the lighter skin closer to the body. It is common, variably distinct, and often asymmetrical.

2 The mediosternal line (MIM 155200) [2] runs across the chest above the nipples (Fig. 1.16). It may be a continuation of the anterior brachial line. Sometimes it takes the form of a band of lighter skin, that is two parallel pigmentary demarcation lines.

Several other lines may be seen [3] including a transpectoral line dipping down to the level of the nipples, a light band down the sternum or just to the side of it and variable lanceolate oblique streaks on the upper chest that are paler and less defined than ash-leaf macules. A line may also be seen on the thigh, extending from the perineum to the medial aspect of the popliteal fossa.

Aetiology

The anterior brachial line fits the general biological observation that dorsal and extensor surfaces are darker than ventral and flexor aspects, perhaps for photoprotection. A more useful observation is that pigmentary demarcation lines correspond anatomically to axial lines of sensory innervation, which separate adjacent areas of skin supplied by non-adjacent areas of the spinal cord (Fig. 1.17). The anterior brachial line separates

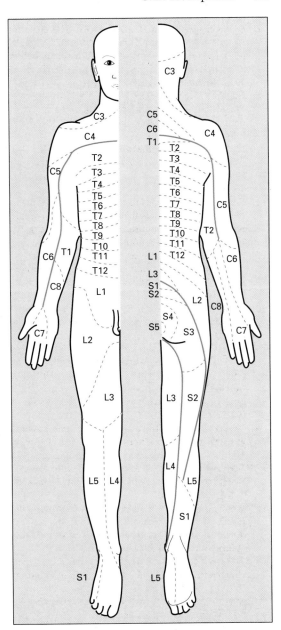

Fig. 1.17 Axial lines (in green) separate areas of skin innervated from non-adjacent spinal segments. They probably coincide with pigmentary demarcation lines and with the longer epidermal naevi.

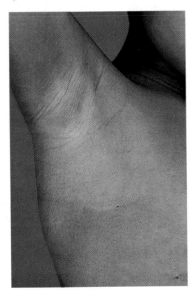

Fig. 1.16 Pigmentary demarcation line around the chest below the axilla.

skin innervated laterally by C4, C5 and C6, and medially by T2 and T1. Similarly, the line on the thigh corresponds to the axial line separating the S2 zone posteriorly from the L1, L2 and L3 zones medially and anteriorly. The mid-sternal line separates skin supplied from different sides of the spinal cord. Pigmentary demarcation lines also coincide with Blaschko's lines, although there are many more of the latter. Since Blaschko's lines are based on the distribution of epidermal naevi it is not surprising that epidermal naevi may follow pigmentary demarcation lines. What is more interesting is that the longest and most well-defined epidermal naevi correspond to the axial lines on the limbs. This is evident from Blaschko's drawings, which show numerous examples of a thin clear line down the posterior medial thigh and of a line arching across the chest above the breast and continuing down the front of the arm.

Finally, there is some correspondence with hair lines: in subjects where both are visible, the point on the anterior upper arm, where hair slope abruptly changes direction, lies, in the author's experience, on Futcher's line.

All these observations suggest that pigmentary demarcation lines are determined by sensory dermatomes, and constitute boundaries to nerve, melanocyte and keratinocyte migration as well as hair growth.

References

1 Futcher PH. The distribution of pigmentation on the arm and thorax of man. *Bull. Johns Hopkins Hosp.* 1940; 67: 372–373.
2 Kisch B, Nasuhoglu A. Mediosternal depigmentation line in negroes. *Exp. Med. Surg.* 1953; 11: 265–267.
3 Selmanowitz VJ, Krivo JM. Pigmentary demarcation lines: comparison of negroes with Japanese. *Br. J. Dermatol.* 1975; 93: 371–377.

Hair patterns

As well as inherited and racial variation in amount of body hair, there are different hair patterns that occur in genetically determined syndromes.

At 18 weeks the fetal face and scalp are uniformly hairy, but subsequently facial hair growth ceases except in the eyebrows and eyelashes. There appear to be periocular zones of hair-growth suppression that may intersect on the upper forehead to produce the 'widow's peak', a feature that may be inherited as an isolated autosomal dominant trait (MIM 194000) or as an X-linked trait associated with ptosis and skeletal anomalies (MIM 314570). This V-shaped downward projection of scalp hair is more prominent in hyperteleorism, when the postulated periocular hair suppression zones intersect lower down the forehead. Furthermore, aberrant hair on the lateral forehead may accompany cryptophthalmos [1].

The direction of the scalp whorl at the vertex appears to be genetically controlled, a clockwise whorl being dominantly inherited (MIM 139400). Slope is probably determined when the follicles are growing downwards between weeks 10 and 16, by relative movements of the dermis and epidermis and the position of the arrector pili muscle. These in turn may be controlled by growth of the underlying tissue. Smith suggested that the slope of hair outwards from the crown is due to the rapid expansion of the brain between 10 and 16 weeks, and supported this with the observation that in microcephaly, where the brain does not grow forwards enough, the forward hair slope correspondingly stops short in a frontal upsweep or 'cowlick' [1]. Abnormalities of scalp hair occur in several mental retardation syndromes. An intriguing abnormality in hair slope is the ridgeback anomaly, in which scalp hair slopes towards the crown coconut-style in an otherwise normal individual [2].

Hair follicles also slope in different directions on different parts of the body, producing a complex pattern of lines and whorls which is fairly constant from person to person [3]. In some sites, particularly the centre of the back and the scalp, the pattern corresponds closely to Blaschko's lines, suggesting that both may be due to the same forces. There may also be some correspondence to pigmentary demarcation lines and axial lines (see pp. 31–32). The predominantly distal- wards direction of hair slope on the limbs may be secondary to growth of the limb, but a further explanation is required for the whorls and abrupt changes of direction often seen on limbs. It may be that an overall pattern due to growth of the fetus is modified by local variations in relative movement of dermis and epidermis, which may have a simple mechanical explanation, or, if one can argue teleologically, may be 'programmed in' according to some evolutionary design to make the body more streamlined.

Abnormal patterns might be expected to accompany defects of limb development, but this has not been reported.

References

1 Jones KL (ed). *Smith's Recognisable Patterns of Human Malformation*, 4th edn. Philadelphia: WB Saunders, 1988; 672–676.
2 Samlaska CP, Benson PM, James WD. The ridgeback anomaly: a new follicular pattern of the scalp. *Arch. Dermatol.* 1989; 125: 98–102.
3 Samlaska CP, James WD, Sperling LC. Scalp whorls. *J. Am. Acad. Dermatol.* 1989; 21: 553–556.

Dermatoglyphics

Dermatoglyphics [1,2], literally meaning skin carvings and so analogous to the word hieroglyphics, is used to describe the fine sculpturing of the surface of the skin. Most interest has centred on the pattern of ridges and furrows, fingerprints on the hands and their equivalent on the feet, of human and other primates. Their legal importance is now equalled by their medical interest.

Development

The surface of the hands and feet is smooth until the 10th week of fetal life. Slight corrugations then appear, first on the inner and later on the outer surface of the epidermis. The differentiation of these ridges and furrows is complete by about 20 weeks.

The precise arrangement, unique to each individual, is in some way linked to the skin tension and curvature caused by volar pads or mounds that appear transiently during the development of the fetal hand and foot. Malformed hands, therefore, are likely to have abnormal fingerprint patterns.

Patterns

Individual epidermal ridges are surmounted by evenly spaced sweat-gland openings. Their arrangement into standard patterns (loops, arches and whorls) is a consequence of the limited number of ways in which a carpet of equidistant fine parallel lines can be fitted over a curved surface. Patterns form like contour lines around a hill, with the centre of the pattern corresponding to the peak of the hill. Parallel ridges stretched over bulbous finger pads form whorls, and over the flattest pads will form arches [3].

Arches can be subdivided into simple or tented: loops into radial or ulnar; and whorls into symmetrical, spiral and double-loop types. Triradii are seen where three systems of ridges meet at angles of more than 90°. The term minutiae is used for the minor irregularities of ridge direction, bifurcations and discontinuities, which are important in fingerprint identification.

Useful measurements of fingerprint pattern include the following.

A ridge count

This is the number of ridges crossed by a straight line joining the core of a loop or whorl to its adjacent triradius. The total ridge count is the sum of this measurement including all of the 10 digits that have loops or whorls. The ridges cut by a line drawn between triradii **a** and **b** on the palms (at the bases of the index and middle fingers) can also be counted.

Pattern frequency

Loops are the most common finger pattern in the UK (70%), followed by whorls (25%) and arches (5%). Whorls are more common in men than women, on right rather than left hands, in Asians than white people and in hypertensives [3]. Certain patterns occur more often on some fingers than on others.

The atd angle

This is the angle, often around 45°, seen when lines are drawn between triradii **a** and **d** (on the palms at the bases of the index and little fingers) and triradius **t** (on the palm overlying the base of the fourth metacarpal).

Genetic control

The high concordance for total ridge count in monozygotic (0.95), as opposed to dizygotic (0.5), twins confirms the importance of inherited factors, which are probably polygenic. However, it has been suggested that a single major autosomal locus with two additive alleles may account for over half the variation in absolute ridge count [4]. The **atd** angle and minutia frequency show less clearcut genetic control. The presence of arches was found to be an autosomal dominant trait in one large kindred [5].

Dermatoglyphic abnormalities

Any disturbance that affects the growth of the hands and feet early in fetal life may distort their dermatoglyphic patterns. This rule applies to environmental agents such as fetal rubella and thalidomide as well as to genetic abnormalities. Fingertip whorls and narrow **atd** angles are associated with raised adult blood pressure; this suggests that important determinants of adult blood pressure act in early gestation. The whorls may have formed in response to fingertips that were unusually bulbous and oedematous at that stage of development [3].

Abnormal dermatoglyphics have been recorded in 26 different types of multiple congenital anomaly [6], most of which include obvious malformations of the hands and feet. Some of these are inherited. Table 1.8 lists some of the single gene disorders that have their main effects on dermatoglyphics.

Chromosomal abnormalities are another important source of dermatoglyphic distortions. Some of the main autosomal associations are given in Table 1.9.

Table 1.8 Some inherited abnormalities of dermatoglyphic pattern

MIM*	Associated features
125540[1]	Patternless ridges
136000[2]	Absence of fingerprints
129200[3]	Ectodermal dysplasia with absent dermatoglyphic pattern
125550[4]	'Ridges-off-the-end', i.e. running vertically off the end of the fingertips
221780[5]	Hypothenar radial arches
221760[6]	Absence of triradius **d**

* First digit of MIM number indicates inheritance:
1 = autosomal dominant; 2 = autosomal recessive;
3 = X-linked.

1 Dondival P. A propos de la dysplasie des cretes epidermiques. *Hum. Genetik* 1972; 15: 20–24
2 Baird HW. Absence of fingerprints in four generations. *Lancet* 1968; ii: 1250.
3 Basan M. Ektodermale Dysplasie. *Arch. Klin. Exp. Dermatol.* 1965; 222: 546–557.
4 David TJ. 'Ridges-off-the-end'—a dermatoglyphic syndrome. *Hum. Hered.* 1971; 21:39–53.
5 Holt SB. The hypothenar radial arch, a genetically determined epidermal ridge configuration. *Am. J. Phys. Anthropol.* 1975; 42: 211–214.
6 Holt SB, Dash Sharma P. Absence of a triradium d on the palms of normal people. *Ann. Hum. Genet.* 1977; 41: 195–197

Table 1.9 Some dermatoglyphic associations of autosomal abnormalities

Condition	Dermatoglyphic associations
Trisomy 13 (Patau syndrome)	Increased **atd** angle. Radial loops on digits 4 and 5
Trisomy 18 (Edward syndrome)	6–10 arches on fingers. Simian crease
Trisomy 21 (Down syndrome)	Ulnar loops on all fingers in 32% (vs. 4% in controls). Increased **atd** angle (over 45%). Simian crease

The dermatoglyphic associations of sex-chromosome abnormalities are more subtle but obey simple rules. They are best detected by total ridge counts and measurements of ridge breadth. Normal males have greater total ridge counts than females (145 vs. 127) [1]. Each extra X chromosome reduces the total ridge count markedly; each extra Y chromosome also reduces it, but to a lesser extent. Similarly males have wider ridges than females; each extra Y chromosome is associated with an increase in ridge breadth.

Associations with skin disease

These may be of interest but are not diagnostic. For example, an increase of digital whorls may be found in psoriatics, and a decrease in ulnar loops on the second digit in alopecia areata [2]. Shallow linear grooves are seen more often on the fingers of patients with atopic dermatitis than in controls with or without other forms of hand dermatitis. These differ from scars by their transience and by not disrupting the ridge pattern [7].

References

1 Penrose LS. Dermatoglyphics and medicine. *Acta Clinica* 1971; 13: 11–36.
2 Verbov J. Clinical significance and genetics of epidermal ridges—a review of dermatoglyphics. *J. Invest. Dermatol.* 1970; 54: 261–271.
3 Godfrey KM, Barker DJP, Peace J, Cloke J, Osmond C. Relation of fingerprints and shape of the palm to fetal growth and adult blood pressure. *BMJ* 1993; 307: 405–409.
4 Spence MA, Elston RC, Namboodiri KK, Pollitzer WS. Evidence for a major gene effect in absolute ridge count. *Hum. Hered.* 1973; 23: 414–421.
5 Anderson MW, Bonne-Tamir B, Carmelli D, Thompson EA. Linkage analysis and the inheritance of arches in a Habbanite isolate. *Am. J. Hum. Genet.* 1979; 31: 620–629.
6 Winter RM, Baraitser M. Abnormal dermatoglyphics. In *Multiple Congenital Anomalies: a Diagnostic Compendium.* London: Chapman and Hall Medical, 1991: 813–814.
7 Cusumano D, Berman B, Bershad S. Dermatoglyphic patterns in patients with atopic dermatitis. *J. Am. Acad. Dermatol.* 1983; 8: 207–210.

2
THE EPIDERMIS
AND ITS DISORDERS

During the last 10 years, much has been published about the molecular biology of epidermal disorders, in particular on the role of keratins in blistering and scaly conditions and the defects underlying pigmentary abnormalities. Identifying the causative mutation in a serious disease is a remarkable and exciting achievement.

Perhaps even more remarkable is the huge number of epidermal disorders still waiting to be matched up to an ever-increasing number of known skin genes. The causes of the numerous ectodermal dysplasias, for example, are completely unknown. Candidates include the genes coding for major structural proteins specific to the epidermis (filaggrin, trichohyalin, loricrin and involucrin as well as the many keratins), to the desmosomes and hemidesmosomes (desmoplakin, desmoglein, desmocollin and plakoglobin) and to the basement membrane zone (collagens, fibronectin, integrins, laminin, nicein, nidogen and thrombospondin) [1]. Rees has drawn attention to skin-specific retinoic acid receptor genes, which have been cloned and characterized though their biological role is unknown [2]. A vast number of jigsaw pieces is waiting to be slotted into place.

If the new technology seems impenetrable to the clinician, it is just as difficult for scientists to understand clinical problems. Physicians and researchers share a background in science but not in medicine. Clinicians must provide the relevant questions for the scientists to answer, bridging the gulf between what is known and what is understood. This should be our aim for the next 10 years.

References

1   Bowden P. Keratins and other epidermal proteins. In *Molecular Aspects of Dermatology.* Priestley GC (ed). Chichester: John Wiley. and Sons, 1993: 19–54.
2   Rees J. The molecular biology of retinoic acid receptors: orphan from good family seeks home. *Br. J. Dermatol.* 1992; 126: 97–104.

Ectodermal dysplasias

Definition

The derivatives of embryonic ectoderm, hair, teeth, nails and sweat apparatus, are affected in a huge variety of conditions. Freire-Maia and Pinheiro, whose book published in 1984 remains an essential reference [1], included 117 and more have been described since. The definition of ectodermal dysplasia (ED) is debatable. Most would agree with the Brazilians in including only those conditions involving two or more ectodermal derivatives, but isolated hypotrichosis (MIM 146550, 241900), anodontia (206780), anonychia (206800) and anhidrosis (206600, 241120) may ultimately prove to belong in this group. However, in the following account we differ from them in not extending the term to conditions with overproduction or overactivity of ectodermal derivatives, such as generalized hypertrichosis or hyperhidrosis, or to conditions where the ectodermal features are inconstant or insignificant compared with other major systemic abnormalities, such as hypomelanosis of Ito. Furthermore, many of the conditions listed by Freire-Maia and Pinheiro were reported in single patients and may represent no more than the chance association of different abnormalities: these again we have excluded, following McKusick. Our final selection might be defended as the common ground shared by Freire-Maia and Pinheiro on the one hand and McKusick on the other, great authorities between whom substantial differences of opinion are apparent in the small print.

Classification

Our ignorance about the pathogenesis of EDs makes it as hard to classify as to define them. A brave attempt was made by Freire-Maia and Pinheiro. In their '1234 system', disorders are assigned a number according to whether there is involvement of hair (1), teeth (2), nails (3) or sweat glands (4) and are numbered within these categories. Unfortunately, there are several drawbacks to this system. First, there is the problem of ascertainment: many authors do not mention minor abnormalities of teeth and nails; and even when looked for, hypohidrosis may be difficult to establish. Secondly, different members of a family, who clearly have the same disorder, may not all show the same features and would be classified differently. Thirdly, conditions that are very different, for example Goltz syndrome and pachyonychia congenita, fall into the same group. However, this system has been used in subsequent dermatology textbooks and diagnostic indices.

In Table 2.1 we number the conditions according to both Freire-Maia and Pinheiro (FM & P) and McKusick (MIM), but group the conditions on the basis of major associated features as follows.

Focal ectodermal dysplasias (a)

In these conditions there are discrete areas of ectodermal dysplasia, the rest of the skin being normal. Goltz syndrome [2] is better known as focal *dermal* dysplasia, but ectodermal derivatives are also deficient in the affected areas. In incontinentia pigmenti and Goltz syndrome, both X-linked dominant disorders, this patchiness probably reflects lyonization. Similarly, female carriers of X-linked recessive ED show focal lack of sweating in Blaschko's lines (see p. 11). The mutation in IP and Goltz syndrome is so serious that affected males, who do not have a normal allele to protect them, are aborted. In contrast, recessive X-linked ED causes a generalized but survivable skin defect in males.

Brauer and Setleis syndromes, which are characterized by focal skin defects on the temples (Fig. 2.1), are probably manifestations of a common developmental anomaly, inherited as an autosomal dominant trait with variable expression [3]. The dermis is deficient as well as the epidermis.

Isolated generalized EDs (b)

This group includes the well-known X-linked recessive hypohidrotic ED dysplasia (see below). These conditions lack major associations (c–h in

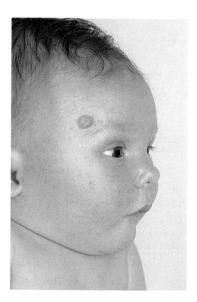

Fig. 2.1 Focal facial dermal dysplasia: the temporal defects may be mistaken for forceps marks.

the table), but there may be facial dysmorphism and other features, some of which are secondary to the ectodermal problems.

Other major associations (c–h)

EDs are frequently associated with sensorineural deafness (c), ocular abnormalities (d), facial clefting (e), and skeletal anomalies, particularly webbing and ectrodactyly (lobster claw) (f). Palmoplantar keratoderma may occur (g). Several other anomalies have been reported in association with ectodermal dysplasias (h). There is considerable overlap between different syndromes; for example, clefting, ectrodactyly and ectodermal dysplasia occur singly and in various combinations. Attempts to lump or split [4] seem fruitless until there is a molecular basis on which to do so.

The only EDs described in detail here are those that have been mapped, namely the X-linked conditions hypohidrotic ED and incontinentia pigmenti. Goltz syndrome is discussed in the section on Blaschko's lines (pp. 17–18).

Table 2.1 Ectodermal dysplasias (EDs)

FM & P	MIM	Name	Associated features
		(a) Focal ED	
1234–3	305600	Goltz focal dermal dysplasia	d, f, h
123–8	308300	Incontinentia pigmenti	d, h
14–1		ED of the head:	
	136500	Brauer	
	227260	Setleis	
		(b) Isolated ED	
1234–1	305100	Christ–Siemens–Touraine	
1234–2	224900	Autosomal recessive hypohidrotic ED	
1234–11	129490	Zanier–Roubicek	
1234–13	129490	Jorgenson syndrome	
123–11	189500	Hypodontia and nail dysgenesis (Witkop's)	
123–27	125640	Dermo-odonto dysplasia	
234–1	104570	Amelo-onychohypohidrotic dysplasia	
		(c) ED with deafness	
1234	125050	Deafness with hypohidrotic ED (HED)	
123–12	200970	Dento-oculocutaneous (Ackerman) syndrome	d
123–24	230740	Growth retardation–alopecia–pseudoanodontia–optic atrophy (GAPO)	d, f, h
12–5	224800	Mikaelian syndrome	h
12–13	243800	Johanson–Blizzard syndrome	h
12–16	147770	Alopecia–anosmia–deafness–hypogonadism	h
23–1	220500	Deafness–onycho-osteodystrophy–mental retardation (DOOR)	f, h
23–3	124480	Robinson syndrome	
—	129510	Tricho-odonto-onychial ED	
—	234580	Deafness, enamel hypoplasia, nail defects	
		(d) ED with ocular anomalies	
1234–10	106260	Ankyloblepharon–ED–cleft lip/palate (AEC)	e
123–1	268400	Rothmund–Thomson syndrome	f, h
123–3	135900	Coffin–Siris syndrome	f, h
123–9	218330	Cranio-ectodermal (Sensenbrenner) syndrome	f, h
123–12	200970	Dento-oculocutaneous (Ackerman) syndrome	c
123–16	278200	Salamon syndrome	
123–18	164200	Oculo-dentodigital (ODD, ODOD)	f, h
123–24	230740	GAPO	c, f, h
124–2	246500	Melanoleucoderma (Berlin's)	h
12–3	234100	Hallermann–Streiff syndrome	h
12–11	211370	Oculo-osteocutaneous syndrome	f, h
13–9	211390	Sabinas brittle hair and mental deficiency	h
23–6	221810	Kirghizian dermato-osteolysis	f
—	262020	Pilodental dysplasia with refractive errors	
—	225280	ED–ectrodactyly–macular dystrophy	f
—	257960	Oculotrichodysplasia (retinitis pigmentosa)	
		(e) ED with clefting	
1234–5	225000	Roselli–Gulienetti syndrome	f, h
1234–8	129400	Rapp–Hodgkin syndrome	h
1234–9	129900	Electrodactyly–ED–cleft lip/palate (EEC)	f, h
1234–10	106260	AEC	d
123–18	164200	Oculo-dentodigital (ODD, ODOD)	d, f
—	225060	Margarita-type ED	f

Continued p. 42

Table 2.1 *continued*

FM & P	MIM*	Name	Associated features
		(f) ED with skeletal anomalies	
1234–3	305600	Goltz syndrome	a, d, h
1234–5	225000	Roselli–Gulienetti syndrome	
1234–9	129900	EEC	e, h
—	129810	Ectrodactyly–ED	
—	225280	ED–ectrodactyly–macular dystrophy	d
123–1	268400	Rothmund–Thomson syndrome	d, h
123–2	129500	Clouston	g, h
123–3	135900	Coffin–Siris syndrome	d, h
123–4	273400	Odontotrichomelic syndrome	h
123–5	190320	Trichodento-osseous (TDO)	
123–9	218330	Cranio-ectodermal (Sensenbrenner) syndrome	d, h
123–13		Trichorhinophalangeal syndrome (TRP I):	
	190350	dominant form	
	275500	recessive form	
	150230	TRP II	
		(Langer–Giedion)	h
123–14	225500	Ellis–van Creveld syndrome	d, h
123–18	164200	Oculodentodigital (ODD, ODOD)	d
123–23	269150	Schinzel–Giedion syndrome	h
123–24	230740	GAPO	c, d, h
12–1	311200	Orofaciodigital (OFD I) Papillon–Leage syndrome	h
12–11	211370	Oculo-osteocutaneous syndrome	d, h
12–15	207780	Acrorenal field defect, ED, lipoatrophic diabetes	h
23–1	220500	DOOR	c, h
23–6	221810	Kirghizian dermato-osteolysis	d
—	225060	Margarita-type ED	e
—	129540	ED with distinctive facies and preaxial polydactyly (feet)	
—	275450	Tricho-odonto-onychial dysplasia	
		(g) ED with keratoderma	
1234–20	257980	Odonto-onychodermal dysplasia	
1234–22	245000	Papillon–Lefevre syndrome	h
123–2	129500	Clouston syndrome	f, h
13–2	104100	Palmoplantar keratoderma and alopecia	
24–1	161000	Naegeli–Franceschetti–Jadassohn syndrome	h
		(h) Other EDs with miscellaneous anomalies	
1234–6	305000	Dyskeratosis congenita	
1234–17	106750	Anonychia and flexural pigment	
1234–19	129550	Odonto-onychohypohidrotic dysplasia with midline scalp defect	
134–6	225050	HED with hypothyroidism	
12–9	261900	Pili torti and enamel hypoplasia	
13–4	258360	Onychotrichodysplasia with neutropenia	
24–3	226750	Amelocerebrohypohidrotic dysplasia	
34–1	129200	Absence of dermal ridges, onychodystrophy, palmoplantar anhidrosis (Basan syndrome)	
—	129510	Tricho-odonto-onychial dysplasia with amastia	
—	129550	ED with adrenal cyst	
—	224750	ED with eccrine tumours	
—	225040	ED, hypothyroidism, agenesis of corpus callosum	

* First digit of MIM number indicates inheritance: 1 = autosomal dominant; 2 = autosomal recessive; 3 = X-linked.

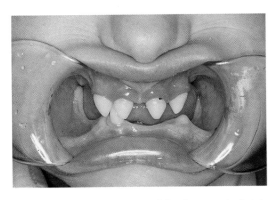

Fig. 2.2 Hypohidrotic ectodermal dysplasia: conical and missing teeth.

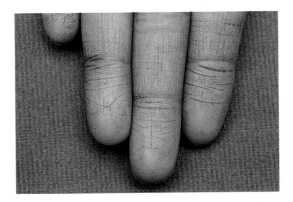

Fig. 2.3 Hypohidrotic ectodermal dysplasia: lack of fingerprints and sweat pores.

X-linked hypohidrotic ED (HED) (Christ–Siemens–Touraine syndrome) (MIM 305100) [5]

Clinical features

This condition manifest in boys is characterized by sparse hair, missing and pointed teeth, dystrophic nails and reduced sweating with hyperpyrexia, which is particularly dangerous in infancy (Figs 2.2 and 2.3). Boys with X-linked HED have a characteristic face with prominent forehead and lips: the shape of the mouth may be related to the lack of teeth. They may be deaf from blockage of the external auditory meati by excessive wax. Recurrent chest infections may be secondary to deficient bronchial secretions and their eczema and other atopic manifestations are perhaps related to abnormal handling of antigens at mucosal surfaces. Female carriers may have mild or patchy manifestations in Blaschko's lines (see p. 11).

Genetic aspects

In 1875 [6] Darwin observed sex-linked inheritance of the condition affecting the 'toothless men of Sind', now known to be X-linked HED. An homologous X-linked disorder occurs in mice (tabby) and cattle [7].

Mapping of this condition on the X chromosome was facilitated by observations in manifesting females with translocations. When a translocation occurs between an X chromosome and an autosome, the normal X chromosome is preferentially inactivated and the translocated X chromosome is active in all cells. This conserves the activity of the translocated autosome, which would otherwise be inactivated along with the fraction of X chromosome to which it was attached. However, if there is a genetic defect at the breakpoint on the X chromosome, this will then affect all cells, and the affected female will manifest a condition normally seen only in males. Using this principle, HED was localized to Xq13.1 from cytogenetic studies on two manifesting females with X-autosome translocations [8,9]. This position was consistent with comparative mapping studies of the homologous mouse tabby locus. Subsequent linkage studies [5] have confirmed the localization to proximal Xq, close to the centromere. A mutation has now been identified [10].

Nothing is yet known of the pathogenesis of the EDs.

References

1 Freire-Maia N, Pinheiro M. *Ectodermal Dysplasias: A Clinical and Genetic Study.* New York: Alan R. Liss, 1984
2 Temple IK, MacDowall P, Baraitser M *et al.* Focal dermal dysplasia (Goltz syndrome). *J. Med. Genet.* 1990; 27: 180–187.
3 Ward KA, Moss C. Evidence for genetic homogeneity of Setleis' syndrome and focal facial dysplasia. *Br. J. Dermatol.* 1994; 130: 645–649.

4   Cambiaghi S, Tadini G, Barbareschi M *et al*. Rapp–Hodgkin syndrome and AEC syndrome—are they the same entity? *Br. J. Dermatol.* 1994; 130: 97–101.

5   Clarke A. Hypohidrotic ectodermal dysplasia. *J. Med. Genet.* 1987; 24: 659–633.

6   Darwin C. *The Variation of Animals and Plants under Domestication*, 2nd edn. London: John Murray, 1875: 319

7   Ohno S. Ancient linkage groups and frozen accidents. *Nature* 1973; 244: 259–262.

8   Turleau C, Niaudet P, Cabanis MO *et al*. X-linked hypohidrotic ectodermal dysplasia and t(X;12) in a female. *Clin. Genet.* 1989; 35: 462–466.

9   Zonana J, Roberts SH, Thomas NST *et al*. Recognition and reanalysis of a cell line from a manifesting female with X-linked hypohidrotic ectodermal dysplasia and an X; autosome balanced translocation. *J. Med. Genet.* 1988; 25: 383–386.

10 Zonana J, Gault J, Davies KJ *et al*. Detection of a molecular deletion at the DXS732 locus in a patient with X-linked hypohidrotic ectodermal dysplasia with the identification of a unique junctional fragment. *Am. J. Hum. Genet.* 1993; 52: 78–84.

Keratinization

Keratinocytes generated in the basal layer progress outwards as prickle cells and granular cells to the

Table 2.2 Desquamation: anatomy, biochemistry and some candidate genes

Cell layer	Structure	Candidate gene
Stratum corneum		
corneocytes	Cornified envelope	Loricrin
	Marginal dense band	Involucrin
	Matrix proteins	Filaggrin
extracellular matrix	Lamellar bilayers	Lipids
		Steroid sulphatase
Granular layer	Lamellar bodies	Steroid sulphatase
	Keratohyaline granules	Profilaggrin
Spinous layer	Tonofilaments	Keratins 1 and 10
	Desmosomes:	Desmoplakins
	plaques	Cadherin
	glue	Desmoglein
		Desmocollin
Basal layer	Tonofilaments	Keratins 5 and 14
	Hemidesmosomes	

stratum corneum to be shed (Table 2.2). The skin's toughness is provided by keratin supporting the living cells from the inside, and the dense matrix proteins and cornified envelope of the dead stratum corneum cells. Waterproofing is provided largely by lipids surrounding the dead corneocytes.

This section covers disorders that result in a thicker epidermis, both those due to hyperkeratosis (increased thickness of the stratum corneum) and acanthosis (increased thickness of the prickle-cell layer). Some of the genes discussed may also undergo mutations that result in a thinner epidermis: those conditions are covered in the section on epidermolysis bullosa (pp. 80–88).

The ichthyoses

The word ichthyosis describes the skin of patients who, in the untreated state, have visible scales that can be removed, in contrast to xeroderma, which means dry skin without scales.

This abnormal desquamation can follow either an increase in cell turnover or an increase in cell cohesiveness, so that the corneocytes stick together and come off in visible clumps rather than discretely (and discreetly). Occasionally epidermal blistering also occurs suggesting, paradoxically, a reduction in cell cohesion.

The palms and soles may be affected; hair, nails and teeth are usually not. In contrast, in the keratodermas only the palmar and plantar skin is involved: it is thickened rather than scaly and the nails are often affected. The erythrokeratodermas resemble the psoriasiform dermatoses more than the ichthyoses in being patchy and migratory rather than generalized and fixed but, by convention, are included here as are the follicular hyperkeratoses.

Defects of keratinization may be due to abnormalities in any of the following (Table 2.2).

1 Keratins, the major structural proteins of the epidermis, which are designated as type I (acidic) and type II (basic) (Table 2.3). A type I and a type II protein form a heterodimer, two of which align to form a tetramer. More than 5000 tetramers join to form a single 10 nm keratin filament. Clusters of keratin genes (*KRT*) have been mapped to chromosomes 12 and 17. The sequences at

Table 2.3 Epidermal keratins

Type I, acidic (kDa)	Type II, basic (kDa)	Site of expression
14 (58)	5 (50)	Basal cells
10 (56.5)	1 (67h, 2e (65.8)	Suprabasal cells
16 (48)	6 (48 and 56)	Hyperproliferative and cultured cells
9 (65)	?4 (59)	Palmoplantar skin only

either end of the gene are highly conserved, and even subtle mutations that do not impair tetramer formation prevent normal filament production [1–3].

2 Constituents of lamellar bodies that are released into intercellular spaces (lipids and enzymes, e.g. steroid sulphatase) [4].

3 Involucrin, which forms the marginal dense band of corneocytes. Expression occurs in the spinous layer and cross-linking to the plasma membrane occurs in the upper granular layer [5].

4 Filaggrin and loricin, matrix proteins that bind keratin filaments within corneocytes [2].

In addition to these structural proteins there are many intermediate filament-associated proteins (IFAPs), well reviewed by Bowden [1]. Other candidates are genes regulating expression of the above-mentoned genes, including retinoic acid-receptor genes [1,6,7].

Classification

The ichthyoses are a diverse group but run true to type within a family. They can be divided broadly into those affecting only the skin (see Table 2.4, p. 46) and those associated with major abnormalities of the skeleton or nervous system (see Table 2.5, p. 51). The clinical features used to classify them include the mode of inheritance, the occurrence of erythroderma and blisters, the involvement of flexures and the morphology of the scales, but they do not always discriminate well enough to make a firm diagnosis.

Other attempts at classification have been made, both to aid management and to elucidate pathogenesis. The ichthyoses have been divided into hyperproliferative and retentive types, but

this is unsatisfactory because sometimes the two types coexist. It is likely that hyperproliferation can lead secondarily to retention because cells entering the stratum corneum in an immature state retain their desmosomal contacts. Conversely, surface abnormalities may lead secondarily to an increased cell turnover.

As biochemical abnormalities have emerged, the ichthyoses have been separated on the basis of whether the defect involves the corneocyte 'bricks' (protein abnormalities) or the 'mortar' between them (lipid abnormalities), but this classification is limited to the minority in which the pathogenesis is known. Until more is learnt, the clinical classification remains the most useful.

Ichthyoses without major involvement of other systems (Table 2.4)

Ichthyosis vulgaris (MIM 146700)

Clinical features

This is the most common form of ichthyosis, affecting 1 in 250 people. Scaling affects predominantly the extensor surfaces of the limbs, and spares the flexures and the face. The trunk may be mildly involved and the palmar creases are exaggerated. The condition may be severe with thick scaling on the limbs, or minimal with just keratosis pilaris on the proximal limbs and hyperlinear palms. In about half the affected individuals it is associated with atopy and cannot be precisely distinguished from the dry skin of atopy.

Genetics

Inheritance is autosomal dominant with high penetrance and variable expressivity.

Pathogenesis

Although the pathogenesis is unknown there is good evidence for a defect of profilaggrin. Histologically, ichthyosis vulgaris is characterized by absence of keratohyaline granules in the upper epidermis. Biochemically, filaggrin and its precur-

Table 2.4 Ichthyoses with no other major system involvement. E, erythema in infancy; F, flexural involvement; B, blisters

MIM*	Disorder	E	F	B	Skin morphology
146700	Ichthyosis vulgaris	−	−	−	Fine, white scales
308100	Steroid sulphatase deficiency	−	−	−	Large, dark scales
113800	Bullous ichthyosiform erthyroderma	+	+	+	Warty hyperkeratosis
242100	Non-bullous ichthyosiform erythroderma	+	+	−	Fine, white scales
242100	Lamellar ichthyosis	−	+	−	Large plates
146750	Lamellar ichthyosis	−	+	−	Large plates
146800	Ichthyosis bullosa of Siemens	−	+	+	Mild flexural hyperkeratosis
242500	Harlequin fetus	−	+	−	Large rigid plates
146590 146600	Ichthyosis hystrix (Curth–Macklin)	−	+	−	Spiky hyperkeratosis.
270300	Peeling skin	−	+	−	Superficial peeling
148370	Oudtshoorn skin	+	+	−	Redness and peeling of palms, soles, and sometimes limbs, worse in winter
256500	Netherton syndrome	+	+	−	Ichthyosis linearis circumflexa with trichorrhexis nodosa
242500	—	−	+	−	Lamellar ichthyosis with split hairs

First digit of MIM number indicates inheritance: 1 = autosomal dominant; 2 = autosomal recessive; 3 = X-linked.

sor profilaggrin, the main component of keratohyaline, are reduced or absent in ichthyosis vulgaris [8]. Profilaggrin and keratohyaline are also absent from keratinocytes cultured from affected skin, and present at intermediate levels in unaffected skin from patients with ichthyosis vulgaris [9]. Therefore, if a reduction in filaggrin is the cause of this ichthyosis, the primary abnormality probably lies in control of expression of the gene rather than in the gene itself. The filaggrin gene has now been cloned and mapped to chromosome 1q21 [10]. The gene encodes a precursor containing numerous tandem filaggrin repeats. A short linker sequence is excised to yield functional molecules. *In situ* hybridization studies showed that expression of the filaggrin gene is tightly regulated at the transcriptional level in terminally differentiating epidermis.

If a defect in filaggrin is the primary abnormality in ichthyosis vulgaris, it is still not clear how this causes scaling. This is a retentive rather than hyperproliferative ichthyosis. It may be that the defective keratohyaline matrix of corneocytes renders the stratum corneum more crumbly and somehow more sticky.

Abnormalities of filaggrin are also found in other disorders including restrictive dermopathy, harlequin fetus and psoriasis.

X-linked recessive ichthyosis (XLRI) (MIM 308100)

Clinical features

This form of ichthyosis affects 1 in 6000 males and is generally similar to ichthyosis vulgaris but more severe, and less likely to affect the palms (Fig. 2.4). It may be associated with deep corneal opacities and cryptorchidism. It is due to steroid sulphatase deficiency [11].

Genetic aspects

Inheritance is X-linked recessive. Like other X-linked recessive disorders, XLRI is not normally manifest in female carriers but if it is, a cytogenetic abnormality must be considered. In Turner syndrome, where there is only one X chromosome, and in X-autosome translocations where there is preferential inactivation of one X chromosome, the

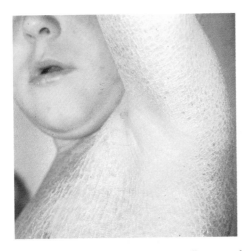

Fig. 2.4 X-linked ichthyosis characteristically spares the flexures.

female is effectively rendered hemizygous rather than heterozygous. If the single active X chromosome carries XLRI, the abnormal allele is no longer compensated for by normal steroid sulphatase production from the other X chromosome so the female is affected as completely as a male.

The steroid sulphatase gene, located at the end of the short arm of the X chromosome, is of particular interest because it is partially resistant to the normal X-inactivation process. Lyonization generally provides 'dosage compensation', that is it ensures that females do not have double the dose of X-linked genes. Steroid sulphatase activity, however, is normally higher in females than in males. The female/male ratio of steroid sulphatase activity in fibroblasts is 1.6, suggesting that the gene partially escapes inactivation, rather than 2, which would indicate that both alleles were active in all female cells.

Point mutations in the steroid sulphatase gene have been found in a few families with XLRI [12] but in 80% of patients the gene is completely deleted. In some families the deletion also affects the adjacent locus for Kallman syndrome (hypogonadotrophic hypogonadism with anosmia) [13]. One patient had XLRI, chondrodysplasia punctata and mental retardation due to a large deletion affecting contiguous genes [14].

Pathogenesis

Shapiro *et al.* [11] made the connection between a low maternal urinary oestriol in pregnancy and XLRI in the offspring. Both are due to lack of steroid sulphatase. The carrier females are unaffected but during pregnancy a placenta belonging to an affected male fetus is unable to convert oestradiol to oestriol; the resultant low maternal oestriol excretion may be misinterpreted as an index of fetoplacental distress.

The ichthyosis of steroid sulphatase deficiency is unexplained but has been attributed to raised cholesterol sulphate and reduced cholesterol levels in the epidermis due to lack of epidermal steroid sulphatase. This would alter the properties of intercellular lipid, affecting cell cohesiveness. Topical application of 10% cholesterol cream is said to improve XLRI [15]; conversely, topical application of cholesterol sulphate to mouse skin causes ichthyosis. However, it is possible that other aspects of epidermal steroid metabolism are also disturbed by steroid sulphatase deficiency and contribute to the ichthyosis. As well as raised plasma cholesterol sulphate, affected males have raised levels of dehydroepiandrosterone sulphate and reduced androstenedione and oestradiol, abnormalities that may be related to the increased incidence of cryptorchidism (12% in one series [16]).

Application of 10% cholesterol cream has been suggested on theoretical grounds, but the improvement is not dramatic. An exciting development is correction of steroid sulphatase deficiency by gene transfer into cultured basal cells of patients with XLRI [17], opening up the possibility of gene therapy.

Bullous ichthyosiform erythroderma (BIE) (MIM 113800)

Clinical features

This rare disorder combines scaliness with blistering and redness. In the neonate, erythema and bullae predominate, with shedding of large clumps of scale made up of almost full-thickness stratum corneum, as if cohesiveness is both increased above and decreased below. Later there is mainly hyperkeratosis and scaling with marked flexural involvement.

Genetic aspects

Inheritance of bullous ichthyosiform erythroderma is autosomal dominant, with full penetrance and uniform expressivity within a family. Many cases are sporadic and assumed to represent new mutations. Of particular interest are families where a child with bullous ichthyosiform erythroderma has a parent with linear ichthyosis hystrix [18]: presumably the parent has undergone somatic mutation and demonstrates cutaneous and gonadal mosaicism.

Family studies have shown linkage to the keratin gene clusters [19], facilitating antenatal diagnosis of this serious disorder, previously possible only by electronmicroscopy of a fetal skin biopsy at 19 weeks. In some families antenatal diagnosis based on gene mutations is now possible [20].

Pathogenesis

Bullous ichthyosiform erythroderma is now known to be due to mutations in the genes for keratins 1 and 10. The first clue came from parallels with epidermolysis bullosa simplex (EBS): both have epidermal blistering and both show tonofilament clumps, particularly around the nuclei, in the suprabasal layers. The tonofilament clumps in EBS can be labelled with antibodies to keratins 5 and 14, while those in BIE label with antibodies to keratins 1 and 10 [21]. Experiments in transgenic mice showed that a truncated keratin 10 gene gives rise to a condition similar to BIE [22]. Several mutations have now been found in keratin 1 and 10 genes in patients with BIE, usually in the highly conserved regions at the ends of the rod domains, which are critical for normal filament assembly [2,20,21,23–25].

Autosomal recessive ichthyosis (MIM 242100)

Clinical features

This category encompasses at least two different disorders [26, 27]
1 Lamellar ichthyosis (Fig. 2.5). This is characterized by large dark plate-like scales with marked involvement of the face and ears. There is no erythroderma. The epidermal proliferation rate is normal and histologically there is hypergranulosis and compact hyperkeratosis.
2 Non-bullous ichthyosiform erythroderma. In contrast to lamellar ichthyosis, this condition is more variable and usually milder with fine white scales on the trunk and some facial tautness. Erythroderma is prominent in childhood but lessens with age. There is increased epidermopoiesis and epidermal thickening. This is the most common cause of a collodion baby (MIM 242300) (Fig. 2.6), a term that is a description rather than a diagnosis.

Genetic aspects

Both are autosomal recessive. However, an autosomal dominant form of lamellar ichthyosis also occurs (MIM 146750) [28].

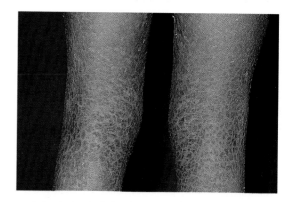

Fig. 2.5 Recessive lamellar ichthyosis, involving the flexures.

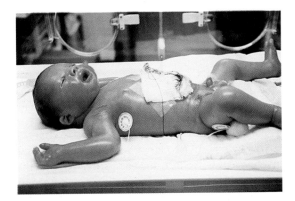

Fig. 2.6 A collodion baby: the shiny, smooth skin looks almost as though it has been painted with collodion.

Pathogenesis

The claim that non-bullous ichthyosiform erythroderma could be distinguished by high levels of *n*-alkanes [27] became untenable when Bortz *et al.* [29] showed, by carbon dating, that alkanes in human skin are predominantly exogenous, acquired, for example, from topical emollients containing petrolatum. Bergers *et al.* [30] suggested that erythrodermic and non-erythrodermic (lamellar) recessive ichthyosis can be distinguished by a relatively low β-glucosidase and phospholipase in scales of the former and low butyrase in the latter. Elias's group found abnormal lamellar bodies in the erythrodermic form and persistence of desmosomes in both [31].

Ichthyosis bullosa of Siemens (MIM 146800)

Clinical features

Mild flexural hyperkeratosis develops during the first year of life. There is superficial blistering but no erythroderma.

Genetic aspects

This dominantly inherited disorder has been found, in a five generation kindred, to be due to a keratin 2e mutation [32].

Harlequin fetus (MIM 242500)

Clinical features

Affected babies usually die shortly after birth but some, given etretinate in the neonatal period, have survived. In many respects it is like a severe form of collodion baby: it is most severe at birth and evolves into an ichthyosis resembling congenital ichthyosiform erythroderma in the survivors. The name probably covers more than one disorder and refers to the large roughly diamond-shaped scales, like the pattern on the traditional harlequin costume.

Genetic aspects

Familial cases suggest autosomal recessive inheritance.

Pathogenesis

Dale *et al.* [33] studied nine harlequin fetuses and found certain common features including reduced keratin filaments in the granular layer, abnormal lamellar granules, lack of lipid lamellae between stratum corneum cells and lipid droplets within an excessive and compact cornified layer. However, they concluded that this was a heterogeneous group, the variable features being a block in the conversion of profilaggrin to filaggrin and the presence of hyperproliferative keratins type 6 and 16. The abnormal stacking of the corneocytes of the harlequin fetus is maintained in cell culture. Subsequent studies [34] suggest that the lamellar granule contents are normal but both lipid and protein constituents are retained in the cell rather than being discharged to the intercellular space. More recently defective protein dephosphorylation has been suggested [35].

Ichthyosis hystrix

Hystrix means porcupine, and the term ichthyosis hystrix indicates spikes of massive hyperkeratosis. The term is a description rather than a diagnosis and is used confusingly by dermatologists to indicate any of the following.

1 A linear epidermal naevus with epidermolytic hyperkeratosis, referred to above as a mosaic form of bullous ichthyosiform erythroderma.

2 Systematized verrucous epidermal naevus.

3 Ichthyosis hystrix gravior (MIM 146600), the generalized spiky ichthyosis reported in the Lambert family of Suffolk who in the 19th century were exhibited in fairs as 'porcupine men'. The condition was originally thought to be Y-linked, but re-analysis of the family data suggested autosomal dominant inheritance [36].

4 Curth–Macklin ichthyosis hystrix (MIM 146590). In this rare autosomal dominant condition there is massive hyperkeratosis and ultrastructurally the tonofilaments show an abnormal arrangement around the nucleus [37]. It is similar to bullous ichthyosiform erythroderma, in which there is hyperkeratosis with abnormal tonofilaments, but in Curth–Macklin ichthyosis hystrix there is no blister formation. Furthermore, Curth–Macklin ichthyosis hystrix is not apparently linked to the keratin gene clusters [38].

Netherton syndrome (MIM 256500)

The clinical features of this autosomal recessive condition are trichorrhexis nodosa, ichthyosis linearis circumflexa and atopy. Some patients have ichthyosis resembling lamellar ichthyosis or congenital ichthyosiform erythroderma. Developmental delay, growth retardation, impaired cellular immunity and aminoaciduria have been reported. The pathogenesis is unknown.

Ichthyoses with major non-cutaneous features

Sjögren–Larsson syndrome (MIM 270200)

Clinical features

This is a rare disorder in which ichthyosis is associated with spastic paraparesis and mental retardation (Fig. 2.7). The ichthyosis is similar to congenital ichthyosiform erythroderma, with marked flexural involvement and sparing of the face. There may be macular 'glistening dots' in the retina.

Genetic aspects

Inheritance is autosomal recessive.

Pathogenesis

The first clue was the observation 25 years ago that dietary fat restriction with supplementation of medium-chain fatty acids led to clinical improvement. Subsequently, reduced metabolism of linoleic acid was found [39]. Rizzo *et al.* [40], investigated fatty alcohol metabolism in Sjögren–Larsson syndrome because it supplies lipid substrate for both the skin and nervous system. They found impaired fatty alcohol oxidation in fibroblasts from affected individuals and intermediate levels in carriers. The condition can now be diagnosed histochemically on skin or jejunal mucosa using hexanol as the substrate: in the presence of fatty alcohol oxidoreductase, tetra-

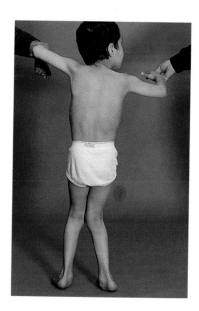

Fig. 2.7 The Sjögren–Larsson syndrome is characterized by spasticity, retardation and an ichthyosis that involves the flexures.

Table 2.5 Ichthyoses with major non-cutaneous features

MIM	Name	Associated features
With neurological involvement		
270200	Sjögren–Larsson syndrome	Retardation, spasticity
242510	Sjögren–Larsson-like	Retardation, spasticity, alopecia, ectropion
266500	Refsum syndrome	Retinitis pigmentosa, neuropathy, ataxia
308200	Rud syndrome	Retardation, hypogonadism, retinitis pigmentosa
275630	Dorfman–Chanarin syndrome	Myopathy, hepatosplenomegaly
148210	Keratitis–ichthyosis–	
242150	Deafness (KID) syndrome	Keratitis, deafness
242170	IBIDS (Tay syndrome)	Brittle hair, impaired intelligence, decreased fertility, short stature
242520	—	Cerebellar degeneration, hepatosplenomegaly
242530	—	Retardation, dwarfism, renal impairment
280000	Zanuch syndrome	Retardation, deafness, ocular coloboma
With skeletal involvement		
272200	Multiple sulphatase deficiency	Retardation, mucopolysaccharidosis
118650		
215100	Conradi–Hunerman syndrome	Dwarfism, short limbs, cataracts
302950	(chondrodysplasia punctata)	
302960		
166740	—	Osteosclerosis, fractures
146720	Ichthyosis–cheek–eyebrow	Full cheeks, sparse eyebrows, kyphoscoliosis and other skeletal defects
	(ICE) syndrome	
308050	CHILD syndrome	Limb reductions

* First digit of MIM number indicates inheritance; 1 = autosomal dominant; 2 = autossomal recessive; 3 = X-linked.

zolium is converted to black formazan, therefore a negative reaction indicates absence of the enzyme [41].

Fatty alcohol oxidoreductase activity is prob-ably due to more than one enzyme. The component most decreased in Sjögren–Larsson syndrome is that which is susceptible to inhibition by palmitoyl CoA [42,43].

Refsum syndrome (MIM 266500)

Clinical features

The essential clinical features are cerebellar ataxia, peripheral neuropathy and retinitis pigmentosa. Scaling most like that of ichthyosis vulgaris is present in 50% of patients.

Genetic aspects

Inheritance is autosomal recessive.

Pathogenesis

Deficiency of α-phytanic acid α-hydroxylase leads to an accumulation of phytanic acid in the epidermis, substituted for essential fatty acids in all subfractions, especially phospholipid. Histologically, there are lipid deposits in the basal cells. Labelling studies show hyperproliferation. Since free cholesterol is normally esterified by phytanic acid in the epidermis, the ichthyosis might be due to reduced levels of epidermal cholesterol, as has been suggested for X-linked ichthyosis.

Multiple sulphatase deficiency (MIM 272200)

Clinical aspects and pathogenesis

Deficiency of several enzymes contributes to the complex phenotype of this disorder. Lack of aryl sulphatase A causes a metachromatic leucodystrophy with psychomotor retardation; lack of aryl sulphatase B leads to a mucopolysaccharidosis of the Maroteaux–Lamy type; the ichthyosis is due to steroid sulphatase (aryl sulphatase C) deficiency; and an absence of other enzymes can produce features of other storage diseases including Hunter's, Sanfillipo A, Morquio A and mucopolysaccharidosis type VIII.

Genetic aspects

Inheritance is autosomal recessive. The genes for these enzymes lie on different chromosomes and how they are jointly regulated is unknown.

Dorfman–Chanarin syndrome (MIM 275630)

This is a very rare autosomal recessive lipid storage disorder with congenital ichthyosis, hepatosplenomegaly, myopathy and vacuolated granulocytes. Patients may subsequently develop cataracts, nystagmus, deafness and ataxia. There is multisystem deposition of triglyceride, possibly due to a defect in fatty acid oxidation.

There are some obvious similarities to Sjögren–Larsson syndrome, now known to be due to a fatty alcohol oxidoreductase deficiency. In both, improvement has been reported with medium-chain triglyceride supplementation.

Rud syndrome (MIM 308200)

This term has been applied to patients with ichthyosis and various neurological abnormalities including epilepsy and retardation. It is not clearly defined and it seems likely that several different conditions have been included in this category.

Tay syndrome, IBIDS, trichothiodystrophy (MIM 242170)

This group of conditions with overlapping features is discussed in detail in the section on trichothiodystrophy (pp. 115–116)

Conradi–Hunerman syndrome (chondrodysplasia puntata)

Clinical features and genetic aspects

There are apparently four types of this disorder, which combines skin and skeletal abnormalities. The diagnostic feature is punctate mineralization of the epiphyses, visible radiologically as stippling in infancy. The skin, when affected, shows an ichthyosis that fades, leaving follicular atrophoderma (Fig. 2.8). Scalp involvement gives rise to abnormal hair or alopecia. The characteristics of the different types are summarized in Table 2.6.

Autosomal dominant (MIM 118650)

There is growth deficiency, scoliosis and limb shortening. Ichthyosis is said to occur in 27% and follicular atrophoderma is also described. The prognosis for survival is good.

Autosomal recessive, rhizomelic type (MIM 215100)

This is a more serious condition with severe

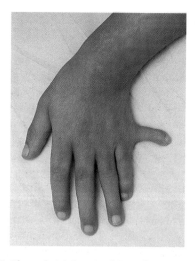

Fig. 2.8 The early ichthyosis of Conradi–Hunerman syndrome is followed by follicular atrophoderma, seen here on the back of the hand.

Table 2.6 Classification of chondrodysplasia punctata (Conradi–Hunerman syndrome)

	AD	AR	XD	XR
Prognosis	Good	Poor	Good	Good
Ichthyosis	All over	All over	Linear	All over
Cataracts	Rare	Common	Sectorial	Common
Central nervous system	Normal	Retarded	Normal	Retarded, deaf
Rhizomelia	Variable	Severe	Asymmetric	Unusual
Short stature	+	++	+	+
Other bony involvement	–	Scoliosis	–	Hypoplasia of nasal bones and distal phalanges
Peroxisomal abnormality	–	+	+ or –	–
Locus	?	?	Distal Xq or mid-Xp	Distal Xp adjacent to steroid sulphatase gene

AD, autosomal dominant; AR, autosomal recessive; XD, X-linked dominant; XR, X-linked recessive.

growth and psychomotor retardation and death before the age of 2 years. There is a symmetrical shortening of proximal limbs, cataracts occur in 72%, and 28% have ichthyosis. The phenotype is similar to warfarin embryopathy. There is an abnormality of peroxisomal enzymes.

X-linked dominant (Happle syndrome) (MIM 302960)

In this predominantly female group, patients have short proximal limbs, cataracts and an ichthyosis present at birth following Blaschko's lines. The ichthyosis resolves in a few weeks, leaving follicular atrophoderma. Intelligence is normal and the prognosis is good. Peroxisomal enzyme activity was decreased in one three-generation family, but is usually normal.

The pattern of the skin involvement has been attributed to lyonization and embryonic clonal migration of cells carrying a lethal gene rescued by mosaicism [44]. The X-linked dominant form has been localized tentatively to either distal Xq or mid-Xp on the basis of homology with the mouse gene 'bare patches' [45]. The condition is assumed to be lethal before birth in the hemizygous males.

However, males with this whorled pattern do occur, and their phenotype is no more severe than that of the females. A possible explanation is somatic mutation at the X-dominant locus producing mosaicism, again manifest as Blaschko's lines. Another possibility is that all males and an equivalent number of females diagnosed as X-linked dominant chondrodysplasia punctata with no family history actually represent mosaicism for a mutation at the autosomal dominant locus. This might be the explanation for the mildly affected female described by Prendiville *et al.* [46] and for exclusion of the entire X-chromosome in one linkage study [47].

X-linked recessive (MIM 302950)

Males with this form have mild skeletal manifestations, sometimes limited to hypoplasia of distal phalanges and nasal hypoplasia, with retardation. The gene has been mapped adjacent to the steroid sulphatase gene on the basis of several males with both conditions who had a deletion at Xp22.32. In these families the ichthyosis was more characteristic of chondrodysplasia punctata than X-linked recessive ichthyosis in the involvement of flexures and hair.

The erythrokeratodermas
Erythrokeratoderma variabilis (MIM 133200)

Clinical features

This disorder is characterized by fixed plaques of scaly erythema as well as migratory non-scaly erythema (Fig. 2.9). The histology is non-specific with acanthosis, compact hyperkeratosis and patchy parakeratosis.

Genetic aspects

Dutch studies of large kindreds have confirmed close linkage to the rhesus blood group on chromosome 1 but the gene has not yet been identified [48].

Symmetrical progressive erythrokeratoderma (Gottron syndrome)

This differs from erythrokeratoderma variabilis in the absence of migratory erythema. The histology is also more specific, with perinuclear lipid-like vacuoles in keratinocytes. Familial cases show autosomal dominant inheritance, but the condition is usually sporadic. In one family it was associated with late-onset ataxia [49] (MIM 133190).

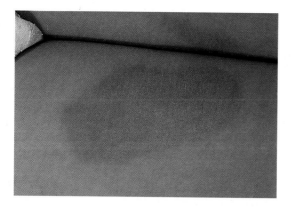

Fig. 2.9 Erythrokeratoderma variabilis showing variable erythema. (Reproduced by kind permission of Dr Julian Verbov.)

The palmoplantar keratodermas

Clinical features and genetic aspects

The conditions in this large and genetically heterogeneous group are distinguished by their distribution (e.g. diffuse or focal), age of onset and associated abnormalities. An erythematous margin and transgrediens pattern (that is extending on to the dorsum of the hands and feet) may simply reflect severity. Keratoderma (or tylosis) is usually an isolated abnormality but numerous associations have been reported. Only those which segregate with the keratoderma within a family are relevant here. The individual conditions have been well reviewed elsewhere [50] and are summarized in Table 2.7, which is an attempt to reconcile the dermatological and genetic terminology. It can be seen that not all the disorders recognized by dermatologists have a MIM number, that not all conditions recognized by McKusick have a dermatological eponym and that there is much uncertainty about the identity of many of these conditions.

Pathogenesis

Palmoplantar skin appears thicker but otherwise histologically similar to the skin elsewhere. Therefore, it seems remarkable that there are more than 30 genetic disorders producing marked palmoplantar keratoderma with no other cutaneous abnormality. Presumably the genetic defects here involve not only keratinization but other special features of palmoplantar skin such as sweating, fingerprint and palmar crease development, hyperkeratotic response to friction and tactile function. The cause of only two of the keratodermas is known: Richner–Hanhart syndrome due to tyrosine amino transferase deficiency and mapped to 16q22.1–22.3, and epidermolytic hyperkeratosis of the palms and soles due to a keratin 9 mutation. Three others have been mapped: sclerotylosis of Huriez to 4q28–31, focal acral hyperkeratosis of Costa to 2p and Thost–Unna palmoplantar keratoderma to 12q.

Table 2.7 The keratodermas

MIM*	Name	Onset	Distribution	Associated features
(a) Diffuse keratodermas				
122440	Corneodermato-osseous syndrome	Child		Corneal dysplasia, brachydactyly, onycholysis, short stature
124500	Vohwinkel mutilating	Infant		Extensor keratoses, deafness, pseudoainhum
129500	Clouston syndrome	Child		Nail dystrophy, alopecia
144200	Vorner syndrome	Child		Epidermolytic hyperkeratosis
148350	—	Child		Deafness
148360	—	Child		Nail dystrophy, neuropathy
148400	Thost–Unna syndrome, Greither syndrome	Child		None
148500	Howel–Evans syndrome	Adult		Oesophageal cancer
148520	—	Child		Clinodactyly
149200	Bart–Pumphrey syndrome	Adult		Knuckle pads, leuconychia, deafness
161000	Naegeli–Franceschetti–Jadassohn syndrome	Child		Pigmentation, nail and dental dystrophy
167200	Jadassohn–Lewandowsky pachyonychia congenita	Child		Nail dystrophy, oral leucokeratosis
167210	Jackson–Lawlor pachyonychia congenita	Child		Nail dystrophy, natal teeth, epidermoid cysts corneal dystrophy
181600	Huriez sclerotylosis	Birth		Scleroatrophy, hypoplastic nails, atopy, deafness
AD	Olmsted syndrome	Child		Perioral keratoderma
221700	—	Child		Atopy, deafness
244850	Norbotten syndrome	Child		None
245000	Papillon le Fevre	Child		Periodontopathia
212360	Cataract–alopecia–sclerodactyly (CASS)	Child		Cataract, alopecia, sclerodactyly
245010	Cochin Jewish disorder	Child		Periodontopathia and onychogryposis
248300	Mal de Meleda	Infant		Atopic eczema, extensor keratotic plaques, nail dystrophy, heart defects
260130	Pachyonychia congenita (recessive)	Child		Nail dystrophy
(b) Focal keratodermas				
AD	Punctate keratoses of palmar creases	Adult	Palmar creases	—
101840	Papulotranslucent acrokeratoderma	Adult	Palms, soles	Fine scalp hair
101850	Costa acrokeratoelastoides Focal acral hyperkeratosis		Palmar creases and margins	—
101900	Hopf acrokeratosis verruciformis	Child	Palms	Warty papules over joints, nail dystrophy
114140	Familial painful callosities	Child	Pressure areas	—
148600	Buschke, Fischer, Brauer syndromes	Adult	Variable	—
148700	Siemens, Wachter syndromes	Child	Striate on palms or areate on soles	Enamel dysplasia
148730	Palmoplantar keratoderma with leucoplakia	Teens Child,	Pressure areas	Thickened nails, gingival hyperkeratosis
175850	Porokeratosis plantaris, palmaris et disseminata	Adult	Palms, soles, disseminated	—
175860	Porokeratosis punctata palmaris et plantaris (Mantoux syndrome)	Adult	Palms, soles,	—

Continued on p. 56

Table 2.7 *continued*

MIM	Name	Onset	Distribution	Associated features
276600	Richner–Hanhart syndrome Tyrosinase aminotransferase deficiency	Child	Pressure areas	Corneal ulcers, retardation
AR	Jakac, Wolf, Touraine syndromes	Child	Disseminated follicular	Dysplastic teeth
309560	Fitzsimmons syndrome	Child	Striate on palms, diffuse on soles	Spastic paraplegia, retardation

* Where there is no MIM number, the inheritance is indicated by AD (autosomal dominatint) or AR (autosomal recessive).

Thost–Unna non-epidermolytic palmoplantar keratoderma

Clinical features

This is the most common form of keratoderma. A uniform yellow hyperkeratosis appears in early childhood on the palms and soles, sharply demarcated by an erythematous margin (Fig. 2.10).

Genetic aspects and pathogenesis

Inheritance of this disorder is autosomal dominant. The gene has been mapped to the keratin gene cluster at 12q11–q13, and there is reduced expression of keratins 6 and 16 in palmoplantar skin [51].

Vorner epidermolytic hyperkeratosis of the palms and soles (MIM 144200)

Clinical features

The appearance is indistinguishable from that of Thost–Unna keratoderma. However, histologically, Vorner's type is distinguished by epidermolytic hyperkeratosis.

Genetic features

This condition is inherited as an autosomal dominant trait with high penetrance. A linkage study in a large German family has mapped the gene to 17q11–23 [52].

Pathogenesis

The chromosomal localization corresponds to that of the acidic (type I) keratin gene cluster. Reis *et al.* proposed as candidate gene keratin 9, a type I keratin expressed only in palmoplantar skin [52]. The same group has now isolated the keratin 9 gene and identified three different mutations in five families with epidermolytic palmoplantar keratoderma [53].

Howel–Evans syndrome (MIM 148500)

Clinical features

The well-known association of tylosis and oesophageal carcinoma has been found in only

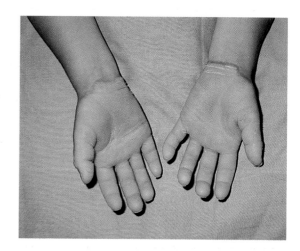

Fig. 2.10 Palmoplantar keratoderma.

three families; two in Liverpool [54] and one in Oxford [55]. The keratoderma differs from the more common, isolated dominant diffuse type (Thost–Unna) only in its later onset. The average age at diagnosis of the cancer was 61 years in the Oxford family and 45 in the Liverpool families.

Genetic aspects

This is inherited as an autosomal dominant trait. Pathogenesis is unknown.

The follicular hyperkeratoses

This is a heterogeneous group (Table 2.8). The conditions vary in the nature and distribution of the follicular abnormality, the development of follicular atrophy, the involvement of non-follicular epidermis and associated non-cutaneous features.

Darier's disease

Clinical features (Figs 2.11–2.13)

The prevalence of this disorder is about 1 in 50 000. Nail changes are the earliest sign and include linear streaks, V-shaped nicks in the free edge of the nail [56] and gross dystrophy [57]. The typical rash consists of greasy papules in seborrhoeic areas and flexures and is exacerbated by light. There are punctate keratoses on the palms and flat warty lesions on the backs of the hands distinguishable from acrokeratosis verruciformis of Hopf only by the histological finding of suprabasal clefting in Darier's disease. The rash is usually improved considerably by treatment with etretinate.

Genetic aspects

The condition is autosomal dominant with complete penetrance and variable expressivity [57].

Table 2.8 Follicular hyperkeratoses

MIM*	Name	Onset	Morphology	Associated features	Distribution
101900	Hopf acrokeratosis verruciformis	Child	Warty papules	Palmar keratoses	Knuckles, knees, elbows
120450	Familial dyskeratotic comedones	Puberty	Comedones	None	Anywhere
124200	Darier keratosis follicularis	Child	Greasy papules	Palmar keratoses, acrokeratosis verruciformis, nail dystrophy	Seborrhoeic areas and flexures
144150	Flegel syndrome	Adult	Small scaly papules	None	Limbs
149500	Kyrle syndrome	Adult	Large scaly plugs	None	Limbs
209700	Ulerythema ophryogenes	Infant	Follicular keratoses and atrophy	None	Eyebrows, cheeks
209700	Atrophoderma vermiculata	Child	Follicular plugs then atrophy	None	Cheeks
308800	Keratosis pilaris spinulosa decalvans	Infant	Follicular plugs then atrophy	None	Face, scalp
308830			Keratosis pilaris	Alopecia, dwarfism, cerebral atrophy	Generalized
115150	Cardiofacio cutaneous	Child	Keratosis pilaris	Noonan-like	Face and scalp

* First digit of MIM number indicates inheritance: 1 = autosomal dominant; 2 = autosomal recessive; 3 = X-linked.

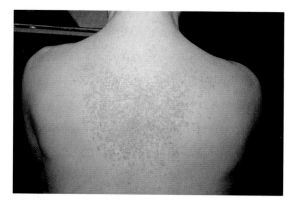

Fig. 2.11 Darier's disease: follicular keratotic papules on the back.

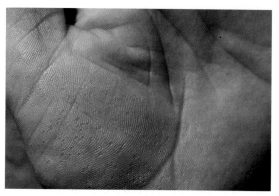

Fig. 2.13 Darier's disease: discontinuities in palmar prints.

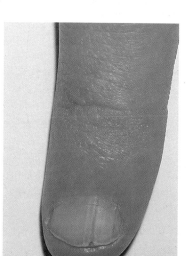

Fig. 2.12 Darier's disease: the typical nail abnormality, seen here in a 12-year-old, is usually the earliest sign.

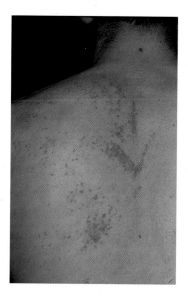

Fig. 2.14 Linear Darier's disease in a patient presumably mosaic for the mutant gene.

Occasionally, Darier's disease is seen in a linear distribution following Blaschko's lines (Fig. 2.14). These patients are thought to be mosaic for the Darier's mutation: they have no antecedent family history but could theoretically produce offspring with generalized Darier's if they have gonadal as well as cutaneous mosaicism [58]. Linkage studies have now mapped this condition to the long arm of chromosome 12 [59,60].

Pathogenesis

The response to retinoids suggests that this may be a disorder of epidermal-cell differentiation. There is loss of cell cohesion as well as hyperkeratosis: these two phenomena coexist in other disorders of keratinization, such as bullous ichthyosiform erythroderma and pachyonychia congenita. Keratin genes seem likely candidates

[61], but the locus on chromosome 12 is distal to that for the type II keratin genes [59,60,62].

Keratosis follicularis spinulosa decalvans (MIM 308800)

Clinical features

This affects the eyes as well as the skin [63]. Follicular hyperkeratosis appears in childhood, particularly of the scalp and eyebrows, and is followed by scarring alopecia. Corneal dystrophy presents as photophobia. The fingernails may show unusually long cuticles.

Genetic aspects and pathogenesis

Males are affected more severely than females who none the less show marked follicular changes, and the pattern of inheritance is X-linked dominant. This disorder has been mapped by linkage studies in a large Dutch family to Xp21.2–22.2 [64] The pathogenesis is unknown.

Cardiofaciocutaneous syndrome (CFC) (MIM 115150)

Clinical features

Patients with this disorder have congenital heart defects, particularly pulmonary stenosis, a typical facial appearance with high forehead, antimongoloid eyes and posteriorly rotated ears, and poorly defined ichthyosis. Usually there is keratosis pilaris but often the skin disorder is not adequately described.

The facial appearance and pulmonary stenosis may be identical to those of Noonan syndrome, a dominant disorder which is sometimes associated with ulerythema ophryogenes (keratosis pilaris with scarring alopecia particularly affecting the eyebrows) [65]. This has led to the suggestion that CFC is in fact the same as Noonan syndrome with ulerythema ophryogenes [66,67] (Fig. 2.15).

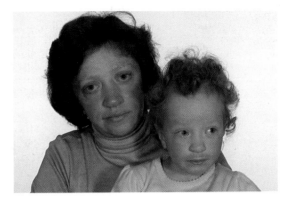

Fig. 2.15 The cardiofaciocutaneous syndrome, seen here in a mother and daughter, may be the same as the Noonan syndrome with ulerythema oophryogenes.

Genetic aspects

CFC is usually sporadic but sometimes dominantly inherited. The cause is unknown.

References

1 Bowden PE. Keratins and other epidermal proteins. In *Molecular Aspects of Dermatology* (Priestley GC ed.) Chichester: John Wiley and Sons, 1993: 19–54.
2 Fuchs E. Genetic skin disorders of keratin. *J. Invest. Dermatol.* 1992; 99: 671–674.
3 Steinert PM. Structure, function and dynamics of keratin intermediate filaments. *J. Invest. Dermatol.* 1993; 100: 729–734.
4 Williams ML. Lipids in normal and pathological desquamation. *Adv. Lipid Res.* 1991; 24: 211–298.
5 Eckert RL, Yaffe MB, Crish JL *et al.* Involucrin—structure and role in envelope assembly. *J. Invest. Dermatol.* 1993; 100: 613–617.
6 Rees J. The molecular biology of retinoic acid receptors: orphan from good family seeks home. *Br. J. Dermatol.* 1992; 126: 97–104.
7 Tomic-Canic M, Sunjevaric I, Freedberg IM, Blumenberg M. Identification of the retinoic acid and thyroid hormone receptor-responsive element in the human K14 keratin gene. *J. Invest. Dermatol.* 1992; 99: 842–847.
8 Sybert VP, Dale BA, Holbrook KA. Ichthyosis vulgaris: identification of a defect in synthesis of filaggrin correlated with an absence of keratohyaline granules. *J. Invest. Dermatol.* 1985; 84: 191–194.
9 Fleckman P, Holbrook KA, Dale BA, Sybert VP. Keratinocytes cultured from subjects with ichthyosis vulgaris are phenotypically abnormal. *J. Invest. Dermatol.* 1987; 88: 640–645.

10 McKinley-Grant LJ, Idler WW, Bernstein IS *et al*. Characterisation of a cDNA clone encoding human filaggrin and localisation of the gene to chromosome region 1q21. *Proc. Natl. Acad. Sci. USA*. 1989; 86: 4848–4852.

11 Shapiro LJ, Weiss R, Buxman MM *et al*. Enzymatic basis of typical X-linked ichthyosis. *Lancet* 1978; ii: 756–757.

12 Basler E, Grompe M, Parenti G *et al*. Identification of point mutations in the steroid sulphatase gene of three patients with X-linked ichthyosis. *Am. J. Hum. Genet.* 1992; 50: 483–491.

13 Paige Da, Emilion GG, Bouloux PMG, Harper JI. A clinical and genetic study of X-linked recessive ichthyosis and contiguous gene defects. *Br. J. Dermatol.* 1994; 131: 622–629.

14 Curry CJR, Magenis RE, Brown M *et al*. Inherited chondrodysplasia punctata due to a deletion of the terminal short arm of an X chromosome. *N. Engl. J.* 1984; 311: 1010–1015.

15 Lykkesfeldt G, Hoyer H. Topical cholesterol treatment of recessive X-linked ichthyosis. *Lancet* 1983; ii: 1337–1338.

16 Lykkesfeldt G, Bennet P, Lykesfeldt AE *et al*. Abnormal androgen and oestrogen metabolism in men with steroid sulphatase deficiency and recessive X-linked ichthyosis. *Clin. Endocrinol.* 1985; 23: 385–393.

17 Jensen TG, Jensen UB, Jensen PKA *et al*. Correction of steroid sulfatase deficiency by gene-transfer into basal cells of tissue-cultured epidermis from patients with recessive X-linked ichthyosis. *Exper. Cell Res.* 1993; 209: 392–397.

18 Paller AS, Syder AJ, Chan Y-M *et al*. Genetic and clinical mosaicism in a type of epidermal naevus. *New Engl. J. Med.* 1994; 331: 1408–1415.

19 Compton JG, DiGiovanna JJ, Santucci SK *et al*. Linkage of epidermolytic hyperkeratosis to the type II keratin gene cluster on chromosome 12q. *Nat. Genet.* 1992; 1: 301–305.

20 Rothnagel JA, Longley MA, Holder RA *et al*. Prenatal diagnosis of epidermolytic hyperkeratosis by direct gene sequencing. *J. Invest. Dermatol.* 1994; 102: 13–16.

21 Ishida-Yamamoto A, McGrath JA, Judge MR *et al*. Selective involvement of keratins K1 and K10 in the cytoskeletal abnormality of epidermolytic hyperkeratosis (bullous congenital ichthyosiform erythroderma. *J. Invest. Dermatol.* 1992; 99: 19–26.

22 Fuchs E, Esteves RA, Coulombe PA. Transgenic mice expressing a mutant keratin 10 gene reveal the likely basis for epidermolytic hyperkeratosis. *Proc. Natl. Acad. Sci. USA* 1992; 89: 6906–6910.

23 McClean WH, Eady RAJ, Doping-Hepenstal PJC *et al*. Mutations in the rod 1A domain of keratins 1 and 10 in bullous congenital ichthyosiform erythroderma (BCIE). *J. Invest. Dermatol.* 1994; 102: 24–30.

24 Rothnagel JA, Dominey AM, Dempsey LD *et al*. Mutations in the rod domains of keratins 1 and 10 in epidermolytic hyperkeratosis. *Science* 1992; 257: 1128–1130.

25 Yang J-M, Constantin C, Chipov JJ *et al*. Mutations in the H1 and 1A domains in the keratin 1 gene in epidermolytic hyperkeratosis. *J. Invest. Derm.* 1994; 102: 17–23.

26 Hazell M, Marks R. Clinical, histologic and cell kinetic discriminants between lamellar ichthyosis and nonbullous congenital ichthyosiform erythroderma. *Arch. Dermatol.* 1985; 121: 489–493.

27 Williams ML, Elias PM. Heterogeneity in autosomal recessive ichthyosis. *Arch. Dermatol.* 1985; 121: 477–488.

28 Melnik B, Kuster W, Hollman J. Autosomal dominant lamellar ichthyosis exhibits an abnormal scale lipid pattern. *Clin. Genet.* 1989; 35: 152–156.

29 Bortz JT, Wertz PW, Downing DT. The origin of alkanes found in human skin surface lipids. *J. Invest. Dermatol.* 1989; 93: 723–727.

30 Bergers M, Traupe H, Dunnwald SC *et al*. Enzymatic distinction between two subgroups of autosomal recessive lamellar ichthyosis. *J. Invest. Dermatol.* 1990; 94: 407–412.

31 Ghadially R, Williams ML, Hou SYE, Elias PM. Membrane structural abnormalities in the stratum corneum of the autosomal recessive ichthyoses. *J. Invest. Dermatol.* 1992; 99: 755–763.

32 McLean WHI, Morley SM, Lane EB *et al*. Ichthyosis bullosa of Siemens (IBS)—a disease involving keratin 2e. *J. Invest. Derm.* 1994; 103: 277–281.

33 Dale BA, Holbrook KA, Fleckman P *et al*. Heterogeneity in harlequin ichthyosis, an inborn error of keratinisation: variable morphology and structural protein expression and a defect in lamellar granules. *J. Invest. Dermatol.* 1990; 94: 6–18.

34 Milner ME, O'Guin M, Holbrook KA, Dale B. Abnormal lamellar granules in Harlequin ichthyosis. *J. Invest. Dermatol.* 1992; 99: 824–829.

35 Dale BA, Kam E. Harlequin ichthyosis: variability in expression and hypothesis for disease mechanism. *Arch. Dermatol.* 1993; 129: 1471–1477.

36 Penrose LS, Stern C. Reconsideration of the Lambert pedigree (ichthyosis hystrix gravior). *Ann. Hum. Genet.* 1958; 22: 258–283.

37 Kanerva L, Karvonen J, Oikarinen A. Ichthyosis hystrix (Curth–Macklin): light and electron microscopic studies performed before and after etretinate treatment. *Arch. Dermatol.* 1984; 120: 1218–1223.

38 Bonifas JM, Bare JW, Chen MA *et al*. Evidence against keratin gene mutations in a family with ichthyosis

hystrix Curth–Macklin. *J. Invest. Dermatol.* 1993; 101: 890–891.

39 Hernell O, Holmgren S, Jagell SF *et al.* Suspected faulty essential fatty acid metabolism in Sjögren–Larsson syndrome. *Pediatr. Res.* 1982; 16: 45–49.

40 Rizzo WB, Dammann AL, Craft DA. Sjögren–Larsson syndrome: impaired fatty alcohol oxidation in cultured fibroblasts due to deficient fatty alcohol : nicotinamide adenine dinucleotide oxidoreductase activity. *J. Clin. Invest.* 1988; 81: 738–744.

41 Judge MR, Lake BD, Smith VV *et al.* Depletion of alcohol (hexanol) dehydrogenase activity in the epidermis and jejunal mucosa in Sjogren–Larsson syndrome. *J. Invest. Dermatol.* 1990; 95: 632–634.

42 Kelson TL, Craft DA, Rizzo WB. Carrier detection for Sjögren–Larsson syndrome. *J. Inher. Metab. Dis.* 1992; 15: 105–111.

43 Rizzo WB, Damman AL, Craft DA *et al.* Sjogren–Larsson syndrome: inherited defect in the fatty alcohol cycle. *J. Pediatr.* 1989; 115: 228–234.

44 Happle R. X-linked dominant chondrodysplasia punctata. *Hum. Genet.* 1979; 53: 65–73.

45 Herman GE, Walton SJ. Close linkage of the murine locus bare patches to the X-linked visual pigment gene: implications for mapping human X-linked dominant chondrodysplasia punctata. *Genomics* 1990; 7: 307–312.

46 Prendiville JS, Zaparackas ZG, Esterley NB. Normal peroxisomal function and absent skeletal manifestations in Conradi–Hunermann syndrome. *Arch. Dermatol.* 1991; 127: 539–542.

47 Traupe H, Muller D, Atherton D *et al.* Exclusion mapping of the X-linked dominant chondrodysplasia punctata/ichthyosis/cataract/short stature (Happle) syndrome: possible involvement of an unstable premutation. *Hum. Genetic.* 1992; 89: 659–665.

48 van der Schroeff JG, van Leeuwen–Cornelisse I, van Haeringen A, Went LN. Further evidence for localisation of the gene of erythrokeratoderma variabilis. *Hum. Genet* 1988; 80: 97–98.

49 Giroux J-M, Barbeau A. Erythrokeratoderma with ataxia. *Arch. Dermatol.* 1972; 106: 183–188.

50 Griffiths WAD, Leigh IM, Marks R. Disorders of keratinisation. In *Textbook of Dermatology*, 5th edn, vol. 2 (Champion RH, Burton JL, Ebling FJG eds) Oxford: Blackwell Scientific Publications, 1992; 1369–1390.

51 Stevens HP, Kelsell DP, Bishop DT *et al.* Mapping of a gene for non-epidermolytic (Unna–Thost) palmoplantar keratoderma (PPK) to 12q with reduced keratin 6 and 16 expression in the palmoplantar epidermis. *Br. J. Dermatol.* 1994; 161: 426.

52 Reis A, Kuster W, Eckardt R, Sperling K. Mapping of a gene for epidermolytic palmoplantar keratoderma to

the region of the acidic gene cluster at 17q12–q21. *Hum. Genet.* 1992; 90: 113–116.

53 Compton JG. Epidermal disease: faulty keratin filaments take their toll. *Nat. Genet.* 1994; 6: 6–7.

54 Howel–Evans W, McConnell RB, Clarke CA, Sheppard PM. Carcinoma of the oesophagus with keratosis palmaris et plantaris (tylosis): a study of two families. *Quart. J. Med.* 1958; 27: 413–429.

55 Shine I, Allison PR. Carcinoma of the oesophagus with tylosis. *Lancet* 1966; i: 951–953.

56 Savin JA, Samman PD. The nail changes in Darier's disease. *Med. Biol. Ill.* 1970; 20: 85–88.

57 Munro CS. The phenotype of Darier's disease: penetrance and expressivity in adults and children. *Br. J. Dermatol.* 1992; 127: 126–30.

58 Munro CS, Cox NH. An acantholytic dyskeratotic epidermal naevus with other features of Darier's disease on the same side of the body. *Br. J. Dermatol.* 1992; 127: 168–171.

59 Bashir R, Munro CS, Mason S *et al.* Localisation of a gene for Darier's disease. *Hum. Molec. Genet.* 1993; 2: 1937–1939.

60 Craddock N, Dawson E, Burge S. The gene for Darier's disease maps to chromosome 12q23–q24.1. *Hum. Molec. Genet.* 1993; 2: 1941–1943.

61 Burge SM. Darier's disease, keratins and proteases: a review. *J. Roy. Soc. Med.* 1989; 82: 673–676.

62 Buxton RS. Yet another skin defect, Darier's disease, maps to chromosome 12q. *Hum. Molec. Genet.* 1993; 2: 1763–1764.

63 van Osch LDM, Oranje AP, Keukens FM *et al.* Keratosis follicularis spinulosa decalvans: a family study of seven male cases and six female carriers. *J. Med. Genet.* 1992; 29: 36–40.

64 Oosterwijk JC, Nelen M, van Zandvoort PM *et al.* Linkage analysis of keratosis follicularis spinulosa decalvans, and regional assignment to human chromosome Xp21.2–p22.2. *Am. J. Hum. Genet.* 1992; 50: 801–807.

65 Burton JL. The genes for Noonan's syndrome, woolly hair and ulerythema ophryogenes. *Postgrad. Med. J.* 1992; 68: 595.

66 Fryer AE, Holt PJ, Hughes HE. The cardio-facio-cutaneous syndrome and Noonan syndrome: are they the same? *Am. J. Med. Genet.* 1991; 38: 548–551.

67 Ward KA, Moss C, McKeown C. The cardio-facio-cutaneous syndrome: a manifestation of the Noonan syndrome? *Br. J. Dermatol.* 1994; 131: 270–274.

Acanthosis nigricans

This widespread thickening and darkening of the epidermis, without ichthyosis, particularly affects the flexures (Fig. 2.16). Sheets of brown velvety

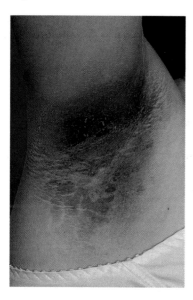

Fig. 2.16 Acanthosis nigricans in a girl with hyper-insulinism.

skin may coexist with numerous small warty lesions showing the same histology. It occurs in several situations, all presumably involving increased epidermal cell turnover. Acanthosis nigricans of adult onset is associated with drugs, obesity, malignancy or endocrinopathy. In children it usually has a genetic basis, being one of three types.

1 A benign, isolated, autosomal dominant condition (MIM 100600).
2 Isolated, secondary to insulin resistance (MIM 147670).
3 Part of a syndrome, perhaps secondary to insulin resistance, e.g.

176270	Prader–Willi syndrome
203800	Alastrom syndrome
208900	Ataxia telangiectasia
210900	Bloom syndrome
269700	Seip syndrome
246200	Leprechaunism (patients with specific insulin receptor mutations are coded 147670.0002, .0003, .0010, .0014, .0020)
277900	Wilson's disease

200170	Muscle cramps, large hands and acanthosis nigricans
147670.0012, .0013	Rabson–Mendenhall syndrome.

4 Part of a syndrome without insulin resistance (MIM 123500, Crouzon's disease).

Pathogenesis of acanthosis nigricans secondary to insulin resistance

Individuals whose cells are resistant to the action of insulin will produce extra insulin to maintain normal glucose metabolism.

High concentrations of insulin stimulate DNA synthesis and cell proliferation via insulin-like growth factor (IGF-1) receptors on keratinocytes. IGF-1 acts like epidermal growth factor, and activation of the IGF-1 receptor is presumed to cause the acanthosis [1].

The insulin-receptor gene has been well characterized: there are 11 exons encoding the α subunit and 11 exons encoding the β subunit. It produces a receptor precursor that undergoes several post-translational changes (e.g. cleavage into separate α and β subunits) before being transported to the cell surface. The mature insulin receptor is a tetramer of two α subunits that are extracellular and bind insulin, and two β subunits that attach to the cell membrane and include the intracellular tyrosine kinase domain. The binding of insulin to the receptor at the cell surface activates the receptor tyrosine kinase, which in turn mediates the effect of insulin. The insulin–receptor complex is then taken into the cell: some of the receptor is recycled and some is degraded.

Mutations of the insulin-receptor gene in patients with acanthosis nigricans fall into the following categories [2]:
1 impaired receptor biosynthesis;
2 impaired transport of receptors to the cell surface;
3 decreased binding affinity for insulin;
4 impaired tyrosine kinase activity;
5 accelerated receptor degradation.

It is not yet clear why different mutations in the same gene produce such dissimilar phenotypes, although one factor is severity of insulin resistance, which is greatest in patients with leprechaunism.

Pathogenesis of insulin resistance in Crouzon's disease

Crouzon's craniosynostosis is due to mutations in a gene encoding a fibroblast growth-factor receptor. The same gene can be alternatively spliced to produce a keratinocyte growth-factor receptor [3]. An activating mutation of this gene may be responsible for the abnormal growth of skin as well as cranial bones (W. Reardon, pers. comm.).

References

1   Cruz PD, Hud JA. Excess insulin binding to insulin-like growth factor receptors: proposed mechanism for acanthosis nigricans. *J. Invest. Dermatol.* 1992; 98: 82S–85S.
2   Accili D, Barbetti F, Cama a *et al.* Mutations in the insulin receptor gene in patients with genetic syndromes of insulin resistance and acanthosis nigricans. *J. Invest. Derm.* 1992; 98: 77S–81S.
3   Reardon W, Winter RM, Rutland P *et al.* Mutations in the fibroblast growth factor receptor 2 gene cause Crouzon syndrome. *Nat. Genet.* 1994; 8: 98–103.

Hair

Many genes interact in a complex but regulated way to produce the estimated 50–100 proteins, belonging to at least 10 different families, that are expressed in the growing hair [1]. Prominent among them are those responsible for hair colour (p. 69), and for the production of hair-specific keratins whose high content of cysteine and disulphide bonds make them harder and tougher than their epidermal counterparts [2].

This complexity is matched by a profusion of genetic abnormalities of hair, most of them uncommon but distinctive, and few, so far, mapped to a known gene. Some feature an excess (Table 2.9) or a lack (Table 2.10) of hair. Others are characterized by an abnormal shape (Table 2.11), colour or distribution of hair. Sometimes the hair abnormality is just one component of a wider disorder, as in the ectodermal dysplasias (p. 39), or reflects an underlying disorder as in trichothiodystrophy or Menkes syndrome (p. 67).

Hair excess

Cornelia de Lange syndrome (MIM 122470)

Clinical features

Abnormalities of hair growth are an important feature of this rare condition and occur in combination with mental retardation, microcephaly and upper limb defects. Hair overgrowth is particularly obvious on the ears, forehead and back but may be generalized. The eyebrows meet in the midline and the eyelashes are unusually long.

Genetic aspects

Most cases are sporadic but the condition has run, apparently as an autosomal dominant trait, in a few families. The gene has been tentatively located to chromosome 3q26.3 [3], and this would fit with the rather similar set of abnormalities seen in partial trisomy 3q.

Trichomegaly

Unusually long eyelashes (MIM 190330) run as an autosomal dominant trait in some families, sometimes in association with other problems such as cataracts. In the Oliver–Macfarlane syndrome (MIM 275400) [4], long eyelashes and brow hair are associated with dwarfism and retinal pigmentary degeneration.

Lack of hair

Androgenetic alopecia (male pattern baldness, MIM 109200)

There have been surprisingly few good studies of affected families. A fair case has been made out

Table 2.9 Some inherited conditions featuring hypertrichosis

MIM*	Name	Associated features
145700[1]	Hypertrichosis universalis	Excessive hairiness over whole body and face
307151[2]	(H. lanuginosa congenita)	Excessive hairiness over whole body and face
139500[3]	Hairy ears	Affects ear rims in Indian men
139600[4]	Hairy elbows	Short stature. Seen in Amish kindred
139650[5]	Hairy palms	Hairy areas on central proximal palms and foot arches
139630	Hairy nose tip	Manifest only in men
157200	Mid-digital hair	—
239840[6]	Central anterior cervical hypertrichosis with peripheral sensory and motor neuropathy	Neck affected plus peripheral neuropathy
239850[7]	Hypertrichotic osteochondroplasia	Cardiomegaly and multiple skeletal abnormalities
135900[8]	Coffin–Siris syndrome	Mental retardation and absent terminal phalanges of fifth fingers
211770	CAHMR syndrome	Cataract and mental retardation
122470	Cornelia de Lange syndrome	See p. 63
135400	Hypertrichosis with gingival fibromatosis	Gingival fibromas
266270	Ramon syndrome	Cherubism, gingival hyperplasia, epilepsy

* First digit of MIM number indicates inheritance: 1 = autosomal dominant; 2 = autosomal recessive; 3 = X-linked.

1 Felgenhauer WR. Hypertrichosis lanuginosa universalis. *J. Genet. Hum.* 1969; 17: 1–44.
2 Macias-Flores MA, Garcia-Cruz D, Rivera H *et al.* A new form of hypertrichosis inherited as an X-linked dominant. *Hum. Genet.* 1984; 66: 66–70.
3 Rao DC. A contribution to the genetics of hypertrichosis of the ear rims. *Hum. Hered.* 1970; 20: 486–492.
4 Macdermot KD, Paton MA, Williams MJH, Winter RM. Hypertrichosis cubiti (hairy elbows) and short stature: a recognisable association. *J. Med. Genet.* 1989; 26: 383–385.
5 Jackson CE, Cassies QC, Krull EA, Mehregan A. Hairy cutaneous malformations of palms and soles: a hereditary condition. *Arch. Dermatol.* 1975; 111:1146–1149.
6 Trattner A, Hodak E, Sagie-Lerman T, David M, Nitzan M, Garty BZ. Familial congenital anterior cervical hypertrichosis associated with peripheral sensory and motor neuropathy—a new syndrome? *J. Am. Acad. Dermatol.* 1991; 25: 767–770.
7 Cantu JM, Garcia-Cruz D, Sanchez-Corona J, Hernandez A, Nazara Z. A distinct osteochrondrodysplasia with hypertrichosis—individualisation of a probable autosomal recessive entity. *Hum. Genet.* 1982; 60: 36–41.
8 Levy P, Baraitser M. Coffin–Siris syndrome. *J Med. Genet.* 1991; 28: 338–341.

[5] for jettisoning the long-accepted view [6] that a single autosomal dominant gene manifests itself as baldness in male homozygotes and heterozygotes (*BB* and *Bb*) but only in female homozygotes (*BB*). However, in one study of 10 families of probands with polycystic ovaries [7], early onset male pattern baldness was found in obligate male carriers. This led to the suggestion that polycystic ovaries and male pattern baldness might be caused by alleles of the same gene affecting the production or action of androgen. A polygenic mode of inheritance would perhaps fit better with the normal distribution pattern of baldness in the population [5].

Table 2.10 Some generalized disorders with alopecia as one component

MIM*	Name	Associated features
190350[1] 150230 275500	Trichorhino-phalangeal syndromes	Sparse hair, pear-shaped nose, swelling of proximal finger joints (p. 65)
250250[3] 250460	Cartilage hair hypoplasia	Sparse, fine, pale hair and short-limbed dwarfism (p. 61)
234100[3] — —	Hallerman–Streiff syndrome Premature ageing syndromes Ectodermal dysplasias	Baldness characteristically following cranial suture lines. Cataracts, bird-like faces
118650[4] 215100	Chondrodysplasia punctata	Patchy cicatricial alopecia; stippled epiphyses
201100	Acrodermatitis enteropathica	Sparse hair, eruption around mouth, inability to absorb zinc adequately
146520	Hypotrichosis simplex	—
146530	Hypotrichosis with light-coloured hair and milia	As given in title
104130	Alopecia with psychomotor epilepsy pyorrhoea and mental subnormality	As given in title
158310	Mucoepithelial dysplasia	Photophobia, cataracts

* First digit of MIM number indicates inheritance: 1 = autosomal dominant; 2 = autosomal recessive; 3 = X-linked.
1 Buhler EM, Buhler VK, Beutler C, Fessler R. A final word on the tricho-rhino-phalangeal syndromes. *Clin. Genet.* 1987; 31: 273–275.
2 Van der Burgt T, Haraldsson A, Oosterwijk JC, Van Essen AJ, Weemaes C, Hamel B. Cartilage hair hypoplasia, metaphyseal chondrodysplasia type McKusick: description of seven patients and review of the literature. *Am. J. Med. Genet.* 1991; 41: 371–380.
3 Cohen MM. Hallermann–Streiff syndrome: a review. *Am. J. Med. Genet.* 1991; 41: 488–499.
4 Bodian EL. Skin manifestations of Conradi's disease. Chondrodysplasia congenita punctata. *Arch. Dermatol.* 1966; 94: 743–748.

Hereditary hypotrichosis (Marie–Unna type) (MIM 146550) [8]

In this rare condition, inherited as an autosomal dominant trait, the scalp hair is either scanty or normal at birth but becomes progressively sparse until it is replaced at the age of about three by thick coarse unruly hair, like horse hair. At puberty this scalp hair is lost over the vertex and round the scalp margins; the pattern of the scarring alopecia and the remaining coarse hair gives a characteristic appearance.

Trichorhinophalangeal syndrome (TRPS)

Clinical features (Figs 2.17 and 2.18)

Patients with type I TRPS (MIM 190350) have a characteristic facies with a bulbous nose, a long philtrum, prominent ears and sparse brittle hair. Their stature is short and their fingers are angulated with cone-shaped epiphyses creating swollen interphalangeal joints. Patients with type II TRPS, also known as the Langer–Giedion syndrome (MIM 150230), have these features too, but in addition are mentally retarded with microcephaly, multiple exostoses and redundant skin.

Genetic aspects

Both types of TRPs are due to deletions in the same area of chromosome 8. Band 8q24.12 is deleted in type I: in type II the deletion is larger (8q24.11–q24.13) with loss of band 8q24.13 being important in the production of exostoses [9,10]. However, the gene for multipe exostoses,

Table 2.11 Some inherited hair-shaft abnormalities

MIM*	Name	Associated features
234050 242170 275550	Trichothiodystrophy	See p. 115
261900	Pili torti	See p. 67
309400	Menkes syndrome	See p. 67
158000 252000	Monilethrix	See p. 68
194300[1] 278150	Woolly hair	Woolly scalp hair Blond in the recessive form
191480[2]	Uncombable hair (pili trianguli et canaliculi)	Hairs, usually triangular in cross-section with longitudinal grooves, look like spun glass
180600[3]	Pili annulati	Alternating light and dark bands on the hair shafts

* First digit of MIM number indicates inheritance: 1 = autosomal dominant; 2 = autosomal recessive; 3 = X-linked.

1 Hutchinson PE, Cairns RJ, Wells RS. Woolly hair: clinical and general aspects. *Trans. St. John's Hosp. Dermatol. Soc.* 1974: 60: 160–177.
2 Herbert AA, Charrow J, Esterly NB, Fretzin DF. Uncombable hair (pili trianguli et canaliculi): evidence for dominant inheritance with complete penetrance based on scanning electron microscopy. *Am. J. Med. Gen.* 1987: 28: 185–193.
3 Ashley LM, Jaques RS. Four generations of ringed hair. *J. Hered.* 1950; 41: 82–84.

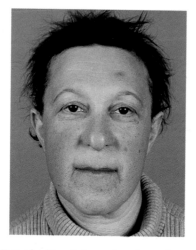

Fig. 2.17 Trichorhinophalangeal syndrome: hypotrichosis and a pear-shaped nose.

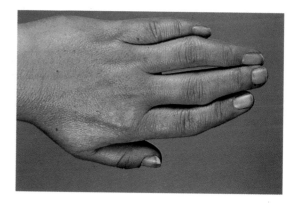

Fig. 2.18 Trichorhinophalangeal syndrome: abnormal knuckles due to cone-shaped epiphyses.

when inherited as an isolated abnormality, does not map to this region [11]. A recessively inherited type also exists (MIM 275500) but its genetic defect has not been identified.

The loose anagen syndrome

This recently described condition has been recorded as running as an autosomal dominant trait in a few families [12]. Its essential feature is the easy and painless extraction, by gentle pulling, of clumps of loose anagen hairs. The pathogenesis is not established but could involve an abnormality of adhesion molecules within the follicles, such as desmogleins or cadherins.

Cartilage–hair hypoplasia (MIM 250250)

Short-limbed dwarfism is associated with sparse

pale hair and inherited as an autosomal recessive trait. A tendency to develop lymphomas and a susceptibility to viral infections reflect defective cellular immunity. The condition is particularly common in Finland [13].

Hair-shaft abnormalities

Pili torti

Clinical features

In most cases only the scalp is involved. Affected hairs have flattened shafts with irregularly spaced runs of up to 10 twists through 180°. These produce a characteristic spangled appearance in reflected light. Such hairs are unruly and lustreless: they are also brittle and tend to break off short, leading to clinical confusion with monilethrix. Microscopy should readily separate the two.

Pili torti can occur as an isolated defect (MIM 261900) or with other ectodermal abnormalities such as keratosis pilaris, widely spaced teeth with hypoplastic enamel and dystrophic nails. In addition a number of rare syndromes include pili torti as one component (Table 2.12). All children with pili torti should be tested early for sensorineural hearing loss (a feature of Bjonstad and Crandall syndromes). The best understood of these associations is with Menkes syndrome, which will be considered separately.

Genetic aspects

Pili torti is clearly not a single genetic entity. The isolated, early-onset type may, for example, be inherited as an autosomal dominant or as a recessive trait. It is not known why it affects females more often than males. The modes of inheritance of pili torti in association with other defects are given in Table 2.12.

Pathogenesis

A failure to cross-link peptide chains in keratin has been confirmed in Menkes' disease and may also be important in other conditions showing pili torti.

Menkes syndrome (kinky hair disease) (MIM 309400)

Clinical features

This X-linked condition is less common than was once thought, probably affecting no more than 1 in 298 000 live births [14]. Affected boys fail to thrive within the first few months of life and usually die by the age of 3 years. Neurological problems predominate and include psychomotor retardation and myoclonic seizures. A combination of depigmentation and pili torti gives the hairs their classical steel-wool appearance.

Table 2.12 Syndromes that may include pili torti

MIM*	Name	Associated features
262000	Bjonstad syndrome	Sensorineural deafness
262000	Crandall syndrome	Sensorineural deafness and hypogonadism
109520	Basex syndrome	Follicular atrophoderma and basal-cell carcinoma
309400	Menkes syndrome	Abnormality of copper metabolism, failure to thrive, cutis laxa and hypopigmentation
305100	Hypohidrotic ectodermal dysplasia	Sparse hair, decreased sweating
167210	Jackson-Lawlor pachyonychia congenita	Nail dystrophy, natal teeth, epidermoid cysts

* First digit of MIM number indicates inheritance: 1 = autosomal dominant; 2 = autosomal recessive; 3 = X-linked.

Genetic aspects

This is an X-linked recessive trait. Carrier females may be clinically normal, but pili torti can be found in as many as half of them if several scalp sites are sampled [15,16]. Mottling has also been found in the skin of some pigmented carriers.

Only a few females have developed Menkes syndrome [17]: some of these have had X-autosome translocations. Studies of breakpoints in these cases suggested that the gene probably lies in band Xq13 [18,19]. Linkage studies in 11 families, each with more than one affected member, confirmed that it lay between Xq12 and Xq13.3 [20]. Fine mapping to sub-band Xq13.3 was suggested by the investigation of a family with a unique rearrangement of the X chromosome [21].

Pathogenesis

The first clues came when a similarity was detected between Menkes syndrome and copper deficiency in sheep [22]. However, Menkes syndrome is not a copper deficiency as such, but rather a disorder of copper handling and distribution. Intestinal absorption is reduced and serum, brain and liver copper levels are low. In contrast, other organs such as the kidneys, muscles and skin have higher than normal levels of copper bound to cysteine-rich metallothioneins. Three groups have now successfully isolated the responsible gene [23], which seems to encode a heavy metal-binding protein similar to a bacterial copper-transporting adenosine triphosphatase.

When Menkes revisited his syndrome in 1988 [24], 25 years after describing it, he saw that many of its features could be accounted for by abnormal functioning of five copper-dependent enzymes (Table 2.13). Confirming this is the success of injections of copper histidinate in reducing pili torti and restoring hair colour [25]. The arrest of the progressive cerebral dysfunction is less certain but may occur if the injections are given early enough [26]. In the mottled brindled mouse model of Menkes syndrome, delaying copper treatment until after

Table 2.13 Copper-dependent enzyme systems whose underactivity leads to many of the features of Menkes syndrome

Copper-dependent enzyme	Effects of underactivity
Lysyl oxidase	Defect in cross-linking in elastin fibres in intima of blood vessels
	Involvement of cerebral vessels leads to neuronal degeneration
	Cutis laxa-like changes
Cytochrome-C oxidase	Tendency to hypothermia
Ascorbic acid oxidase	Skeletal abnormalities like those of scurvy
Tyrosinase	Abnormally pale hair and skin
Enzymes involved in cross-linking in keratin	Pili torti: reduced disulphide bonds plus increased sulphydryl content of hairs

postnatal day 7 leads to irreversible brain changes [27].

Prenatal diagnosis [28] and genetic counselling

Prenatal diagnosis based on increased ^{64}Cu uptake by cultured amniotic cells is unreliable because of variation with fetal age [28]. Similarly, attempts to use this type of test to detect carriers are hampered by a considerable overlap with values obtained in normal controls.

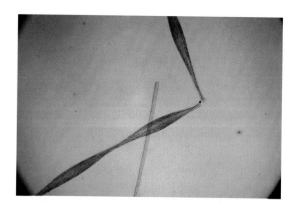

Fig. 2.19 The regular nodes and internodes of the hair in monilethrix.

Monilethrix

Clinical features (Fig. 2.19)

The classical beaded hairs usually appear during the first few months of life, and are most obvious on the occiput where a stubble of broken hairs shows up against a background of follicular plugging. The condition is usually limited in extent, but occasionally all scalp and body hairs are affected.

Genetics

Careful studies of affected families show that monilethrix is usually inherited as an autosomal dominant trait with high penetrance and variable expressivity. Mild examples may be missed and this could account for the apparently recessive inheritance pattern of some families [29]. Evidence from linkage studies suggests that the monilethrix gene may lie on chromosome 14q32–33, close to an immunoglobulin-heavy gene cluster [30] and a protease inhibitor [31].

CHANDS (MIM 214350)

This is a rarity whose initials stand for *c*urly *h*air, *a*nkyloblepharon, *n*ail *d*ysplasia *s*yndrome. Its inheritance seems to be as an autosomal recessive with pseudodominance [32].

Hair colour

Although racial and familial differences are obvious, surprisingly little is known about their genetic control. Much of our present knowledge has flowed from mouse to human.

In mice, more than 50 genetic loci have been identified that affect coat colour. Other mammalian species have been shown to conform to the overall mouse pattern of control, and similar gene complexes are likely to be important in the control of human pigmentation. They can be divided into four major groups [33,34].

1 *Those affecting the migration, proliferation and survival of melanocytes.* Mutations of the corresponding human genes have been found in piebaldism (p. 75) and Waardenburg syndrome (p. 77).

2 *Those controlling the amount of melanin produced.* In humans these include genes encoding tyrosinase (see tyrosinase-negative albinism on p. 74). Dopachrome tautomerase also controls melanogenesis: its murine 'slaty' mutation has so far found no human equivalent, nor have mutations in the genes responsible for the regulatory factors tyrosinase-related protein and melanocyte protein mel 17 (on human chromosome 12).

3 *Those that determine the kind of melanin synthesized.* In mice, two loci (extension and agouti) are involved in the regulation of eumelanin vs. phaeomelanin. The melanin-synthesizing hormone receptor has tentatively been mapped to the extension locus in mice but the agouti locus does not seem to exist in humans.

4 *Those influencing the shape and ultrastructure of melanocytes and melanosomes.* Mutations of the human homologue of the mouse pink-eye dilution factor are responsible for some examples of tyrosinase-positive albinism (p. 74). Mutations of the murine 'pallid' locus lead to changes similar to those seen in Chediak–Higashi disease.

In humans the picture remains confused. Phaeomelanins and eumelanins are found in various proportions in all hairs, whatever their colour. Tyrosinase activity is especially high in the follicles of red-haired individuals: their melanocytes contain spherical phaeomelanic melanosomes and sometimes also 'mosaic' melanosomes with features both of eumelanosomes and phaeomelanosomes. With age, both red and blond hairs tend to darken. Genes affecting the proportion of eumelanin to phaeomelanin and melanosome shape are presumably involved in these changes.

Factors responsible for black and brown hair tend to override (are epistatic to) those for red and blond hair. Red hair (MIM 266300) seems to be epistatic to blond hair (MIM 210750) and a major gene for red human hair is linked to the MN blood group locus on chromosome 4q28.2–q31.1 [35]. Homozygotes for a red hair gene may have red hairs only while heterozygotes have a mixture of red and dark hairs [36]. Brown hair colour (MIM

113750) appears to be linked to green eye colour (MIM 227240) [37].

Premature greying of the hair (MIM 139100) may have many causes but has been recorded in five generations of one family [38]. With premolar aplasia and hyperhidrosis, it forms part of the Book syndrome (MIM 112300).

References

1 Rogers GE, Powell BC. Organization and expression of hair follicle genes. *J. Invest. Dermatol.* 1993; 101: 50S–55S.
2 Yu J, Yu D, Checkla DM, Freedberg IM, Bertolino AP. Human hair keratins. *J. Invest. Dermatol.* 1993; 101: 565–595.
3 Ireland M, English C, Cross I, Houlsby WT, Burn J. A *de novo* translocation t (3:17) (q26.3; q23.1) in a child with Cornelia de Lange syndrome. *J. Med. Genet.* 1991; 28: 639–640
4 Oliver GL, Macfarlane DC. Congenital trichodystrophy with associated pigmentary degeneration of the retina, dwarfism and mental retardation. *Arch. Ophthalmol.* 1965: 74: 169–171.
5 Küster W, Happle R. The inheritance of common baldness: two B or not two B? *J. Amer. Acad. of Dermatol.* 1984; 11: 921–926.
6 Osborn D. Inheritance of baldness. *J. Hered.* 1916; 7: 347–355.
7 Carey AH, Chan KL, Short F, White D, Williamson R, Frank S. Evidence for a single gene effect causing polycystic ovaries and male pattern baldness. *Clin. Endocrinol.* 1993; 38: 653–658.
8 Peachey RDG, Wells RS. Hereditary hypotrichosis (Marie–Unna type). *Trans. St. John's Hosp Dermatol. Soc.* 1971; 57: 157–166.
9 Ludecke H-J, Johnson C, Wagner MJ et al. Molecular definition of the shortest region of deletion overlap in the Langer–Giedion syndrome. *Am. J. Hum. Genet.* 1991: 49: 1197–1206.
10 Yamamoto Y, Oguro N, Miyao M Yanagisawa M. Tricho-rhino-phalangeal syndrome type I with severe mental retardation due to interstitial deletion of 8q23.3–24.13. *Am. J. Med. Genet.* 1989; 32: 133–135.
11 Le Merrer M, Ben Othane K Stanescu V et al. The gene for hereditary multiple exostoses does not map to the Langer–Giedion region (8q23–q24). *J. Med. Genet.* 1992; 29: 713–715.
12 Baden HP, Kvedar JC, Magro CM. Loose anagen hair as a cause of hereditary hair loss in children. *Arch. Dermatol.* 1992; 128: 1349–1353.
13 Makitie O. Cartilage–hair hypoplasia in Finland: epidemiological and genetic aspects of 107 patients. *J. Med. Genet.* 1992; 29: 652–655.
14 Tønnesen T, Kleijer WJ, Horn N. Incidence of Menkes' disease. *Hum. Genet.* 1991; 86: 408–410.
15 Collie WR, Moore CM, Goka TJ, Howell RR. Pili torti as marker for carriers of Menkes' disease. *Lancet* 1978; i: 607–608.
16 Moore CM, Howell R. Ectodermal manifestations in Menkes' disease. *Clin. Genet.* 1985; 28: 532–540.
17 Gerdes AM, Tønnesen T, Horn N et al. Clinical expression of Menkes' syndrome in females. *Clin. Genet.* 1990; 38: 452–459.
18 Kapur S, Higgins JV, Delp K, Rogers SB. Menkes' syndrome in a girl with X-autosome translocation. *Am. J. Med. Genet.* 1987; 26: 503–510.
19 Varga V, Hall BK, Wang SR, Johnson S, Higgins JV, Glover TW. Localization of the translocation breakpoint in a female with Menkes' syndrome to Xq13.2–q13.3 proximal to PGK-1. *Am. J. Hum. Genet* 1991; 48: 1133–1138.
20 Tønnessen T, Petterson A, Kruse TA, Gerdes AM, Horn N. Multipoint linkage analysis in Menkes' disease. *Am. J. of Hum. Genet.* 1992; 50: 1012–1017.
21 Tumer Z, Tommerup N Tønnessen T, Kreuder J, Craig IW, Horn N. Mapping of the Menkes locus to Xq13.3 distal to the X-inactivation center by an intrachromosomal insertion of the segment Xq13–q21.2. *Hum. Genet.* 1992; 88: 668–672.
22 Danks DM, Campbell PE, Stevens BJ, Mayne V, Cartwright E. Menkes' kinky hair syndrome. An inherited defect in copper absorption with widespread effects. *Pediatrics* 1972; 50: 188–201.
23 Davies K. Cloning the Menkes disease gene. *Nature* 1993: 361: 98.
24 Menkes JH. Kinky hair disease: twenty-five years later. *Brain Develop.* 1988: 10: 77–79.
25 Tomita Y, Kondo Y, Ito S et al. Menkes' disease: report of a case and determination of eumelanin and pheomelanin in hypopigmented hair. *Dermatology* 1992; 185: 66–68.
26 Nadal D, Baerlocher K. Menkes' disease: longterm treatment with copper and D-penicillamine. *Eur. J. Paediatr.* 1988; 147: 621–625.
27 Fujii T Ito M, Tsuda H, Mikawa H. Biochemical study on the critical period for treatment of the mottled brindled mouse. *J. Neurochem.* 1990; 55: 885–889.
28 Horn N. Menkes X-linked disease: prenatal diagnosis and carrier detection. *J. Inher. Metab. Dis.* 1983: 6 (Suppl. 1): 59–62.
29 Hamm H, Echternacht-Happle K, Happle R. Monilethrix: ausschiesslicher Befall der Korperbehaarung. *Z. Hautler* 1984; 59: 1177–1178.
30 Renwick JH, Izatt MM. Linkage data on monilethrix. *Cytogenet. Cell Genet.* 1988; 47: 108.
31 Spence MA, Sparkes RS, Curtis RK, Tideman S, Sparkes MC, Crist M. Linkage analysis of one large pedigree segregating autosomal dominant monilethrix. *Cytogenet. Cell Genet.* 1979; 25: 108

32 Toriello HV, Lindstrom JA, Waterman DF. Re-evaluation of CHANDS. *J. Med. Genet.* 1989; 16: 316–317.

33 Hearing VJ. Unravelling the melanocyte. *Am. J. Hum. Genet.* 1993; 52: 1–7.

34 Ortonne J-P, Prota G. Hair melanins and hair colour: ultrastructural and biochemical aspects. *J. Invest. Dermatol.* 1993; 101: 82S–89S.

35 Eiberg H, Morh J. Major locus for red hair colour linked to MNS blood groups on chromosome 4. *Clin. Genet.* 1987; 32: 125–128.

36 Nicholls EM. Microspectrophotometry in the study of red hair. *Ann. Hum. Genet.* 1968; 32: 15–26.

37 Eiberg M, Mohr J. Major genes for eye and hair colour linked to LU and SE. *Clin. Genet.* 1987; 31: 186–191.

38 Hare HJH. Premature whitening of hair. *J. Hered.* 1929; 20: 31–32.

Nails

The size and shape of normal nails [1] and their proportion of proteins with high and low sulphur contents [2] have a hereditary basis. Beyond this, genetic abnormalities of the nail fall into three main groups [3] as follows.

1 *Abnormalities of the nail matrix.* These may lead to the formation of nails of abnormal size (ranging from hypoplastic nails to anonychia (MIM 107000), of abnormal composition as in trichothiodystrophy (p. 115), of abnormal position or of abnormal colour (e.g. the white nails of leukonychia totalis (MIM 151600) and the Bart–Pumphreys syndrome (MIM 149200). The nail changes in the ectodermal dysplasias (p. 39) fit into this group also.

2 *Abnormalities of the nail bed.* The most striking example of this is pachonychia congenita (p. 72) in which the heaped up nails are due to an excessive production of keratin by the distal nail bed. Hereditary koilonychia (MIM 149300) has been described.

3 *Defects associated with mesodermal abnormalities.* Nails *en raquette* (brachydactyly type D, MIM 113200) are a common abnormality, usually affecting only the thumb nails, and inherited as an autosomal dominant trait with penetrance that is complete in females and incomplete in males [4]. The nail abnormality is secondary to short distal phalanges. In addition, absent nails with defects of the terminal phalanx are seen in many other conditions (e.g. the Coffin–Siris syndrome). The nail–patella syndrome is discussed below. The nail changes in familial clubbing (MIM 119900) and pachydermoperiostosis (MIM 167100) are also presumably secondary to the underlying mesodermal abnormalities.

The nail–patella syndrome (hereditary osteo-onychodysplasia; HOOD) (MIM 161200) (Fig. 20.2)

Clinical features

The main features of the syndrome are:
1 nail dystrophy;
2 absent or hypoplastic patellae;
3 subluxation of the radial heads;
4 exostoses ('horns') of the iliac crests;
5 nephropathy.

The nail changes are usually present at birth and are most obvious on the thumbs, less obvious on the fingers and seldom seen on the toes. They range from total absence, through partial loss of the nail plate, to small nails with thinning and cracking. Lunulae, if visible, tend to be triangular with their apices pointing distally.

Genetic aspects

The nail–patella syndrome is inherited as an auto-

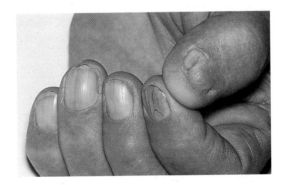

Fig. 2.20 The nail dystrophy of the nail–patella syndrome is most severe on the thumbs.

somal dominant trait with high penetrance but variable expressivity. The gene lies on chromosome 9q34 and is linked to the genes for the ABO blood group and for adenylate kinase-1 (AK-1) [5]. Perhaps more important to understanding the pathogenesis of the condition is the mapping of the COL5A1 gene to the same chromosomal region [6]. Type V collagen is widely distributed as a component of the extracellular matrix and consists of one pro-α2 (V) and two pro-α1 (V) chains. The latter are encoded by the COL5A1 gene, mutations of which may be responsible for the nail–patella syndrome and possibly also for a Goltz-like syndrome [7].

It is not yet clear whether there are two allelic forms; one associated with nephropathy and one without. Overall, the child of a person with the nail–patella syndrome has about a 1 in 4 chance of developing nephropathy and a 1 in 10 chance of going on to renal failure [8].

Pachyonychia congenita (MIM 167200, 167210, 260130)

Clinical features

This rare syndrome is popular with those who like to split rather than lump. Only 168 cases were recorded in the literature between 1904 and 1985, but these have been subdivided into four types [9]. All share the characteristic nail changes, palmoplantar hyperkeratosis, follicular keratoses and a tendency to oral leukokeratosis. Variable additional findings include the presence of teeth at birth, steatocystoma multiplex, blisters, excessive sweating of the palms and soles, hair abnormalities and cataracts.

The nail changes develop within the first few months of life. Subungual hyperkeratosis then forces the distal nail plate up to form the typical wedge-shaped profile (Fig. 2.21)

Genetic aspects

Usually transmitted as an autosomal dominant trait with high penetrance. There have also been examples of an apparently recessive mode of inher-

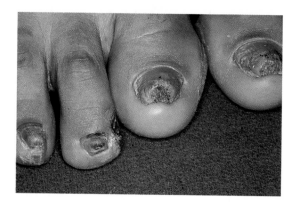

Fig. 2.21 Pachyonychia congenita: tubular nails with massive subungual hyperkeratosis.

itance. The gene in one family with associated epidermal cysts has been provisionally mapped to the keratin gene locus on chromosome 17q [10].

Pathogenesis

The linkage data, involvement of nails and hair follicles, and the association with blistering strongly implicate a keratin gene.

References

1 Hamilton JB, Terada H, Mestler GE. Studies of growth throughout the lifespan in Japanese: growth and size of nails and their relationship to age, sex, heredity, and other factors. *J. Gerontol.* 1955; 10: 401–415.
2 Marshall RC. Genetic variation in the proteins of human nail. *J. Invest. Dermatol.* 1980; 75: 264–269.
3 Telfer NR, Barth JH, Dawber RPR. Congenital and hereditary nail dystrophies—an embryological approach to classification. *Clin. Exp. Dermatol.* 1988; 13: 160–163.
4 Gray E, Hurt VK. Inheritance of brachydactyly type D. *J. Hered.* 1984; 75: 297–299.
5 Ferguson-Smith MA, Aitken DA, Turleav C, de Grouchy J. Localization of the human ABO: N.P.-1: AK-1 linkage group by regional assignment of AK-1 to 9q34. *Hum. Genet.* 1976; 34: 35–43.
6 Greenspan DS, Byers MD, Eddy RL *et al.* Human collagen gene COL5A1 maps to the q34.2–q34.3 region of chromosome 9, near the locus for nail–patella syndrome. *Genomics* 1992; 12: 836–837.
7 Ghiggeri GM, Caridi II, Altieri P, Pezzolo A, Gimelli G, Zuffardi O. Are the nail–patella syndrome and the autosomal Goltz-like syndrome the phenotypic expres-

sions of different alleles at the COL5A1 locus? *Human Genet.* 1993; 91: 175–177.

8   Looij BJ, Te Slaa RL, Hogewind BL, van de Kamp JJ. Genetic counselling in hereditary osteo-onychodysplasia (HOOD, nail–patella syndrome) with nephropathy. *J. Med. Genet.* 1988; 25: 682–686.

9   Feinstein A, Friedman J, Schewach-Millet M. Pachyonychia congenita. *J. Am. Acad. Dermatol.* 1988; 19: 705–771.

10 Munro CS, Carter S, Bryce S *et al.* A gene for pachyonychia congenita is closely linked to the keratin gene cluster on 17q12–q12. *J. Med. Genet.* 1994; 31: 675–678.

Pigmentation

The remarkable number of genetic disorders showing pigmentary abnormalities reflects the complexity of the pigmentary system and the number of points at which it can go wrong. Neural crest cells differentiate into melanoblasts, which migrate out to populate the skin where they become melanocytes, in a density that varies from region to region. Melanin production is regulated not only quantitatively by tyrosinase but also qualitatively by several other factors that divert the production of simple eumelanin into other pigments. The packaging of melanin into melanosomes and its dispersal and transfer to keratinocytes are also carefully regulated processes. Errors might be expected to occur in any of these functions.

In the mouse, more than 150 different mutations at 50 distinct genetic loci have been identified that affect pigmentation [1,2]. Cooperation between biologists working on mice and those studying humans has facilitated an understanding of several conditions. Once a human disorder has been mapped by linkage studies or by a cytogenetic abnormality the homologous mouse locus can be studied for candidate genes. Conversely, once a mouse pigment gene has been identified, the homologous locus in humans can be studied for linkage with pigmentary disorders. There are now several mouse pigment genes awaiting the identification of a corresponding human disease.

The most well-researched disorder of pigmentation is tyrosinase-negative albinism: dozens of mutations have been identified in the tyrosinase gene. Some patients with tyrosinase-positive albinism have mutations in the *P* gene affecting the transport of tyrosine. To albinism can now be added the melanocyte migratory disorders piebaldism and Waardenburg syndrome, and McCune–Albright syndrome in which pigment production is permanently switched on via the adenyl cyclase system. On the horizon are neurofibromatosis, tuberous sclerosis and hypomelanosis of Ito.

Oculocutaneous albinism (OCA) (MIM 203100, 203200, 203280, 203290)

Clinical features

In albinism, little or no melanin is made in the skin and eyes (oculocutaneous albinism), or in the eyes alone (ocular albinism—not discussed further here). The prevalence of albinism of all types ranges from about 1 in 20 000 in the USA and UK to 5% in some inbred communities [3].

The obvious ocular features are a lack of pigment in the iris and fundus with photophobia. In addition, misrouting of optic nerve fibres and a poorly formed or absent foveal pit lead to decreased visual acuity and nystagmus.

Normal numbers of melanocytes are present in the skin and hair, but little melanin is produced. The appearance of the skin depends on the type of albinism, the degree of sun exposure and the racial background of the individual. Without the protection afforded by melanin, albinos in tropical climates do poorly and develop squamous-cell carcinomas and even melanomas [4], usually of amelanotic type, at an early age.

Classification

The tyrosinase test [5] gave the first clue to genetic heterogeneity. Epilated albino hairs put into a solution of L-tyrosine for 24 hours do not accumulate melanin in tyrosinase-negative albinism but do in tyrosinase-positive cases. This finding explains how children with two albino parents could themselves be normally pigmented

[6], the genes being complementary in the double heterozygote.

The tyrosinase-positive (type II) (MIM 203200) and tyrosine-negative (type I) (MIM 203100) types of OCA can often be distinguished clinically. In the former, some pigment appears with age and the skin and hair may be yellowish. Pigmented freckles appear in sun-exposed areas and pigmented cellular naevi may occur [7]. Visual acuity is less severely affected. Tyrosinase-negative patients have snow-white hair, a pink-eyed appearance and no pigmented freckles or naevi (Fig. 2.22). Tyrosinase-positive OCA is slightly the more common in the USA but marginally less so in the UK [87].

Other clinical variations exist. Yellow mutant (type 1B) albinism was first found in the Amish [9]—testing for tyrosinase may be weakly positive. In temperature-sensitive albinism, pigment is absent at birth but hairs on cooler areas of the skin, for example on the legs, darken with age [10]. A platinum or minimal pigment (MIM 203280) type [11] and a brown type (MIM 203290) [12], have also been described.

Genetic aspects [13]

Type I. The tyrosinase gene lies on chromosome 11q14–q21 [14]: it contains five exons and spans more than 50 kb of DNA. A related gene containing only exons 4 and 5 also exists, on 11p. Allelic

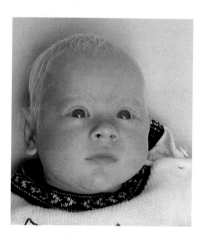

Fig. 2.22 Type 1 (tyrosinase-negative) oculocutaneous albinism.

variants at the tyrosinase locus are now recognized as the cause of tyrosinase-negative (type I) OCA, and also of the yellow mutant (type IB) variety [15]. Some 22 allelic variations, single-base substitutions or frame-shift mutations, are now known at this locus, most clustering within relatively small regions that are likely to represent functionally important sites within the enzyme [16]. Two of these involve copper-A and copper-B binding sites [17]. Prenatal diagnosis can be made as early as 20 weeks [18], but may not be justifiable in view of the good prognosis.

Type II. The genes responsible for tyrosinase-positive (type II) OCA are now being mapped. Studies of a case with a familial translocation suggested a locus either on 2q31.1 or 4q31.2 [19]. However, in the mouse, mutations at the pink-eyed dilution (p) locus cause a reduction of eumelanin. The corresponding human *P* gene lies on chromosome 15q11–q13. It encodes an 838 amino acid polypeptide probably involved in the transport of tyrosine across melanosomal membranes. Mutations of this gene may be responsible for a significant fraction of all cases of tyrosinase-positive OCA. Brown and minimal pigment OCA may be allelic to type-II OCA, and point mutations of the *P* gene may be associated with a wide range of clinical abnormalities ranging from a severe OCA to milder ocular albinism [20].

About 1% of patients with Prader–Willi and Angelman syndromes have tyrosinase-positive OCA [20,21], the result of hemizygosity for inherited mutant alleles of the *P* gene. Many more have milder hypopigmentation and may be hemizygous for non-pathological polymorphisms of the P polypeptide that only slightly reduce its function [20].

Phenylketonuria (MIM 261600)

Clinical features

Phenylketonuria is found in about 1 in 10 000 births [22]. Efficient neonatal screening and early treatment with a diet low in phenylalanine have ensured that it is no longer a cause of major mental handicap. Nevertheless, although children treated early fall into the broad range of normal ability, their mean IQs remain significantly below those of unaffected siblings [23]. The main skin changes are pigment dilution, with paler skin and hair than other family members, and a tendency to eczema.

Genetic aspects

Phenylketonuria is inherited as an autosomal recessive trait, and is due to a deficiency of the hepatic enzyme phenylalanine hydroxylase except in the 1–2% who have defective metabolism of tetrahydrobiopterin [24].

The phenylalanine hydroxylase gene has been mapped to chromosome 12q24.1 and over 40 different mutations have been identified [25]. There are probably many still to be discovered and most affected subjects, therefore, are compound heterozygotes rather than homozygotes.

Prenatal diagnosis is now possible for families with an existing child with phenylketonuria, but has seldom been used as the results of early dietary treatment are so good.

Pathogenesis

Phenylalanine hydroxylase converts phenylalanine to tyrosine, a precursor of melanin. Deficiency leads to an accumulation of phenylalanine and its metabolites in the blood, urine and tissues, but it is still not known precisely how this inhibits myelin synthesis, causing mental defect. Nevertheless, recent work has gone far to explain the wide range of clinical and biochemical severity found in phenylketonuria. Using viral vectors, phenylalanine hydroxylase genes with different mutations can be inserted in pairs into hepatoma cells which themselves lack hydroxylase activity. The enzyme activity of the modified cells can then be assessed. It correlates well with the clinical severity of the same combinations of mutations occurring in patients [26].

Abnormalities in the genes encoding two other enzymes can also lead to the phenylketonuria phenotype. Both enzymes (4a-carbinolamine dehydratase and dihydropterine reductase) play a part in synthesizing tetrahydrobiopterin, a cofactor essential for the conversion of phenylalanine to tyrosine [24].

Successful gene therapy has already been achieved in an inbred strain of mice with phenylalanine hydroxylase deficiency. Using virus vectors, the gene was inserted into liver cells cultured from the mutant mouse. These were then reimplanted and remained healthy within the liver, correcting the biochemical defect for the normal lifespan of the mouse [25].

Piebaldism (MIM 172800)

Clinical features

This rare disorder is characterized by congenital, non-progressive depigmentation, the pattern of which is so constant that it has been recognized since Ancient Greek times. A white forelock arising above a triangle of white skin on the forehead may be the only manifestation, but there is usually also a diamond-shaped area on the front of the trunk, while the mid-portions of the limbs

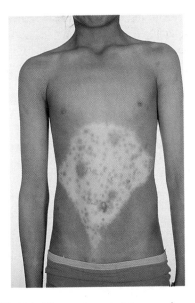

Fig. 2.23 Piebaldism: a characteristic area of hypopigmentation, with pigmented macules, on the front of the abdomen.

have a hypopigmented 'sleeve' of varying length (Fig. 2.23). The lack of pigment affects hair as well as the underlying skin. The white areas usually have pigmented macules within them. Histologically, melanocytes are usually absent from the hypopigmented skin, but sometimes abnormal melanocytes are found [27].

In piebaldism, in contrast to Waardenberg syndrome, there are usually no associated abnormalities. However, deafness has been described and there are two families with piebaldism, retardation, motor incoordination and sensorineural deafness (MIM 172850).

Genetic aspects

Piebaldism is inherited as an autosomal dominant trait with full penetrance. More precisely, it is incompletely dominant. Mendel defined a dominant character as one with identical expression in the heterozygote and the homozygote. A presumed homozygous patient has been described whose parents, first cousins, both had piebaldism [28]. This patient had total lack of pigment as well as retardation, deafness and dysmorphic facies.

Piebaldism was provisionally mapped to 4q12 on the basis of patients with chromosome deletions [29].

Pathogenesis

A pigmentary anomaly in the mouse provided the key to the pathogenesis of piebaldism. Dominant white spotting (W), characterized by depigmentation on the forehead, belly, tail and paws, results from a mutation in the *kit* protooncogene [30]. The human *kit* gene lies on the long arm of chromosome 4, an area implicated in piebaldism by the cytogenetic data mentioned above, so this was an obvious candidate gene. Spritz and others have now found mutations in the *kit* gene in several patients with piebaldism [31–35].

Exactly how the molecular defect produces the pigmentary pattern is not yet known. The pattern of dominant white spotting in mice is consistent with a failure of migrating melanocytes to reach sites furthest from the neural crest, although this does not explain the sparing of the hands and feet

in humans or the freckling within the white areas. The *kit* protooncogene encodes a growth-factor receptor on certain stem cells (the tyrosine–kinase transmembrane cellular receptor for mast-/stem-cell growth factor) without which they cannot respond to the normal signals for development and migration. Mice homozygous for dominant white spotting lack skin pigment, have macrocytic anaemia and are infertile, so the gene product is obviously important for the development of haemopoietic stem cells, germ cells and melanoblasts in the mouse.

The 976 amino acid *kit* polypeptide consists of three parts: an extracellular ligand-binding domain, a transmembrane domain and an intracellular tyrosine-kinase domain. The ligand that binds to this receptor has not yet been identified but is probably encoded by the mouse gene 'steel', defects of which produce a phenotype similar to dominant white spotting. The homologue for the steel locus has been identified in humans but no disorder has yet been associated with it. Ligand binding leads to dimerization of the *kit* receptor and this is apparently a crucial step in signal transduction.

Spritz *et al.* [34] have correlated the mutations in different families with the clinical picture. Patients with complete deletion of the *kit* gene or a mutation producing a severely truncated nonfunctional gene have a relatively mild phenotype, even though the amount of receptor produced by their normal allele can be only 50% of normal. On the other hand, patients with single-point mutations in the intracellular tyrosine-kinase domain have much more extensive piebaldism. This apparent paradox can be explained by a negative dominant effect as follows. When only the intracellular portion of the receptor is abnormal, the extracellular ligand binding site can still function, thus dimerization can occur in the normal way. However, the product is non-functional, even if the abnormal receptor pairs up with a normal one (a non-functional heterodimer). If abnormal receptor monomers dimerized only with other abnormal monomers and the normal receptors likewise dimerized with each other, the functional result would be the same as if the gene were completely deleted, that is 50% of normal function. However, if abnormal monomers dimerize with normal monomers, they reduce the availability of normal receptors to less than 50%.

A third type of mutation is recognized that produces a *kit* polypeptide truncated at the intracellular end and associated with a phenotype that is very variable even within a family. It is suggested that the stability of this receptor is variable, hence it may either not dimerize at all (leaving 50% function) or it may produce non-functional heterodimers (leaving less than 50% function).

No mutations have yet been found in the extracellular ligand-binding domain, perhaps because it is pentarepetitive and therefore an amino acid substitution may not significantly reduce *kit*-dependent signal transduction.

Treatment

Patients who apparently have melanocytes in the white areas may be helped by phototherapy [36], although this must be used with caution. The ambitious approach of autologous melanocyte transplant has been reported in single patients: Lerner *et al.* [37] cultured melanocytes from a normally pigmented area and transplanted them into suction blisters raised on a white area, resulting apparently in normal pigmentation of the surrounding skin.

Waardenburg syndrome (MIM 193500)

Clinical features

In this syndrome cochlear deafness and hypertelorism are accompanied by pigmentary anomalies including a white forelock, heterochromia iridis, white eyelashes and sometimes depigmented areas of skin as in piebaldism. Some patients have Hirschsprung disease (aganglionic megacolon).

Genetic aspects

This is inherited in an autosomal dominant manner. An early suggestion of linkage to the ABO locus could not be confirmed. The first breakthrough was the finding of a *de novo* paracentric inversion on the long arm of chromosome 2 in a sporadic case of Waardenburg syndrome,

the breakpoints being at 2q35 and 2q37.3 [38]. Subsequently, linkage was found to the placental alkaline phosphatase locus at 2q37 suggesting that the distal breakpoint was the Waardenburg locus [39]. However, some families do not show linkage to the 2q markers, therefore multiple genes may be involved [40].

Pathogenesis

The pathogenesis of Waardenburg syndrome has emerged as a result of ideas being bounced back and forth between geneticists studying mouse and humans. On the basis of the cytogenetic and linkage data mentioned above, the Waardenburg locus was identified at 2q37 and is homologous to a region on mouse chromosome 1 containing the splotch locus. This patchy pigment mutation is accompanied by malformation of the central nervous system and inner ear in homozygotes. In one case a deletion involving the splotch locus also included the murine placental alkaline phosphatase locus. Subsequently, close linkage was found between splotch and the paired-box gene *pax*-3, and deletions in *pax*-3 were found in splotch mice, confirming that *pax*-3 is the splotch gene [41]. The human homologue of the mouse *pax*-3 gene is *hup*-2. Tassabehji [42] found mutations in *hup*-2 in 6 out of 17 unrelated Waardenburg syndrome patients, and the variant bands showed perfect linkage to Waardenburg syndrome in the families studied, confirming that the *hup*-2 gene is responsible for this syndrome at least in these families.

hup-2 and *pax*-3 play key organizational roles in normal development, particularly in migration of neural crest derivatives.

McCune–Albright syndrome (MIM 174800,139320.0008,9)

Clinical features

Patients with this condition classically have abnormalities in three systems. The bones show polyostotic fibrous dysplasia. Endocrine overactivity includes hyperthyroidism, growth hormone excess, Cushing's syndrome and precocious puberty in 50% of females. The skin shows discrete areas of hyperpigmentation, the edges of which tend to follow Blaschko's lines although the lesions themselves form large blocks rather than lines. The bony and cutaneous lesions are strikingly asymmetrical.

Genetics

This is a sporadic disorder. Happle has demonstrated that the skin lesions may follow Blaschko's lines and suggested mosaicism due to a dominant somatic mutation, the pigmented patches of skin representing the abnormal cell line [43,44]. Because generalized skin involvement is never seen, he postulated that the mutation is lethal, and patients with McCune–Albright syndrome survive because their mutant cells are 'rescued' by the normal ones [43,44].

Pathogenesis

The endocrine abnormalities of McCune–Albright syndrome are all disorders of hypersecretion—this is the key to the pathogenesis.

Trophic hormones such as growth-hormone releasing hormone (GHRH) use cAMP as a second

messenger to stimulate hormone release. The activity of hormone-sensitive adenylate cyclase is regulated by two guanine-nucleotide-binding proteins termed G_s (stimulatory) and G_i (inhibitory). These proteins are heterotrimers with identical β and γ subunits but unique α subunits. The gene for the α subunit of G_s termed GNAS1 (MIM 139320), mapped to 20q12–13.3 [45], spans 20 kb and is composed of 13 exons and 12 introns [46]. Four different types of RNA can be generated by differential use of certain parts of the GNAS1 gene (splice variants) producing G_s proteins that may regulate different functions [47].

The cause of McCune–Albright syndrome was discovered during work on pituitary tumours. In certain growth-hormone-secreting pituitary tumours G_s was found to be maximally activated [48]. Two years later, in 1989, Landis *et al.* [49] found activating (oncogenic) mutations in the gene for the α subunit of G_s in pituitary tumours, and in 1991 Weinstein *et al.* [50] found similar mutations in affected endocrine organs of patients with McCune–Albright syndrome. Subsequently, Schwindinger *et al.* [51] found the mutation in a higher proportion of skin cells from pigmented than from non-pigmented skin, supporting Happle's hypothesis that this is a mosaic disorder.

Table 2.14 Miscellaneous pigmentary disorders

MIM*	Condition
(a) *Increased pigmentation*	
145100	Hyperpigmentation of eyelids
145250	Hyperpigmentation of wrists, hands and neck
145250	Familial progressive hyperpigmentation
155800	Universal melanosis
179850	Dowling–Degos reticular pigmentation of flexures
(b) *Decreased pigmentation*	
179500	Raindrop hypopigmentation of the upper chest
227010	Black locks, albinism, deafness syndrome (BADS)
256710	Neuroectodermal melanolysosomal disease (hypopigmentation, retardation, fits)
257790	Preus syndrome (oculocerebral syndrome with hypopigmentation)
257800	Cross syndrome (oculocerebral syndrome with hypopigmentation)
(c) *Increased and decreased pigmentation*	
154000	Congenital hypopigmented and hyperpigmented macules
270750	Spastic paraplegia with pigmentary abnormalities

* First digit of MIM number indicates inheritance: 1 = autosomal dominant; 2 = autosomal recessive; 3 = X-linked.

The effect of these mutations on melanocytes in McCune–Albright syndrome has not yet been studied. However, adenyl cyclase is known to be involved in the regulation of melanogenesis, and the activating mutation would be expected to increase pigment production. This is consistent with the histological finding of normal numbers and size of melanocytes with enlarged melanosomes in the melanotic macules of McCune–Albright syndrome.

Reduced expression of GNAS1 occurs in patients with pseudohypoparathyroidism (Albright's hereditary osteodystrophy). McKusick pointed out that it seems to be poetic justice that two conditions described by Fuller Albright should have a defect in the same gene, one producing deficiency and the other producing excess.

Miscellaneous disorders of pigmentation

There are many more inherited conditions with abnormal pigmentation. Some of them are listed in Table 2.14.

Reference

1 Hearing VJ. Unraveling the melanocyte (editorial). *Am. J. Hum. Genet.* 1993; 52: 1–7.

2 Mishima Y, Noris DA (eds). Molecular and biological control of melanogenesis and melanoma. *J. Invest. Dermatol.* 1993; 100 (Suppl.): 133S–191S.

3 Stout DB. Further notes on albinism among the San Blas Cuna, Panama. *Am. J. Phys. Anthropol.* 1946; 4: 483.

4 Okoro AN. Albinism in Nigeria. *Br. J. Dermatol.* 1975; 92: 485–492.

5 Kugelman TP, Van Scott EJ. Tyrosinase activity in melanocytes of human albinos. *J. Invest. Dermatol.* 1961; 37: 73–76.

6 Trevor-Roper PD. Marriage of two complete albinos with normally pigmented offspring. *Br. J. Ophthalmol.* 1952; 36: 107–110.

7 Akiyama M, Shimizo H, Sugiura M, Nishikawa T. Do pigmented naevi in albinism provide evidence of tyrosinase positivity? *Br. J. Dermatol.* 1992; 127: 649–653.

8 Jay B, Witkop CJ, King RA. Albinism in England. *Birth Defects* 1982; 18; 319–325.

9 Nance WE, Jackson CE, Witkop CJ. Amish albinism: a distinctive autosomal recessive phenotype. *Am. J. Hum. Genet.* 1970; 22: 578–586.

10 King RA, Townsend D, Detting W, Summers CG, Olds DP, White JG, Spritz RA. Temperature–sensitive tyrosinase associated with peripheral pigmentation in oculocutaneous albinism. *J. Clin. Invest.* 1991; 87: 1046–1053.

11 King RA, Wirtschafer JD, Olds DP, Brumbaugh J. Minimal pigment: a new type of oculocutaneous albinism. *Clin. Genet.* 1986; 29: 42–50.

12 King RA, Rich SS. Segregation analysis of brown oculocutaneous albinism. *Clin. Genet.* 1986; 29: 496–501.

13 Oetting WS, King RA. Molecular basis of oculocutaneous albinism. *J. Invest. Dermatol.* 1994; 103: 131S–136S.

14 Barton DE, Kwon BS, Francke U. Human tyrosinase gene, mapped to chromosome 11 (q14–q21) defines second region of homology with mouse chromosome 7. *Genomics* 1988; 3: 17–24.

15 Giebel LB, Strunk KM, Jackson CE *et al.* Tyrosinase mutations in patients with type IB ('yellow') oculocutaneous albinism. *Am. J. Hum. Genet.* 1990; 47 (Suppl.): A156.

16 Tripathi RK, Strunk KM, Giebel LB, Weleber RG, Spritz RA. Tyrosinase gene mutations in type I (tyrosinase-deficient) oculocutaneous albinism define two clusters of missense substitutions. *Am. J. Med. Genet.* 1992; 43: 865–871.

17 King RA, Mentink MM, Detting WS. Non-random distribution of missense mutations within the human tyrosinase gene in type I (tyrosinase-related) oculocutaneous albinism. *Molec. Biol. Med.* 1991; 8: 19–29.

18 Eady RAJ. Prenatal diagnosis of oculocutaneous albinism: implications for other hereditary disorders of pigmentation. *Semin. Dermatol.* 1984; 3: 241–246.

19 Walpole IR, Mulchahy MI. Tyrosinase positive albinism with familial 46, XY.. (2:4) (q31.2; q31.22) balanced translocation. *J. Med. Genet.* 1991; 28: 482–484.

20 Lee S-T, Nicholls RD, Bundey S *et al.* Mutations of the P-gene in oculocutaneous albinism, ocular albinism and the Prader–Willi syndrome plus albinism. *N. Engl. J. Med.* 1994; 330: 529–534.

21 Rinchnik EM, Bultman SJ, Horsthemke B *et al.* A gene for the mouse pink-eyed dilution locus and for human type II oculocutaneous albinism. *Nature* 1993; 361: 72–76.

22 Smith I, Cook B, Beasley M. Review of neonatal screening for phenylketonuria. *BMJ* 1991; 303: 333–335.

23 Koch R, Azen C, Friedman EG, Williamson ML. Paired comparison between early treated phenylketonuria children and their matched sibling controls on intellectual and school achievement test results at eight years. *J. Inher. Metab. Dis.* 1984; 7: 86–90.

24 Citron BA, Kaufman S, Milstein S *et al.* Mutation in the 4a-carbinolamine reductase gene leads to mild hyperphenylalaninemia with defective cofactor metabolism. *Am. J. Hum. Genet.* 1993; 53: 768–774.

25 Medical Research Council Working Party on Phenylketonuria. Phenylketonuria due to phenylalanine hydroxylase deficiency: an unfolding story. *BMJ* 1993; 306: 115–119.

26 Okano Y, Eisensmith RC, Guttler F *et al.* Molecular basis of phenotypic heterogeneity in phenylketonuria. *N. Engl. J. Med.* 1991; 324: 1232–1238.

27 Mosher DB, Fitzpatrick TB. Piebaldism (editorial). *Arch. Dermatol.* 1988; 124: 364–365.

28 Hulten MA, Honeyman MM, Mayne AJ, Tarlow MJ. Homozygosity in a piebald trait. *J. Med Genet.* 1987; 24: 568–571.

29 Lin AE, Garver KL, Diggans G *et al.* Interstitial and terminal deletions of the long arm of chromosome 4: further delineation of phenotypes. *Am. J. Med. Genet.* 1988; 31: 533–548.

30 Chabot B, Stephenson DA, Chapman VM *et al.* The proto-oncogene c-kit encoding a transmembrane tyrosine kinase receptor maps to the mouse W locus. *Nature* 1988; 335: 88–89.

31 Fleischman RA, Saltman DL, Stastny V, Zneimer S. Deletion of the c-kit protooncogene in the human developmental defect piebald trait. *Proc. Natl. Acad. Sci. USA* 1991; 88: 10885–10889.

32 Giebel LB, Spritz RA. Mutation of the KIT (mast/stem cell growth factor receptor) protooncogene in human piebaldism. *Proc. Natl. Acad. Sci. USA* 1991; 88: 8696–8699.

33 Spritz RA, Giebel LB, Holmes SA. Dominant negative and loss of function mutations of the c-kit (mast/stem cell growth factor receptor) protooncogene in human piebaldism. *Am. J. Hum. Genet.* 1992; 50: 261–269.

34 Spritz RA, Holmes SA, Ramesar R *et al.* Mutations of the KIT (mast/stem cell growth factor receptor) protooncogene account for a continuous range of phenotypes in human piebaldism. *Am. J. Hum. Genet.* 1992; 51: 1058–1065.

35 Spritz RA, Holmes SA, Itin P *et al.* Novel mutations of the KIT (mast/stem cell growth factor receptor) protooncogene in human piebaldism. *J. Invest. Dermatol.* 1993; 101: 22–25.

36 Hayashibe K, Mishima Y. Tyrosine-positive melanocyte distribution and induction of pigmentation in human piebald skin. *Arch. Dermatol.* 1988; 124: 381–386.

37 Lerner AB, Halaban R, Klaus S, Moelmann GE. Transplantation of human melanocytes. *J. Invest. Dermatol.* 1987; 89: 219–224.

38 Ishikiriyama S, Tonoki H, Shibuya Y *et al.* Waardenburg syndrome type I in a child with *de novo* inversion (2)(q35q37.3). *Am. J. Med Genet.* 1989; 33: 505–507.

39 Foy C, Newton V, Wellesley D *et al.* Assignment of the locus for Waardenburg syndrome type I to human chromosome 2q37 and possible homology to the Splotch mouse. *Am. J. Hum. Genet.* 1990; 46: 1017–1023.

40 Grundfast K, Farrer L, Amos J *et al.* Waardenburg syndrome is caused by defects at multiple loci, one of which is tightly linked to ALPP on chromosome 2—first report of the WS consortium (Abstract). *Am. J. Hum. Genet.* 1991; 49 (Suppl.): 17.

41 Epstein DJ, Vekemans M, Gros P. Splotch (Sp–2H), a mutation affecting development of the mouse neural tube, shows a deletion within the paired homeodomain of PAX-3. *Cell* 1991; 67: 767–774.

42 Tassabehji M, Read AP, Newton VE *et al.* Waardenburg syndrome patients have mutations in the human homologue of the PAX-3 paired box gene. *Nature* 1992; 355: 635–636.

43 Happle R. The McCune–Albright syndrome: a lethal gene surviving by mosaicism. *Clin. Genet.* 1986; 29: 321–324.

44 Happle R. Lethal genes surviving by mosaicism: a possible explanation for sporadic birth defects involving the skin. *J. Am. Acad. Dermatol.* 1987; 16: 899–906.

45 Levine MA, Modi WS, O'Brien SJ. Mapping of the gene encoding the alpha subunit of the stimulatory G protein of adenyl cyclase (GNAS1) to 20q13.2–q13.3 in humans by *in situ* hybridisation. *Genomics* 1991; 11: 478–479.

46 Kozasa T, Itoh H, Tsukamoto T, Kaziro Y. Isolation and characterisation of the human G(s)–alpha gene. *Proc. Natl. Acad. Sci. USA* 1988; 85: 2081–2085.

47 Mattera R, Graziano MP, Yatani A *et al.* Splice variants of the alpha subunit of the G protein G(8) activate both adenylate cyclase and calcium channels. *Science* 1989; 243: 804–807.

48 Vallar L, Spada A, Giannattasio G. Altered Gs and adenylate cyclase activity in human GH-secreting pituitary adenomas. *Nature* 1987; 330: 566–568.

49 Landis CA, Masters SB, Spada A *et al.* GTP-ase inhibiting mutations activate the alpha chain of G(s) and stimulate adenylate cyclase in human pituitary tumours. *Nature* 1989; 340: 692–696.

50 Weinstein LS, Shenker A, Gejman PV *et al.* Activating mutations of the stimulatory G protein in the McCune–Albright syndrome. *N. Engl. J. Med.* 1991; 325: 1688–1695.

51 Schwindinger WF, Francomano CA, Levine MA. Identification of a mutation in the gene encoding the alpha subunit of the stimulatory G protein of adenylyl cyclase in McCune–Albright syndrome. *Proc. Natl. Acad. Sci. USA* 1992; 89: 5152–5156.

Epidermal adhesion

The term epidermolysis bullosa (EB) covers a group of conditions that can be divided broadly into simplex, dystrophic and junctional types, in which blisters occur respectively in the epidermis, dermis or at the dermo-epidermal junction [1]. Although the name brings together a group of disparate disorders and is strictly accurate only for the simplex form, it is well established and useful because sufferers share serious and unusual problems requiring special expertise for their management [2].

This is also one of the most exciting areas of skin biology in terms of our understanding of the molecular basis of disease [3] and the potential for gene therapy.

Since the 1960s, electronmicroscopists have succeeded in identifying the ultrastructural constituents of the dermo-epidermal junction, and their abnormalities in the blistering disorders. Later, monoclonal antibodies were developed to various components, and immunoelectronmicroscopy has further improved diagnostic precision. Newer techniques such as immunoblotting have established the molecular basis of these antigens, and candidate genes have been tested in transgenic mice. As a result, several specific gene mutations responsible for different types of EB are now known. The current state of knowledge is summarized in Figure 2.24.

At present EB can be treated only symptomatically, but gene therapy, at least for the simplex forms, seems only a short step away from the transfection experiments already being performed in animals. If the normal gene can be inserted *in vitro* into keratinocytes from EB simplex (EBS) patients, the corrected cells could be cultured and monolayers grafted on to blistered areas using techniques already available [4].

Epidermolysis bullosa simplex (EBS)

Clinical features

EBS affects about 1 in 50 000 of the population. Disorders in this group share a tendency to blister formation, particularly in response to trauma (Fig. 2.25). There is no scarring.

EBS subtypes differ with regard to severity, distribution of the blisters and associated features, and are listed in Table 2.15. The classification will no doubt be revised as their molecular basis becomes clearer.

Genetic aspects

Most forms of EBS are inherited as autosomal dominant traits, but some rarer forms are

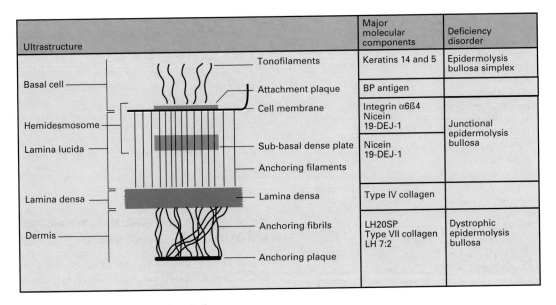

Ultrastructure		Major molecular components	Deficiency disorder
Basal cell	Tonofilaments	Keratins 14 and 5	Epidermolysis bullosa simplex
	Attachment plaque	BP antigen	
Hemidesmosome	Cell membrane	Integrin α6ß4 Nicein 19-DEJ-1	Junctional epidermolysis bullosa
Lamina lucida	Sub-basal dense plate	Nicein 19-DEJ-1	
	Anchoring filaments		
Lamina densa	Lamina densa	Type IV collagen	
Dermis	Anchoring fibrils	LH20SP Type VII collagen LH 7:2	Dystrophic epidermolysis bullosa
	Anchoring plaque		

Fig. 2.24 Summary of epidermolysis bullosa.

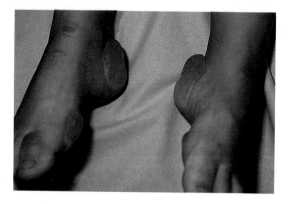

Fig. 2.25 Friction blisters in epidermolysis bullosa simplex.

automal recesive. In general, there is no extracutaneous involvement in the dominant forms except in patients with the Dowling–Meara variant who may have nail dystrophy and oral and oesophageal erosions.

Pathogenesis
The blisters form within the basal and suprabasal

layers of the epidermis. The major structural protein of the epidermis is keratin, so perhaps it is not surprising that several forms of EBS are due to mutations in keratin genes.

In 1982, Anton-Lamprecht [5] showed clumping of keratin tonofilaments in the basal cells of patients with Dowling–Meara EBS, and noted that this change preceded blister formation. She concluded that EBS was likely to arise from structural defects in keratin. In 1989, abnormal keratin filaments were found in cultured EBS keratinocytes [6].

The paired keratins expressed in basal keratinocytes are K14 and K5, and subsequent animal work has focussed on mutant K14 and K5 genes *in vitro* and *in vivo*. Cultured normal keratinocytes transfected with a K14 mutation show the same perturbed keratin network as cultured Dowling–Meara EBS keratinocytes [7]. Furthermore, mutant K14 or K5 genes introduced into transgenic mice produce blistering identical to that in Dowling–Meara EBS [8]. The nature of the mutation determines the degree of abnormal-

Table 2.15 Subtypes of epidermolysis bullosa simplex (EBS)

MIM*	Name	Pattern of blisters	Associated features
Dominant types			
131760 148066.0002† 148066.0003†	Dowling–Meara	Herpetiform	Nail dystrophy Oral and oesophageal blisters Keratoderma
131800‡	Weber–Cockayne	Hands and feet	None
131880	—	Hands and feet	Galactosylhydroxylysyl deficiency
131900 148066.0001†	Koebner	Generalized	None
131950	Ogna	Koebner-like	Bruising tendency
131960	Gedde–Dahl	Koebner-like	Mottled pigmentation
Recessive types			
—	Kallin	Hands, feet, oral	Hypodontia Nail dystrophy Alopecia
226670	'Letalis'	Generalized‡ oral	Neuromuscular disease (limb girdle muscular dystrophy; myasthenia gravis)

* First digit of MIM number indicates inheritance: 1 = autosomal dominant; 2 = autosomal recessive; 3 = X-linked.
† MIM 148066 denotes the K14 gene. These three subtypes represent families with EBS due to specific mutations of the K14 gene.
‡ McKusick assigns the same number to dominant EBS (Weber–Cockayne) and dominant dystrophic EB (Cockayne–Touraine).

ity in keratin filament assembly, which in turn correlates with the severity of the phenotype in transgenic mice [9].

Further work has confirmed the relevance of these findings in EBS patients. In Dowling–Meara EBS the tonofilament clumps are recognized by antibodies to K14 and K5 [10]. Linkage studies in several Koebner and Weber–Cockayne families confirm that the genetic defect maps to chromosomes 17 and 12, corresponding to loci for types I and II keratin gene clusters [11,12]. There are now several reports of K5 and K14 mutations in patients with Dowling–Meara [13,14], Weber–Cockayne and Koebner EBS [11]. Furthermore, one of these point mutations, genetically engineered into normal human K14 cDNA and transfected into human keratinocytes, produced shortened keratin filaments exactly like those seen in Dowling–Meara EBS [13].

Most of the mutations so far found in EBS lie in the highly conserved end domains of the keratin gene, as do those in the K10 and K1 genes in epidermolytic hyperkeratosis (autosomal dominant bullous ichthyosiform erythroderma) [15].

Junctional epidermolysis bullosa (JEB)

Clinical features

JEB is characterized by blistering with atrophic scarring of skin and mucosae, nail dystrophy and loss (Fig. 2.26), and abnormal dental enamel.

Babies with the lethal Herlitz form (MIM 226700) usually die in infancy (Fig. 2.27). If they survive the first few months they often develop chronic crusted erosions of the central face, which may be helped by autologous keratinocyte grafts [16]. They rarely live beyond the age of 2 years.

The mitis and inverse forms cannot be distinguished from the lethal form in infancy either clinically or histologically, but improve with age. The inverse form settles in the flexures. In the localized and progressive variants, the onset of blistering is later. Three patients have been reported with a cicatricial form of junctional epidermolysis bullosa. The different forms of JEB are listed in Table 2.16.

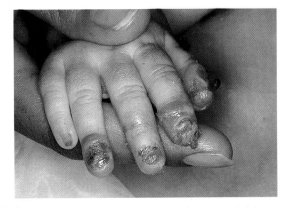

Fig. 2.26 Severe periungual inflammation and nail loss in junctional epidermolysis bullosa.

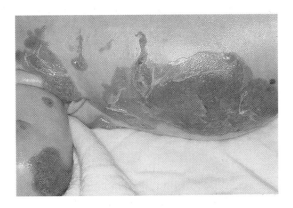

Fig. 2.27 Extensive skin loss in Herlitz-type junctional epidermolysis bullosa.

Table 2.16 Subtypes of junctional epidermolysis bullosa

MIM*	Name	Associated features
226700	Lethal Herlitz	Death in infancy
226730	—	Herlitz-like + pyloric atresia
226650	Mitis, Disentis	Like Herlitz, but non-lethal
—	Inverse	Like Mitis but flexural
—	Localized	Later onset
226500†	Progressive	Later onset of progressive skin atrophy with deafness
—	Cicatricial	Like Herlitz, with scarring alopecia

* First digit of MIM number indicates inheritance : 1 = autosomal dominant; 2 = autosomal recessive ; 3 = X-linked.
† McKusick refers to this as dystrophic.

Genetic aspects

All forms of JEB show autosomal recessive inheritance.

Pathogenesis

Ultrastructurally the split is within the lamina lucida, and the hemidesmosomes are variably abnormal [17]. Diagnosis is confirmed by absent or reduced staining with the monoclonal antibodies GB3 [18] and 19-DEJ-1 [19]. Absence of 19-DEJ-1 is highly sensitive for JEB but does not distinguish the lethal and non-lethal forms and is also found in dystrophic EB. Absent GB3 is more often associated with lethal than non-lethal disease but is not highly specific [20].

These antigens have not yet been defined but are constituents of the anchoring filaments. The GB3 antigen, also called BM600 nicein (after the city of Nice), is related to laminin, kalinin and epiligrin, and is synthesized by normal human keratinocytes [21]. BM600 nicein is a glycoprotein consisting of three subunits, the genes for which are located at 1q25, 1q32 and 18q11. The 19DEJ-1 antigen has not yet been identified. Bullous pemphigoid antigen, which is localized to the attachment plaque within the basal cells, is expressed normally in JEB [22]. Another candidate molecule is integrin $\alpha6$-$\beta4$, the only member of the integrin superfamily of adhesion molecules exclusively associated with keratinocyte–basement membrane adhesion. It is located in hemidesmosomes [23]. However, there have been conflicting results in JEB: Fine *et al.* [24] reported that it was normal, while Jonkman *et al.* [25] found patchy separation of the intra- and extacellular epitopes of integrin $\alpha6$-$\beta4$ in JEB, suggesting a defect in this molecule or its ligand. Talin, a protein present at adherens junctions, is another candidate molecule [21]. Mutations in these different proteins probably account for the heterogeneity of JEB [26].

Patients have been described with a pseudojunctional form of epidermolysis bullosa, which is clinically like the JEB mitis, with absent staining for GB3 and 19-DEJ-1, although the level of the split is in the basal layer not in the lamina lucida.

The recently described laryngo-onychocutaneous syndrome may be another subtype of JEB [27].

Dystrophic epidermolysis bullosa (DEB)

Clinical features (Figs 2.28–2.30)

Patients with the classical Hallopeau–Siemens recessive DEB develop spontaneous as well as traumatic blisters, which heal with scarring and milia formation. The fingers and toes become fused by scar tissue leading to mitten deformities (pseudosyndactyly). Blistering in the mouth and oesophagus leads to microstomia and oesophageal

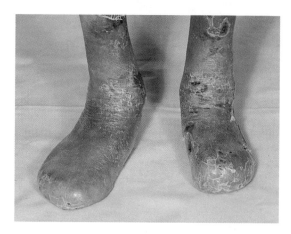

Fig. 2.28 Recessive dystrophic epidermolysis bullosa: skin fragility and acral 'cocoon' formation.

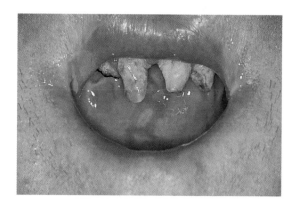

Fig. 2.29 Microstomia, oral ulceration and dental defects contribute to malnutrition in patients with dystrophic epidermolysis bullosa.

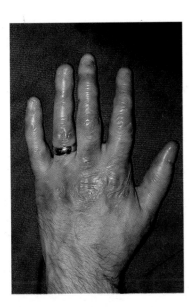

Fig. 2.30 Dominant dystrophic epidermolysis bullosa showing nail loss and skin fragility, but no cocoon formation.

stricture. Cornea, nails and teeth are also involved. Growth deficiency and anaemia are usual. Squamous-cell carcinoma may arise later in chronically eroded areas.

The other forms of DEB are less severe and are listed in Table 2.17.

Genetic aspects

Both milder dominant and more severe recessive forms occur (Table 2.17).

Pathogenesis

Blisters in DEB form in the upper dermis. Twenty years ago, Anton-Lamprecht suggested, on electronmicroscopic evidence in dominant DEB, that there was a defect in the anchoring fibrils [28], and subsequently postulated a defect in the structural gene for anchoring fibrils [29]. Attention was then diverted to collagenase in recessive DEB.

In 1978, Bauer found increased synthesis of collagenase in recessive DEB fibroblasts, and suggested treatment with phenytoin, which inhibits collagenase [30]. The human collagenase gene was mapped to chromosome 11q11–23 in 1987 [31]. However, it gradually emerged that the primary defect did not lie in collagenase: phenytoin was not helpful clinically, and not all patients showed elevated levels of collagenase. Most conclusively, Hovnanian [32] found increased collagenase mRNA in only 2 of 3 affected siblings with recessive DEB and excluded linkage to the collagenase locus in this family.

Table 2.17 Subtypes of dystrophic epidermolysis bullosa

MIM	Name	Associated features
Dominant		
131705	Transient bullous dermolysis of the newborn	Transient neonatal blisters
131750	Pasini	Generalized; albopapuloid lesions
131800*	Cockayne–Touraine	Generalized; milder than Pasini
—	Localized, Minimis	
131850	Pretibial	
—	Centripetal	
132000	Bart syndrome	Generalized + acral aplasia cutis
Recessive		
226600	Hallopeau–Siemens	Severe; pseudosyndactyly; mucous membrane involvement
—	Mitis	Milder; sometimes localized
226450	Inverse	Flexural involvement; otherwise similar to Hallopeau–Siemens
—	Centripetal	Acral, with progressive centripetal spread

* McKusick assigns the same number to dominant epidermolysis bullosa simplex (Weber–Cockayne) and dominant dystrophic epidermolysis bullosa (Cockayne–Touraine).

Most recently attention has swung back to the anchoring fibrils. In 1986, type VII collagen was identified as their major structural component [33]. It is synthesized by keratinocytes as well as by fibroblasts. Immunofluorescence studies have shown reduced or absent type VII collagen in unblistered skin from patients with recessive DEB [34]. In 1991, Ryynanen *et al.* [35] found close linkage between dominant DEB and the gene for type VII collagen (*COL7A1*) at 3p21, and this has been confirmed in other families. Mutations in *COL7A1* have now been found in affected individuals [36].

However, DEB is not simply a collagen VII deficiency disease: the situation is more complex [37,38]. The production of normal collagen VII by recessive DEB keratinocytes [39] and overexpression of collagen VII in some patients with RDEB [40] show that the primary defect is not necessarily a mutation in the *COL7A1* gene. In some cases there may be excessive proteolysis by collagenase, perhaps secondary to a structural abnormality in collagen. The transient neonatal form of DEB may be due to delayed transport of collagen VII from keratinocytes to the dermis [41]. Generalized dominant DEB (Pasini type) shows accumulation of collagen VII and increased collagen VII mRNA in cultured keratinocytes [42]. DEB may prove to be even more heterogeneous at the molecular level than might be suspected clinically.

References

1 Fine J-D, Bauer EA, Briggaman RA *et al.* Revised clinical and laboratory criteria for subtypes of inherited epidermolysis bullosa. *J. Am. Acad. Dermatol.* 1991; 24: 119–135.

2 Priestley GC, Tidman MJ, Weiss JB, Eady RAJ (eds). *Epidermolysis Bullosa: a Comprehensive Review of Classification, Management and Laboratory Studies.* Crowthorne: DEBRA, 1990.

3 Uitto J, Bauer EA, Moshell AN. Symposium on EB: molecular biology and pathology of the cutaneous basement membrane zone. *J. Invest. Dermatol.* 1992; 98: 391–400.

4 O'Connor NE, Gallico GG, Compton C *et al.* Grafting of burns with cultured epithelium prepared from autologous epidermal cells. II. Intermediate term results on three paediatric patients. In *Soft and Hard Tissue Repair*, Vol. 2. (Hunt TK, Heppenstall KB, Pines E, Rovee D eds). New York; Praeger, 1984; 283–292.

5 Anton-Lamprecht I, Schnyder VW. Epidermolysis bullosa herpetiformis Dowling–Meara: report of a case and pathogenesis. *Dermatologica* 1982; 164: 221–235.

6 Kitajima Y, Inoue S, Yaoita H. Abnormal organisation of keratin intermediate filaments in cultured keratinocytes of epidermolysis bullosa simplex. *Arch. Dermatol. Res.* 1989; 281: 5–10.

7 Coulombe P, Chan Y-M, Albers K, Fuchs E. Deletions in epidermal keratins that lead to alterations in filament organisation and assembly: *in vivo* and *in vitro* studies. *J. Cell Biol.* 1990; 111: 3049–3064.

8 Vassar R, Coulombe PA, Degenstein L *et al.* Mutant keratin expression in transgenic mice causes marked abnormalities resembling a human genetic skin disease. *Cell* 1991; 64: 365–380.

9 Coulombe PA, Hutton ME, Vassar R, Fuchs E. A function for keratins and a common thread among different types of epidermolysis bullosa simplex diseases. *J. Cell Biol.* 1991; 115: 1661–1674.

10 Ishida-Yamamoto A, McGrath JA, Chapman SJ *et al.* Epidermolysis bullosa simplex (Dowling–Meara type) is a genetic disease characterised by an abnormal keratin filament network involving keratins K5 and K14. *J. Invest. Dermatol.* 1991; 97: 959–968.

11 Bonifas JM, Rothman AL, Epstein EH. Epidermolysis bullosa simplex: evidence in two families for keratin gene abnormalities. *Science* 1991; 254: 1202–1205.

12 Ryynanen M, Knowlton RG, Uitto J. Mapping of epidermolysis bullosa simplex mutation to chromosome 12. *Am. J. Hum. Genet.* 1991; 49: 978–984.

13 Coulombe PA, Hutton ME, Letai A *et al.* Point mutations in human keratin 14 genes of epidermolysis bullosa simplex patients: genetic and functional analyses. *Cell* 1991; 66: 1301–1311.

14 Lane EB, Rugg EL, Navsaria H *et al.* A mutation in the conserved helix termination peptide of keratin 5 in hereditary skin blistering. *Nature* 1992; 356: 244–246.

15 Fuchs E, Coulombe P, Cheng J *et al.* Genetic basis of epidermolysis bullosa simplex and epidermolytic hyperkeratosis. *J. Invest. Dermatol.* 1994; 103: 25S–30S.

16 Carter DM, Liu AN, Varghese M *et al.* Treatment of junctional epidermolysis bullosa with epidermal autografts. *J. Am. Acad. Dermatol.* 1987; 17: 246–250.

17 Tidman MJ, Eady RAJ. Hemidesmosome heterogeneity in junctional epidermolysis bullosa revealed by morphometric analysis. *J. Invest. Dermatol.* 1986; 86: 51–56.

18 Heagerty AHM, Kennedy AR, Eady RAJ *et al.* GB3 monoclonal antibody for diagnosis of junctional epidermolysis bullosa. *Lancet* 1986; I: 860.

19 Fine JD, Horiguchi Y, Couchman JR. 19-DEJ-1, a hemidesmosomal-anchoring filament complex associated monoclonal antibody, defines a new skin basement membrane antigenic defect in junctional and recessive dystrophic epidermolysis bullosa. *Arch. Dermatol.* 1989; 125: 520–523.

20 Fine J-D, Daniels A, Zeng Li. Comparative analysis of the sensitivity and specificity of 19-DEJ-1 and GB3 monoclonal antibodies for diagnosis and sub-classification of junctional epidermolysis bullosa subsets (Abstract). *J. Invest. Dermatol.* 1993; 100: 530.

21 Kaiser HW, Ness W, Offers M *et al.* Talin: adherens junction protein is localised at the epidermal-dermal interface in skin. *J. Invest. Dermatol.* 1993; 101: 789–793.

22 Heagerty AHM, Kennedy AR, Eady RAJ. Lethal junctional epidermolysis bullosa: a disorder of hemidesmosome formation but not bullous pemphigoid antigen? (Abstract). *J. Invest. Dermatol.* 1986; 87: 144.

23 Stepp MA, Spurr-Michaud S, Tisdale A *et al.* Alpha 6 beta 4 integrin hetrodimer is a component of hemidesmosomes. *Proc. Natl. Acad. Sci. USA*, 1990; 87: 8970–8974.

24 Fine JD, Quaranta V, Horiguchi Y *et al.* Relative expression of four hemidesmosome-associated proteins in junctional epidermolysis bullosa, a disease of epithelial dysadhesion with known abnormal hemidesmosomes (Abstract). *J. Cell Biol.* 1991; 115: 34a.

25 Jonkman MF, de Jong MCJM, Heeres K, Sonnenberg A. Expression of integrin alpha 6 beta 4 in junctional epidermolysis bullosa. *J. Invest. Dermatol.* 1992; 99: 489–496.

26 Gil SG, Brown TA, Ryan MC *et al.* Junctional epidermolysis bullosa: defects in expression of epiligrin/nicein/kalinin and integrin B4 that inhibit hemidesmosomet formation. *J. Invest. Dermatol.* 1994; 103: 31S–38S.

27 Phillips RJ, Strobel S, Gibbs M, Atherton DJ. Laryngo-onycho-cutaneous syndrome: a new form of junctional epidermolysis bullosa? In *Proceedings of the British Paediatric Association Conference* (Abstract G96), 1992: p. 69.

28 Anton-Lamprecht I, Schnyder UW. Epidermolysis bullosa dystrophica dominans—ein Defekt der anchoring fibrils? *Dermatologica* 1973; 147: 289–298.

29 Anton-Lamprecht I, Hashimoto I. Epidermolysis bullosa dystrophica dominans (Pasini)—a primary structural defect of the anchoring fibrils. *Hum. Genet.* 1976; 32: 69–76.

30 Bauer EA, Cooper TW, Tucker DR, Esterly NB. Phenytoin therapy of recessive dystrophic epidermo-ysis bullosa: clinical trial and proposed mechanism of action on collagenase. *N. Engl. J. Med.* 1980; 303: 776–781.

31 Gerhard DS, Jones C, Bauer EA *et al.* Human collagenase gene is localised to 11q (Abstract). *Cytogenet. Cell Genet.* 1987; 46: 619.

32 Hovnanian A, Duquesnoy P, Amselem S *et al.* Exclusion linkage between the collagenase gene and generalised recessive dystrophic epidermolysis bullosa phenotype. *J. Clin. Invest.* 1991; 88: 1716–1721.

33 Sakai, LY, Keene DR, Morris NP, Burgeson RE. Type VII collagen is a major structural component of anchoring fibrils. *J. Cell Biol.* 1986; 103: 1577–1586.

34 Leigh IM, Eady RAJ, Heagerty AHM *et al.* Type VII collagen is a normal component of epidermal basement membrane which shows altered expression in recessive dystrophic epidermolysis bullosa. *J. Invest. Dermatol.* 1988; 90: 639–642.

35 Ryynanen M, Knowlton RG, Parente MG *et al.* Human type VII collagen: genetic linkage of the gene (COL7A1) on chromosome 3 to dominant dystrophic epidermolysis bullosa. *Am. J. Hum. Genet.* 1991; 49: 797–803.

36 Uitto J, Pulkinen L, Christiano AM. Molecular basis of the dystrophic and junctional forms of epidermolysis bullosa: mutations in the Type VII collagen and kalinin (laminin 5) genes. *J. Invest. Dermatol.* 1994; 103: 39S–46S.

37 Burgeson RE. Type VII collagen, anchoring fibrils and epidermolysis bullosa. *J. Invest. Dermatol.* 1993; 101: 252–255.

38 McGrath JA, Ishida-Yamamoto A, O'Grady A *et al.* Structural variations in anchoring fibrils in dystrophic epidermolysis bullosa: correlation with type VII collagen expression. *J. Invest. Dermatol.* 1993; 100: 366–372.

39 Jenison M, Fine J-D, Gammon WR, O'Keefe EJ. Normal molecular weight of type VII collagen produced by recessive dystrophic epidermolysis bullosa keratinocytes. *J. Invest. Dermatol.* 1993; 100: 93–96.

40 Konig A, Winberg J-O, Gedde-Dahl T, Bruckner-Tuderman L. Heterogeneity of severe dystrophic epidermolysis bullosa: overexpression of collagen VII by cutaneous cells from a patient with mutilating disease. *J. Invest. Dermatol.* 1994; 102: 155–159.

41 Fine JD, Horiguchi Y, Stein DH *et al.* Intraepidermal type VII collagen: evidence for abnormal intracytoplasmic processing of a major basement membrane protein in rare patients with dominant and possibly recessive forms of dystrophic epidermolysis bullosa. *J. Am. Acad. Dermatol.* 1990; 22: 188–195.

42 Konig A, Raghunath M, Steinmann B *et al.* Intracellular accumulation of collagen VII in cultured keratinocytes from a patient with dominant dystrophic epidermolysis bullosa. *J. Invest. Dermatol.* 1994; 102: 105–110.

Other blistering disorders

The other inherited disorders in which blistering is a major feature are listed below.

Hailey–Hailey syndrome (MIM 169600)

Clinical features

Persistent rawness and blistering of the axillae,

neck and groins begin in early adult life, sometimes precipitated by bacterial infection.

Genetic aspects

This trait shows autosomal dominant inheritance. It has not yet been mapped.

Pathogenesis

There are clinical and histological similarities to Darier's disease, with less scaling. The intraepidermal blistering and acantholysis reflect loss of intercellular adhesion, which can be demonstrated in clinically normal skin as a reduction in the time taken for suction blisters to form [1].

Weary–Kindler syndrome (MIM 173650, 173700)

Acral blisters in infancy are followed by generalized poikiloderma and keratoses on the extremities. This disorder may be confused with Rothmund–Thomson syndrome and epidermolysis bullosa simplex with mottled pigmentation.

Macular bullous dystrophy (MIM 302000)

Clinical features

This is characterized by blistering, alopecia, nail dystrophy, dwarfism and mental retardation.

Genetics

It is inherited as an X-linked dominant trait, lethal early in life in males. It has been reported in just one Dutch family.

Reference

1   Burge SM, Millard PR, Wojnarowska F. Hailey–Hailey disease: a widespread abnormality of cell adhesion. *Br. J. Derm.* 1991; 124: 329–332.

3
THE DERMIS
AND ITS DISORDERS

The dermis is a complex structure with its own equally complex set of genetic disorders. Its main components fall into two groups. The first consists of insoluble fibres in the form of collagen which resists tensile forces, and elastic fibres, which return the skin to its normal state when stretching stops. The second is an amorphous ground substance, made up of soluble macro-molecules that bind large amounts of water and so help to resist compression: its important constituents are polysaccharides (glycosaminoglycans), which are linked to proteins forming proteoglycans.

For convenience this chapter will also cover some genetic disorders of dermal blood vessels and subcutaneous fat.

Connective tissue

Collagen

The characteristic feature of a collagen molecule is a triple-stranded rope-like helical domain made up of three intertwining polypeptide chains. These so-called α chains consist of repeating triplets of amino acids. Every third residue is glycine and the other two places are usually occupied by proline or glycine.

Currently, 14 types of collagen are recognized, of which only eight are known to be present in the skin. They differ in the structure of their α chains and in the degree to which these are interrupted by non-helical domains. At the ends of the chains are short non-helical domains where adjacent molecules are cross-linked to form fibres. It has been estimated that at least 25 genes code for the polypeptide components of the different collagens. The hydroxylation of proline and lysine residues, aldehyde formation for cross-linking, and glycosylation are other important steps.

In the dermis, types I and II collagen predominate with type V a minor constituent. Type IV collagen is present in basement membranes, and type VII collagen forms anchoring fibrils important in dermo-epidermal adhesion.

Not surprisingly, the complexity of the processes involved is matched by the large number of genetically determined collagen disorders. These include Ehlers–Danlos syndrome , Menkes syndrome (p. 67), focal dermal hypoplasia (p. 17), familial cutaneous collagenoma (p. 129), dystrophic epidermolysis bullosa (p. 84) and the nail–patella syndrome (p. 71)

Ehlers–Danlos syndrome (EDS)

Clinical features

The term EDS covers a heterogeneous group of inherited conditions that share some or all of the following features.
1 Variable degrees of hypermobility of the joints.
2 Variable degrees of hyperelasticity of the skin (Fig. 3.1).
3 Poor wound healing and atrophic scars.
4 Vascular fragility with easy bruising and haematoma formation. In children this may lead to a mistaken diagnosis of physical abuse. The rupture of aortic and cerebral aneurysms is a special risk in type IV.
5 Blue sclerae.

This complicated subject has earned its own scientific group, which continuously updates its classification and molecular biology [1]. Eleven types are currently recognized and their most important distinguishing features are listed in

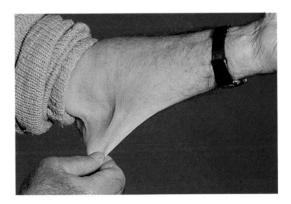

Fig. 3.1 Stretchy skin in Ehlers–Danlos syndrome.

Table 3.1. Some patients overlap these groups and cannot be classified easily.

Genetic aspects

The different modes of inheritance are listed in Table 3.1.

Pathogenesis

All types of EDS are likely to be based on mutations in genes important in the formation or modification of collagen and the extracellular matrix. The first to be identified was the lysyl hydroxylase deficiency found in some type VI patients [2]. The enzyme catalyses the formation of hydroxylysine in collagens. The gene has now been cloned and in affected individuals may show large areas of duplication [3].

In type IV EDS, mutations occur in the gene for type III collagen (*Col*3A1), lying on chromosome 2q31 [4]. At least 20 different mutations have been identified and interesting attempts are being made to correlate the position of the mutation with the clinical phenotype. Mutations at the 3′ end of the gene, for example, seem to lead to acrogeric features [5].

In type VII EDS, the polypeptide chains of type I collagen may have structural defects near the N-protease cleavage site, due to point mutations in either the α1 (1) or α2 (1) genes [6]. This seems to prevent cleavage by procollagen N protease. Other patients with dermatosparaxis (type VII C) may be deficient in the enzyme itself [7]. Decreased action of the copper-dependent enzyme lysyl oxidase is important in type IX EDS.

Prolidase (peptidase D) deficiency (MIM 170100)

Clinical features

In this very rare disorder the skin is fragile and multiple leg ulcers may appear at an early age, raising the differential diagnosis of haemolytic anaemia, Werner's disease and artefacts. Mental defect and a characteristic face (hypertelorism and saddle nose) complete the picture.

Table 3.1 Ehlers–Danlos syndrome

MIM*	Type	Associated features	Underlying biochemical defects
130000	I	Severe classical type: premature rupture of membranes, papyraceous scars; may rupture large vessels or bowel	Not known
130010	II	Similar to, but milder than, type I	Not known
130020	III	Major joint hypermobility—minor skin involvement	Not known
130050 225350	IV	Arterial type: skin particularly thin and translucent; bruises easily; risk of aortic aneurysms, rupture of large arteries, cerebral aneurysm	In type III collagen
305200	V	Like type II	Not known
225400	VI	Ocular type with keratoconus, eye haemorrhages and retinal detachment	Lysyl hydroxylase deficiency
225410	VII	Extreme joint hypermobility; congenital hip dislocation	Abnormal excision of amino-terminal propeptide from type 1 collagen
130080	VIII	Periodontitis	Not known
304150	IX	Occipital horns; related to Menkes disease	Copper-related decrease in lysyl oxidase activity
225310	X	Bruising; defective platelet aggregation	In fibronectin
147900	XI	Large-joint hypermobility	Not known

* First digit of MIM number indicates inheritance: 1 = autosomal dominant; 2 = autosomal recessive; 3 = X-linked.

Genetic aspects

Although classified by MIM number as an autosomal dominant, inheritance as an autosomal recessive has also been recorded [8]. The PEPD gene is located at 19 cen-q13.11 and comprises 15 exons and 14 introns, spanning more than 130 kb [9]. Several types of mutation are known [10,11].

Pathogenesis

Prolidase cleaves iminodipeptides with C-terminal proline or hydroxyproline and so plays an important part in the metabolism of collagen, which is rich in both proline and hydroxyproline. Prolidase deficiency can be detected in fibroblasts and red cells; however, the failure of attempts at enzyme replacement using matched red cells suggests that the enzyme exists within them in an inactivated form, which can be reversed by exposure to manganese ions [12].

Restrictive dermopathy (MIM 275210)

Clinical features

Babies born with this rare lethal disorder are severely growth retarded with generalized rigidity of the skin, causing joint contractures, and an abnormal facies with a small mouth and ectropion.

Genetic aspects

Most cases are sporadic, but reports of affected siblings suggest autosomal recessive inheritance.

Pathogenesis

Histologically there is hyperkeratosis and lack of rete ridges, with an abnormal arrangement of collagen bundles in the dermis. There may be abnormal integrin expression [13]. It seems likely that the dermal abnormality has a secondary effect on epidermopoiesis and that the other abnormalities result from the rigid skin [14]

Elastosis perforans (MIM 130100)

Clinical features (Fig. 3.2)

Small, red, scaly papules appear in serpiginous lines or rings, spreading outwards to leave atrophic areas of skin, usually on the neck.

Genetic aspects

Elastosis perforans is usually sporadic but appears occasionally in families as an autosomal dominant trait [15]. It is associated with certain inherited disorders of connective tissue (see below).

Pathogenesis

This condition is probably a manifestation of a collagen or elastin defect. Histologically there appears to be extrusion of elastic debris through an area of epidermal hyperplasia. It is seen in Ehlers–Danlos type IV (collagen III abnormality), Down's syndrome (which probably involves collagen VI genes) and pseudoxanthoma elasticum. Furthermore, it may be induced by D-penicillamine therapy [16], which is known to damage collagen cross-links.

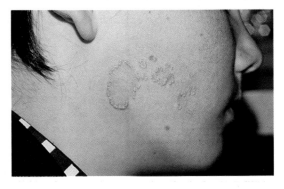

Fig. 3.2 Elastosis perforans serpiginosa.

Reactive perforating collagenosis (MIM 216700)

Clinical features

Keratinous umbilicated papules on the limbs may be precipitated by inflammation and cold, and resolve spontaneously in a few weeks.

Genetic aspects

This disorder is seen sporadically and in families [17]. Occurrence in siblings and in consanguineous families [18] suggests recessive inheritance.

Pathogenesis

Superficial collagen appears to be engulfed and extruded by focal epidermal hyperproliferation. This condition, like other transepithelial elimination disorders (perforating elastosis, Kyrle's disease and perforating folliculitis), may be seen in patients with diabetes and chronic renal failure. It is not clear whether this represents primarily a disorder of collagen, or of the overlying epidermis.

Elastic fibres

Electron microscopy shows that these have two components. Elastin molecules are aligned on a scaffolding of microfibrils made of fibrillin, a large glycoprotein the chains of which are linked together by disulphide bonds.

Elastin itself is a protein. The numerous complex lysine-derived cross-links between its polypeptide chains seem to contribute to its rubber-like qualities. A copper-dependent enzyme, lysyl oxidase, is important in the formation of desmosines. The elastin gene has been mapped to chromosome 7q11.2 Deletion of the elastin gene occurs in Williams syndrome, in which vascular and CNS changes are much more obvious than those in the skin [19].

Abnormalities of fibrillin are important in Marfan syndrome and elastin in pseudoxanthoma elasticum (p. 95), the Buschke–Ollendorf syndrome (p. 130) and in cutis laxa (p. 96).

Marfan syndrome (MS) (MIM 154700)

Clinical features

These fall into three main groups.
1 *Skeletal*—increased height with disproportionately long limbs and digits (arachnodactyly); joint laxity; chest and vertebral column deformities; high arched palate.
2 *Ocular*—subluxation of the lenses, myopia and retinal detachments.
3 *Cardiovascular*—dilatation of the aortic root and aortic regurgitation, mitral valve prolapse and regurgitation may lead to an early death.

In contrast, the skin changes are minor and inconstant. Wound healing may be poor; stretch marks may be severe; and there is an association with perforating elastoma.

Those with MS tend to die young, mainly from the complications of aortic root dilatation. Their mean age at death lies in the mid-30s [20].

Therapeutic strategies that can be used to reduce the high mortality and morbidity include regular cardiac and ophthalmological assessments and perhaps the administration of β-blockers from early childhood in an attempt to slow down aortic root dilatation. Prophylactic aortic root replacement may be worthwhile if annual echocardiograms show that significant dilatation is taking place.

Genetic aspects

MS is inherited as an autosomal dominant trait, with variable expression and almost complete penetrance. Its estimated prevalence is about 1 in 10 000 and about a quarter of affected cases arise as new mutations.

The gene for MS was first mapped by linkage analysis to chromosome 15 [21] and then more precisely to a locus between the markers D15S1 and D15S48 on its long arm [22], subsequently shown to be the locus for one of the genes responsible for fibrillin production [23]. Several gene defects coding for a shortened fibrillin molecule have now been described in MS [24] but most Marfan families seem to carry their own private mutations.

The fibrillin gene has now been analysed fully [25]. It is relatively large and highly fragmented, with 65 exons. It contains numerous cystein-rich sequences homologous to those found in epidermal growth factor. All of the five characterized missense mutations have occurred within these repeats [26].

In one affected family a prenatal diagnosis was made at 11 weeks using linkage analysis with fibrillin-specific markers [27].

Pathogenesis

Fibrillin was first identified in 1986 [28]. It is a large glycoprotein that is an important component of the elastin-containing microfibrils found in many tissues. In the context of MS, it is noteworthy that microfibrils in the suspensory ligament of the lens as well as in periosteum and in blood vessel walls contain fibrillin.

Soon after its discovery, the fibrillin component of the skin of Marfan sufferers was shown to be reduced [29,30], and Marfan fibroblasts were found to have defective fibrillin production [31]. One fibrillin gene was then mapped to chromosome 15q21.1 and linkage with MS was established [23].

The clinical features of MS fit well with what might be expected from a fibrillin defect. Interestingly, another gene important in fibrillin production has been mapped to chromosome 5 [32] and linked to congenital contractural arachnodactyly (MIM 121050) in which the loose-jointedness of MS is replaced by flexion contractures but which may also be associated with mitral valve and aortic abnormalities.

Pseudoxanthoma elasticum (PXE) (MIM 177850, 264800)

Clinical features (Fig. 3.3)

This rare condition affects an estimated 1 in 160 000 in the UK. Its first manifestations are usually in the skin, beginning in the teens. Plaques made up of small yellowish papules appear symmetrically, most often on the sides of the neck, in the armpits and groin and on the abdomen. The skin may be generally lax with a

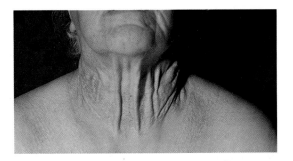

Fig. 3.3 Extensive pseudoxanthoma elasticum.

chicken-skin appearance. The eye changes include mottling of the retina, angioid streaks and, later on, retinal haemorrhages. The cardiovascular changes are similar to those of generalized arteriosclerosis but occur at an unusually early age.

Major and minor diagnostic criteria have now been defined [33], and a tentative classification has been proposed as follows [34].
Category I: classic manifestations including angioid streaks and skin changes.
Category II: those with limited evidence of PXE; for example, angioid streaks only.
However, with time, all patients tend to merge into a single classical phenotype involving the skin, eyes and cardiovascular system, but with considerable variation in expression [33]. Clearly this classification will have to be revised when gene markers for PXE are identified.

Genetic aspects

Although autosomal dominant inheritance may occur [35], most cases are inherited through an autosomal recessive mode [33]. No combination of clinical features can reliably distinguish between these forms of the disease.

Pathogenesis

The underlying pathology is that of fragmentation and calcification of elastic structures, with an accumulation of disorganized elastotic material [36]. Fibrillin, a glycoprotein in elastin-containing fibrils, contains several calcium-binding domains, and abnormalities in one of the several fibrillin genes may be important in PXE. Several patients with PXE have had perforating elastomas on affected skin. These are also found in Ehlers–Danlos syndrome type IV and some PXE patients have a reduction in collagen III (Pope FM, pers. comm., 1992).

The following candidate genes for PXE have been suggested [34]: an elastin gene on chromosome 7q11.2; three fibrillin genes (on chromosomes 15q15–21, 5q23.3–31.2 and 17q); and lysyl oxidase (on 5q23–31). In fact, mutations in several genes may explain the genetic heterogeneity of PXE [37]. In one family, linkage with the elastin gene was excluded [38].

Cutis laxa (MIM 123700, 219100)

Clinical features

Sagging skin folds sometimes beginning in infancy give the appearance of premature ageing (Fig. 3.4). Elastic recoil after stretching is poor and this differentiates the condition from the Ehlers–Danlos syndrome. The defects are not always confined to the skin. Associated herniae, diverticulae of gut and bladder, dislocations of the hips and pulmonary emphysema are most common in the autosomal recessive types. Cosmetic surgery may improve the facial appearance.

Genetic aspects

Autosomal dominant [39] and recessive [40] types exist. Internal manifestations may be more common in the recessive type.

Pathogenesis

Elastic fibres in the skin are sparse and fragmented. There are several possible reasons for this. In acquired cutis laxa, leucocyte elastases are responsible and, mirroring this, elevated serum elastase-like metalloproteinase activity has been found in one patient with the autosomal recessive type [41]. A marked reduction in elastin gene expression has been found in fibroblasts from patients with the recessive type [42].

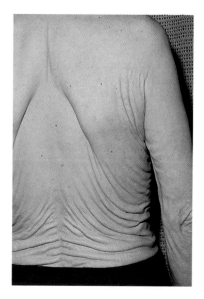

Fig. 3.4 Sagging skin in cutis laxa.

The ground substance

Glycosaminoglycans are polysaccharide chains made up of repeating disaccharide units consisting of a uronic acid and a hexosamine. The main ones in the dermis are hyaluronic acid and dermatan sulphate; heparan and chondroitin sulphates are also present in smaller quantities. Glycosaminoglycans make up only about 1% of the dry weight of the skin but are able to bind water up to 1000 times their own weight. Proteoglycans are formed when glycosaminoglycans become bound to a protein core.

The mucopolysaccharidoses, which characteristically show thickening of the skin, are genetic disorders in which glycosaminoglycans accumulate through inadequate degradation.

The mucopolysaccharidoses (MIM 252700–253230, 309900)

Clinical features

Many different types exist: all are rare and their combined prevalence in the population is no more than 1 in 20 000. Hypertrichosis, cuta-

Table 3.2 Other disorders of connective tissue

MIM*	Name
177350	Pseudoatrophoderma colli
218040	Costello syndrome
167100	Pachydermoperiostosis
173700	Hereditary sclerosing poikiloderma
181750	Familial scleroderma
184900	Stiff skin syndrome
260530	Parana hard skin syndrome
228020	Fascial dystrophy
185200	Familial striae
278250	Wrinkly skin
219300	Cutis verticis gyrata + mental retardation
304200	Cutis verticis gyrata + mental retardation and thyroid hypoplasia
221790	Dermatoleukodystrophy

* First digit of MIM number indicates inheritance: 1 = autosomal dominant; 2 = autosomal recessive; 3 = X-linked.

neous nodules or thickening, and a coarse facies are part of several of the syndromes. More important features include mental defect and cardiac involvement often leading to an early death.

Genetic aspects and pathogenesis

Each clinical syndrome is based on a defect in a different lysosomal enzyme involved in the breakdown of glycosaminoglycans, such as dermatan and heparan sulphate, which then accumulate in the tissues. Abnormalities in 11 such enzymes have so far been described, and the genes responsible for five of them have been mapped.

All are inherited as autosomal recessive traits except mucopolysaccharidosis type II (Hunter syndrome), which is an X-linked recessive condition due to a defect in the gene for iduronate sulphatase on chromosome Xq28 [43]. Other important conditions include Hurler syndrome (deficiency of α-L-iduronidase on chromosome 4p16.3 [44] and the Morquio syndrome type A (deficiency in galactosamine-6-sulphatase mapped to chromosome 16q24.3 [45]). A detailed description of these conditions is beyond the scope of this book, but for some, techniques are available for prenatal diagnosis. Bone marrow transplantation has had variable success.

Other familial disorders of connective tissue

Many more dermal abnormalities are familial: some of them are listed in Table 3.2.

References

1 Beighton P, de Paepe A, Danks D *et al*. International Nosology of Inherited Disorders of Connective Tissue. *Am. J. Med. Genet.* 1988; 29; 581–584.

2 Pinnell SR, Krane SM, Kenzora JE, Glimcher MJ. Heritable disorder with hydroxylysine-deficient collagen. *N. Engl. J. Med.* 1972; 286: 1013–1020.

3 Hautala T, Heikkinen J, Kivirikko KI, Myllyla R. A large duplication in the gene for lysyl hydroxylase accounts for the type VI variant of Ehlers–Danlos syndrome in two siblings. *Genomics* 1993; 15: 399–404.

4 Byers PH. Ehlers–Danlos syndrome: recent advances and current understanding of the clinical and genetic heterogeneity. *J. Invest. Dermatol.* 1994; 103: 47S–52S.

5 Pope FM, Narcisi P, Johnson P, Richards AJ. Molecular abnormalities of the Col 3A1 gene in vascular Ehlers–Danlos syndrome. *Br. J. Dermatol.* 1993; 129 (Suppl. 42): 43.

6 Pope FM, Nicholls AC, Palan A, Kwee ML, de Groot WP, Hausmann R. Clinical features of an affected father and daughter with Ehlers–Danlos syndrome type VIIB. *Br. J. Dermatol.* 1992; 126: 77–82.

7 Nusgens BV, Verellen-Dumoulin C, Hermanns LT *et al*. Evidence for a relationship between Ehlers–Danlos type VII C in humans and bovine dermatosparaxis. *Nat. Genet.* 1992; 1: 214–217.

8 Ogata A, Tanaka S, Tomoda T. Autosomal recessive prolidase deficiency. *Arch. Dermatol.* 1981; 117: 689–697.

9 Tanoue A, Endo F, Matsuda I. Structural organisation of the gene for human prolidase (peptidase D) and demonstration of a partial gene deletion in a patient with prolidase deficiency. *J. Biol. Chem.* 1990; 265: 11306–11311.

10 Boright AP, Scriver CR, Lancaster GA, Choy F. Prolidase deficiency: biochemical classification of alleles. *Am. J. Hum. Genet.* 1989; 44: 731–740.

11 Endo F, Matsuda I. Molecular basis of prolidase (peptidase D) deficiency. *Molec. Biol. Med.* 1991; 8: 117–127.

12 Hechtman P, Richter A, Corman N, Leong Y-M. *In situ* activation of human erythrocyte prolidase: potential for enzyme replacement therapy in prolidase deficiency. *Pediatr. Res.* 1988; 24: 709–712.

13 Dean JCS, Gray ES, Stewart KN *et al*. Restrictive dermopathy—a disorder of skin differentiation with

abnormal integrin expression. *Clin. Genet.* 1993; 44: 287–291.

14 Welsh KM, Smoller BR, Holbrook KA. Restrictive dermopathy: report of two affected siblings and a review of the literature. *Arch. Dermatol.* 1992; 128: 228–231.

15 Ayala F, Donofrio P. Elastosis perforans serpiginosa: report of a family. *Dermatologica* 1983; 166: 32–37.

16 Sahn EE, Maize JC, Garen PD *et al*. D-penicillamine-induced elastosis perforans serpiginosa in a child with juvenile rheumatoid arthritis. *J. Am. Acad. Dermatol.* 1989; 20: 979–988.

17 Nair BKH, Sarojini PA, Basheer AM, Nair CHK. Reactive perforating collagenosis. *Br. J. Dermatol.* 1974; 91: 399–403.

18 Kanan MW. Familial reactive perforating collagenosis and intolerance to cold. *Br. J. Dermatol.* 1974; 91: 405–414.

19 Christiano AM, Uitto J. Molecular pathology of the elastic fibres. *J. Invest. Dermatol.* 1994; 103: 53S–57S.

20 Marsalese DL, Moodie DS, Vacante M *et al*. Marfan syndrome: natural history and long-term follow-up of cardiovascular involvement. *JACC* 1989; 14: 422–428.

21 Kainulainen K, Pulkkinen L, Savolainen A, Kaitila I, Peltonen L. Localisation on chromosome 15 of the gene defect causing Marfan syndrome. *N. Engl. J. Med.* 1990; 323: 935–939.

22 Sarfarazi M, Tsipouras P, Del Mastro R *et al*. A linkage map of 10 loci flanking the Marfan syndrome locus on 15q: results of an international consortium study. *J. Med. Genet.* 1992; 29: 75–80.

23 Lee B, Godfrey M, Vitale E *et al*. Linkage of Marfan syndrome and a phenotypically related disorder to two different fibrillin genes. *Nature* 1991; 352: 330–334.

24 Godfrey M. From fluorescence to the gene: the skin in Marfan syndrome. *J. Invest. Dermatol.* 1994; 103: 58S–62S.

25 Pereira L, D'Alessio M, Ramirez F *et al*. Genomic organization of the sequence coding for fibrillin, the defective gene product in Marfan syndrome. *Hum. Molec. Genet.* 1993; 2: 961–968.

26 Dietz HC, Saraiva JM, Pyeritz RE, Cutting GR, Francomano CA. Clustering of fibrillin (FBNI) missense mutations in Marfan syndrome patients at cysteine residues in EGF-like domains. *Hum. Mutat.* 1992; 1: 366–374.

27 Godfrey M, Vandermark N, Wang M, Velinov M *et al*. Prenatal diagnosis and a donor splice mutation in fibrillin in a family with Marfan syndrome. *Am. J. Hum. Genet.* 1993; 53: 472–480.

28 Sakai L, Keene DR, Engvall E. Fibrillin, a new 350 KD glycoprotein is a component of extracellular microfibrils. *J. Cell Biol.* 1986; 103: 2499–2509.

29 Godfrey M, Olson S, Burgio R *et al*. Unilateral microfibrillar abnormalities in a case of asymmetric

Marfan syndrome. *Am. J. Hum. Genet.* 1990; 46: 661–671.

30 Hollister DW, Godfrey M, Sakai LY, Pyeritz RE. Immuno-histologic abnormalities of the microfibrillar-fiber system in the Marfan syndrome. *N. Engl. J. Med.* 1990; 323: 152–159.

31 McGookey DJ, Pyeritz RE, Byers PH. Marfan syndrome: altered synthesis, secretion or extracellular matrix incorporation of fibrillin. *Am. J. Hum. Genet.* 1990; 47: A67.

32 Tsipouras P, Del Mastro R, Sarfarazi M *et al*. Genetic linkage of the Marfan syndrome, ectopia lentis, and congenital contractural arachnodactyly to the fibrillin genes on chromosomes 15 and 5. *N. Engl. J. Med.* 1992; 326: 905–909.

33 Lebwohl M, Neldner K, Pope M *et al*. Classification of pseudoxanthoma elasticum: report of a consensus conference. *J. Am. Acad. Dermatol.* 1994; 30: 103–107.

34 Christiano AM, Lebworth MG, Boyd CD, Uitto J. Workshop on pseudoxanthoma elasticum: molecular biology and pathology of the elastic fibers. *J. Invest. Dermatol.* 1992; 99: 660–663.

35 Neldner KH. Pseudoxanthoma elasticum. *Clin. Dermatol.* 1988; 6: 1–159.

36 Neldner KH. Pseudoxanthoma elasticum. *Int. J. Dermatol.* 1988; 27: 98–100.

37 Pope FM. Historical evidence for the genetic heterogeneity of pseudoxanthoma elasticum. *Br. J. Dermatol.* 1975; 92: 493–509.

38 Raybould MC, Birley A, Moss C *et al*. Exclusion of an elastin gene mutation as the cause of pseudoxanthoma elasticum in a recessive family. *Clin. Genet.* 1994; 45: 48–51.

39 Damkier A, Brandrup F, Starklint H. Cutis laxa: autosomal dominant inheritance in five generations. *Clin. Genet.* 1991; 39: 321–329.

40 Goltz RW, Hult AM, Goldfarb M, Gorlin RJ. Cutix laxa, a manifestation of generalized elastolysis. *Arch. Dermatol.* 1965; 92: 373–387.

41 Anderson LL, Oikarinen, AI, Ryhanen L *et al*. Characterization and partial purification of a neutral protease from the serum of a patient with autosomal recessive pulmonary emphysema and cutis laxa. *J. Lab. Clin. Med.* 1985; 105: 537–546.

42 Olsen DR, Fazio MJ, Shamban AT, Rosenbloom J, Uitto J. Cutis laxa: reduced elastin gene expression in skin fibroblast cultures. *J. Biol. Chem.* 1988; 263: 6465–6467.

43 Wilson PJ, Suthers GK, Callen DF *et al*. Frequent deletions of Xq28 indicate genetic heterogeneity in Hunter syndrome. *Hum. Genet.* 1991; 86: 505–508.

44 Scott HS, Ashton LJ, Eyre HJ *et al*. Chromosomal localization of the human alpha-L-iduronidase gene to 4p16.3. *Am. J. Hum. Genet.* 1990; 47: 802–807.

45 Baker E, Guo XH, Orsborn AM *et al.* The Morquio syndrome gene maps to 16q24.3. *Am. J. Hum. Genet.* 1993; 52: 96–98.

Blood vessels

Hereditary haemorrhagic telangiectasia (MIM 187300)

Clinical features (Fig. 3.5)

This affects about 1 in 50 000 and must always be considered in cases of recurrent nasal or gut bleeding. The multiple small telangiectatic lesions, most obvious on the lips, tongue, face and hands, are surprisingly easy to overlook and indeed may not appear until the second or third decades. Internal angiodysplasias occur rarely in several organs such as the liver and brain. Best known are the pulmonary arteriovenous fistulae which are found in about 5% [1], causing a variable mixture of symptoms and signs including dyspnoea, cyanosis with secondary polycythaemia, high output cardiac failure and brain abscesses. Hereditary benign telangiectasia (MIM 187260) has similar skin lesions but lacks internal involvement.

Often no treatment is required. Recurrent nose bleeds may lead to chronic anaemia requiring iron therapy or transfusions. Minor nasal lesions can be treated by cautery or laser therapy. Skin grafts to the nasal septum may be needed in severe cases [2].

Genetic aspects

The condition is inherited as an autosomal dominant trait with variable expressivity. Penetrance for at least one manifestation of the condition is 97% [3]. In some, but not all affected families there is linkage to markers on the long arm of chromosome 9 [4,5] and the collagen V, α I gene has been mentioned as a possible candidate. Occasional associations with von Willebrand disease have been recorded but genetic linkage has not been found [1].

Angiokeratoma corporis diffusum (Anderson–Fabry disease) (MIM 301500)

Clinical features (Fig. 3.6)

The skin lesions of this rare disorder appear before puberty as punctate bluish or dark-red angiomas, often in groups on the umbilicus, scrotum and thighs. Some, but not all, have a keratotic surface. Similar skin lesions can be seen in other lysosomal disorders (e.g. α-L-fucosidase deficiency, type II fucosidosis and aspartylglycosaminuria), but a few patients with Anderson–Fabry disease have no skin lesions.

Internally, the main problems stem from involvement of the kidneys (progressive renal failure causing early death), eyes (corneal dystrophy and tortuosity of retinal vessels) and the autonomic nervous system (severe burning pains particularly of the limbs, bouts of high fever, and vasomotor instability).

Genetic aspects

This is an X-linked recessive condition with its most severe manifestations in males. The Fabry (*GLA*) gene has been localized to Xq22. It is about 12 kb long and has been cloned and characterized

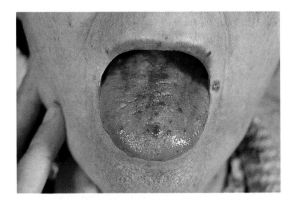

Fig. 3.5 Oral lesions of hereditary haemorrhagic telangiectasia.

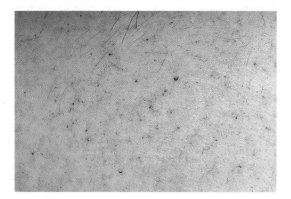

Fig. 3.6 Angiokeratomas in α-galactosidase deficiency (Fabry's disease).

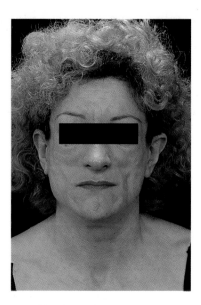

Fig. 3.7 Partial lipodystrophy (with a naevus sebaceous on the chin).

[6]. Several mutations based on different amino acid substitutions have been described [7].

Pathogenesis

The Anderson–Fabry (*GLE*) gene encodes the α-galactosidase A subunit. Alpha-galactosidase is a lysosomal enzyme that normally cleaves the terminal galactose from ceremide trihexoside as part of the breakdown of gangliosides. Defects lead to metabolic byproducts of glycosphingolipids being deposited in the lysosomes of vascular endothelium and also in other sites such as the cornea and glomeruli. These lipid inclusions are birefringent and show a characteristic lamellar structure on electron microscopy.

The diagnosis, therefore, can be made by detecting lipid inclusions in skin biopsies, or in cells found in urinary sediment. Decreased levels of plasma and leucocyte α-galactosidase are also present. Carrier females may show intermediate levels of the enzyme and may have corneal dystrophy demonstrable on slit-lamp microscopy. However, a rapid method is now available using the polymerase chain reaction to identify gene rearrangements in affected hemizygotes and to determine heterozygosity in at-risk females in affected families [8].

Renal transplants may be appropriate in the stage of chronic renal failure but do not, as had been hoped, reliably raise plasma α-galactosidase A activity [9].

References

1 Iannuzzi MC, Hidaka N, Boehnke M *et al.* Analysis of the relationship of Von Willebrand disease and hereditary haemorrhagic telangiectasia and identification of a potential type IIa vWD mutation (ile 865-to-thr). *Am. J. Hum. Genet.* 1991; 48: 757–763.
2 Ulso C, Vase P, Stoksted P. Long term results of dermatoplasty in the treatment of hereditary haemorrhagic telangiectasia. *J. Laryngol. Otol.* 1983; 97: 223–226.
3 Plauchu H, de Charevian JP, Bideau A, Robert J-M. Age-related clinical profile of hereditary haemorrhagic telangiectasia in an epidemiologically recruited population. *Am. J. Med. Genet.* 1989; 32: 291–297.
4 Macdonald MT, Papenberg KA, Glatfelter AA *et al.* A disease locus for hereditary haemorrhagic telangiectasia maps to chromosome 9q33–34. *Nature Genet.* 1994; 6: 197–204.
5 Shovlin CL, Hughes JM, Tuddenham EG *et al.* A gene for hereditary haemorrhagic telangiectasia maps to chromosome 9q3. *Nature Genet.* 1994; 6: 205–209.
6 Bishop DF, Kornreich R, Desnick RJ. Structural organisation of the human alpha-galactosidase A gene:

further evidence for the absence of a 3-prime untranslated region. *Proc. Nat. Acad. Sci. USA* 1988; 85; 3903–3907.

7 Yokoi T, Shinoda K, Ohno I *et al.* A 3-prime splice site consensus sequence mutation in the intron of the alpha-galactosidase A gene in a patient with Fabry's disease. *Jap. J. Hum. Genet.* 1991; 36: 245–250.
8 Kornreich R, Desnick RJ. Fabry disease: detection of gene rearrangements in the human alpha-galactosidase A gene by multiplex PCR amplification. *Hum. Mutat.* 1993; 2: 108–111.
9 Morgan SH, Crawfurd MD. Anderson–Fabry disease: a commonly missed diagnosis. *BMJ* 1988; 297: 872.

Fat

Lipodystrophies

A full description of the various clinical patterns and their suggested modes of inheritance is beyond the scope of this book. Loss of subcutaneous fat (Fig. 3.7) and diabetes are two consistent features in this group of disorders, which are summarized in Table 3.3.

Table 3.3 The inheritance of the lipodystrophies

MIM*	Name	Inheritance
269700	Total lipoatrophy and acromegaloid gigantism (Lawrence–Seip or Berardinelli syndrome)	Autosomal recessive
308980	Familial partial lipodystrophy	X-linked dominant with lethality in the hemizygous male conceptus
151600	Reverse partial lipodystrophy	Autosomal dominant
151680	Partial lipodystrophy with Rieger anomaly	Autosomal dominant

* First digit of MIM number indicates inheritance: 1 = autosomal dominant; 2 = autosomal recessive; 3 = X-linked.

4
CANCER AND
PREMATURE AGEING

Oncogenesis [1]

Perhaps 5–10% of common cancers occur in familial clusters due to genetic susceptibility [2]. This chapter deals with dermatological examples: but the subject cannot be understood without looking first at the genetic changes found within tumour cells.

Most cancers arise from a single cell, which has acquired a heritable growth advantage often after damage by a genotoxic agent such as a chemical carcinogen or irradiation. The accumulation within a cell of a complete set of the critical mutations that lead to cancer depends on a mixture of environmental and inherited factors [3]. Those who have already inherited one or more of these critical mutations through the germ line will be especially liable to develop cancer. In other words, some cancers arise from the interaction of germ cell and somatic mutations.

A clear-cut example of this is retinoblastoma. Inherited tumours occur earlier than sporadic ones and often affect both eyes. In affected families one critical mutation is inherited in the germ line but is by itself harmless. Nevertheless, only one more mutation (a second 'hit') is required for a tumour to form. The probability of two mutations affecting the same cell by chance is low and sporadic retinoblastomas are therefore rare and unilateral. The principle is clear enough but it is still not known how or when it applies to skin tumours.

Changes in three broad classes of gene may be involved in the transition from a normal cell into a malignant one: these are oncogenes, tumour-suppressor genes and DNA repair genes. Thereafter, for metastases to occur genes concerned in cell motility and adhesion or in the production of tissue metalloproteinases [4] are likely to be important.

Oncogenes

Some viruses can transform the cells they infect in such a way that tumours occur. Cellular genes (c-onc), homologous to the viral ones (v-onc) responsible for this, have been identified in the human genome and named after the viruses in which they were first found. Hence the H-*ras* oncogene is named after the rat sarcoma virus (Harvey strain) and the *myc* oncogene after the avian myelocytomatosis virus.

The name oncogene is unfortunate as it is now known that these are normal regulatory genes (proto-oncogenes), which become oncogenic only if abnormally activated. Perhaps less than 100 of the 50 000 human genes are potential oncogenes. Their normal roles include encoding growth factors or growth-factor receptors, mediating changes in intracellular metabolism in response to signals from cell-surface receptors (signal transducers) and binding to DNA and thereby controlling the transcription of genes. Proto-oncogenes can be activated by point mutations or chromosomal translocations leading to an abnormal protein product, or by amplification.

Tumour-suppressor genes

Hybrids between tumour and normal cells do not behave malignantly because the normal cells contain tumour-suppressor genes. Their usual function is to regulate growth: their loss or inactivation may be associated with the development of malignancy.

Loss of heterozygosity in a particular chromosomal region in tumour cells, as compared to normal cells, implies the presence in that region of one or more tumour-suppressor genes. A tumour-suppressor gene important in melanoma has been traced in this way to the short arm of chromosome 1.

Mutations in the p53 gene on chromosome 17 p13 are the commonest genetic alterations in human cancers [5]. It encodes a 53 kDa protein that regulates entry into the cell cycle. Wild-type (normal) p53 has a half life of less than 30 minutes and is not detectable by immunohistochemistry. However, mutant p53 protein accumulates and can be detected in the nuclei of some malignant melanomas but not of benign melanocytic naevi [6]. It can also be found in some squamous-cell carcinomas and keratoacanthomas [7], conforming to the general rule that there is no absolute association between any oncogene or tumour-suppressor gene and any one type of tumour. In addition, there is no consistent evidence that activation of any one oncogene correlates with either a good or a poor prognosis.

References

1 Poole S, Fenske NA. Cutaneous markers of internal malignancy I. Malignant involvement of the skin and genodermatoses. *J. Am. Acad. Dermatol.* 1993; 28(1): 1–13.
2 Ponder BAJ. Molecular genetics of cancer. *BMJ* 1992; 304: 1234–1236.
3 Yuspa SH, Dugosz AA, Cheng CK *et al.* Role of oncogenes and tumour suppressor genes in multistage carcinogenesis. *J. Invest. Dermatol.* 1994; 103: 90S–95S.
4 Waxman J, Wasan H. The architecture of cancer. *BMJ* 1992; 305: 1306–1307.
5 Bassett-Séguin N, Moies J-P, Mils V *et al.* TP53 tumour suppressor gene and skin carcinogenesis. *J. Invest. Dermatol.* 1994; 103: 102S–106S.
6 McGregor JM, Yu CC, Dublin EA *et al.* P53 immunoreactivity in human malignant melanoma and dysplastic naevi. *Br. J. Dermatol.* 1993; 128: 606–611.
7 McGregor JM, Yu CC, Dublin EA, Levison DA, MacDonald DM. Aberrant expression of p53 tumoursuppressor protein in non-melanoma skin cancer. *Br. J. Dermatol.* 1992; 127 : 463–469.

Tumour-prone skin disorders

Skin malignancy

Naevoid basal-cell carcinoma syndrome (NBCCS) (Gorlin syndrome) (MIM 109400)

Clinical features [1]

The syndrome is uncommon (minimum prevalence of 1 in 57 000) [2] but is seen more often in patients who have had a basal-cell carcinoma (1 in 200), and especially in those who develop one before the age of 15 (1 in 5) [3].

Basal-cell carcinomas occur in about 85% of those affected, usually appearing around the time of puberty as unimpressive, small, skin-coloured, shiny, domed papules looking rather like cellular naevi, hence the name naevoid (Fig. 4.1). The

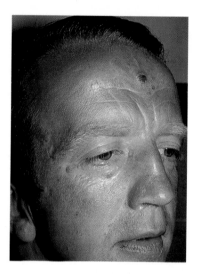

Fig. 4.1 Multiple basal-cell carcinomas in Gorlin syndrome.

numbers vary from one or two to over 100. Many remain static but some, particularly on the face, can become as invasive as the sporadic type of basal-cell carcinoma. For this reason, early treatment is needed but should not include radiotherapy as this encourages the formation of more tumours in the area.

Other skin manifestations include the appearance, usually during the second decade, of pits on the palms and soles of up to 75% of patients. These are shallow, 2–3 mm in diameter, with vertical sides and a reddish base. Dermal calcinosis and epidermoid cysts may also be seen.

Many other organs may be involved: the features are listed in Table 4.1. Jaw cysts are perhaps the best known.

Genetic aspects [4–6]

This is a fully penetrant, autosomal dominant trait with variable expressivity.

NBCCS has been mapped to 9q22.3–q31 by analysis of linkage to DNA polymorphisms, mostly multiallelic microsatellites, using polymerase chain amplification. The region is not yet well characterized and no obvious candidate gene has been reported within it. Genetic homogeneity is likely, as all kindreds studied from several countries have shown this linkage.

Table 4.1 Some features that may be associated with the naevoid basal-cell carcinoma syndrome

System	Clinical feature
Skin	Naevoid basal-cell carcinoma
	Palmar and plantar pits
	Epidermoid cysts
	Subcutaneous calcification
Skeleton	Characteristic facies with hypertelorism, frontal bossing and prognathism
	Bifid ribs
	Kyphoscoliosis
	Marfanoid habitus
	Pectus excavatum
	Short fourth metacarpals
Central nervous system	Mental retardation
	Agenesis of corpus callosum
	Hydrocephalus
	Calcification of falx cerebri
Tumours	Medulloblastoma
	Fibrosarcoma of jaw
	Ovarian fibroma
Reproductive	Male hypogonadism
	Bicornuate uterus

Pathogenesis

The NBCCS gene seems likely to function normally as a tumour suppressor, controlling cell growth and active in all three embryonic germ layers. It is of interest that allelic loss from several loci on chromosome 9 can be demonstrated in tissue from sporadically occurring basal-cell carcinomas [7].

In Gorlin syndrome, cells containing a mutant gene need a further stimulus to form a naevoid basal-cell carcinoma, and perhaps another one for this to become invasive. Examples of such stimuli include radiotherapy, which can cause multiple skin tumours to appear locally a few months after the treatment of a medulloblastoma, and sunlight, leading to the excess of tumours in exposed areas.

Multiple self-healing squamous epitheliomas (Ferguson–Smith) (MIM 132800)

Clinical features

This is rare and not to be confused with familial multiple keratoacanthomas (MIM 148390). Lesions usually begin to appear in the late teens or 20s and most are on the face where sun exposure is a predisposing factor. Each skin lesion goes through a characteristic sequence. Minute reddish papules, some with a horny plug, enlarge over a few weeks and then ulcerate. Later, the ulcers heal but leave pitted scars with irregular overhanging edges, which can be ugly if numerous.

Genetic aspects

Inheritance is as an autosomal dominant trait and the tendency to investigate it must be familial too. The condition was first described by J. Ferguson-Smith, a dermatologist, in 1934 [8]. Gene mapping was achieved by his son, M.A. Ferguson-Smith, in 1993 [9]. Most of the known families originated in western Scotland and the responsible mutation is thought to have occurred before 1790 [10].

Linkage to the ABO blood group attracted attention to chromosome 9, and 18 affected families were investigated using polymorphic DNA markers [9]. The gene proved to be tightly linked to the marker D9S53 (9q31). The gene predisposing to Gorlin syndrome lies in this region too, raising the possibility that these two clinically distinct conditions may be due to different mutations on the same gene.

Pathogenesis

The interest here lies in the spontaneous resolution of lesions, which histologically are squamous carcinomas. Further information about the precise nature of the genetic defect may well help our understanding both of the development and of the control of malignancy. A hint that immunological mechanisms may be involved comes from the lymphocytic infiltration of the tumours.

Follicular atrophoderma and basal-cell carcinomas (Basex syndrome) (MIM 109520)

Clinical features

This is unrelated to NBCCS but shares with it a

tendency for multiple naevoid basal-cell carcinomas to appear in early adult life. The characteristic pitted appearance of the skin on the backs of
the hands, elbow points and face, is due to the
presence of exaggerated follicular funnels [11].
Scalp hairs are sparse and may show marked
twisting and flattening [12]. Associated hypohidrosis may be generalized or confined to the
head and neck.

Genetic aspects

Male to male transmission has never been
recorded and in one study all daughters of an
affected male were also affected [11]. This has
raised the possibility of an X-linked dominant
mode of inheritance but too few pedigrees have
been published for this to be firmly established
and autosomal dominant inheritance remains
possible.

Porokeratosis

Little is known about the genetics of this group of
conditions all of which show atrophic areas sur-
rounded by a keratotic rim. The Mibelli (MIM
175800), palmoplantar (MIM 175850, 175860)
and disseminated superficial actinic (MIM 175900)
types may occur sporadically or be inherited as an
autosomal dominant trait. Underlying clonal chromosomal abnormalities have been found, mainly
of chromosome 3 [13]. This chromosomal instability may be a factor in the known tendency to
develop squamous-cell carcinoma. A linear pattern
might be due to a somatic mutation affecting a
porokeratosis locus [14].

**Dysplastic naevus syndrome and hereditary
cutaneous malignant melanoma
(MIM 155600)**

Clinical features (Fig. 4.2)

Dysplastic naevi tend to be numerous, larger than
5 mm in diameter with indistinct, irregular or
notched borders and variable pigmentation. Some
are pink. However, many naevi that are clinically

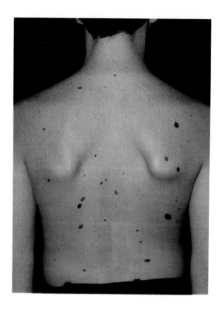

Fig. 4.2 Atypical naevi in the dysplastic naevus
syndrome.

atypical do not have the histology of a true dysplastic naevus. The presence of dysplastic naevi
signals an increased risk of a malignant
melanoma developing, especially if there is a personal or family history of previous melanomas. In
one study of 23 melanoma-prone families [15],
the risk of members with dysplastic naevi developing a melanoma was 85 times higher than
normal, but there was no excess of cancer other
than melanoma. In another study, dysplastic
naevi were found in 10.5% of patients with single
melanomas and 47.8% of those with multiple
melanomas [16]. In contrast, some melanoma-
prone families have no dysplastic naevi [17].

Patients with dysplastic naevi should avoid
excessive sun exposure, and those with a personal or family history of malignant melanomas
should be under regular surveillance by a
dermatologist.

Genetic aspects

Dysplastic naevi may occur sporadically or run
in families as an autosomal dominant trait,
with incomplete penetrance, affecting several
generations.

Evidence of linkage with the rhesus blood group on chromosome 1p [18] was later followed up by linkage analysis using 26 polymorphic markers on 1p in six families with a predisposition to melanomas. A gene for susceptibility to melanoma was mapped to chromosome 1p36 [19]. Loss of heterozygosity at loci on distal 1p has been found in DNA samples from melanomas and their metastases, but occurs as a late event and is also seen in other tumours of neuro-ectodermal origin [20]. However, the 1p locus is important only in a subset of melanoma families [21], as linkage to it has been excluded in several other studies, from Holland, Utah and Australia, of families prone to melanoma, both with and without dysplastic naevi [22,23,24].

Other melanoma tumour-suppressor genes lie elsewhere. One may exist on chromosome 6q [25], but attention has now shifted to the short arm of chromosome 9 where loss of heterozygosity is regularly found in melanoma cell lines [26]. Another pointer to this area came from studies of a woman with an unbalanced translocation involving the short arm of chromosome 9 who developed multiple melanomas [27]; and several large melanoma-prone families show linkage to a locus on chromosome 9p13–p22 [28,29].

Systemic malignancy

Gardner syndrome (GS) (MIM 175100)

Clinical features

GS is familial polyposis of the colon with additional extra-intestinal features including the following.
1 Multiple epidermoid or sebaceous cysts.
2 Fibrous tissue (desmoid) tumours, occurring spontaneously or at incision sites; for example, after colectomy.
3 Fifty percent of affected individuals develop multiple osteomas, most often of the maxilla or mandible.
4 Areas of congenital hypertrophy of the retinal pigment epithelium (CHRPE's) can be a valuable clue to the diagnosis long before other features

develop. Bilateral and multiple lesions are a good clinical marker for GS.

GS is present in between 1 in 8000 and 1 in 16 000 births [30]. Its importance lies in the risk of the colonic polyps becoming malignant. They arise during the second decade but malignant change may be delayed until 10–20 years later.

Proctosigmoidoscopy will not detect proximal lesions and some recommend air-contrast barium enemas every 2 years. Colonic ultrasonography after the retrograde instillation of fluid into the colon is another possibility [31]. Early prophylactic colectomy may be reasonable in those with many polyps.

Genetic aspects

GS is inherited as an autosomal dominant trait with high penetrance and variable expressivity. In 1986, a patient was described with a presumed contiguous gene syndrome including polyposis coli, severe mental retardation and a number of congenital abnormalities [32]. The presence of an interstitial deletion on chromosome 5q led to a search for linkage with RFLP (see Glossary) markers there [33] and the gene was later mapped to 5q22 [34].

GS and familial polyposis of the colon without extra-intestinal manifestations are thought to be allelic [33]. The gene for adenomatous polyposis of the colon has now been characterized and several different mutations identified [35,36]. The mouse multiple intestinal neoplasia gene may be a useful animal model for further studies. It has been mapped to mouse chromosome 18, which shares extensive homologies with human chromosome 5.

Linkage studies using DNA probes allow a presymptomatic diagnosis to be made with a high degree of probability [37]. An integrated risk analysis can be based on a combination of colonic, ophthalmic, genotypic and perhaps radiographic studies [38].

Pathogenesis

This is not fully understood. The gene encodes an

unusually large protein and is expressed in many tissues [39]. Studies of skin fibroblasts show an increased susceptibility to retrovirus transformation [40] and it has also been suggested that the gene may be important in the programmed senescence of normal human fibroblasts [41].

The colonic polyps are multiclonal [42] and loss of heterozygosity for markers on chromosome 5 is a frequent finding in sporadic colonic cancers [43].

Peutz–Jeghers syndrome (MIM 175200)

Clinical features

The two classical features are pigmented macules (Fig. 4.3) and multiple hamartomatous intestinal polyps.

Characteristic pigmented macules are found on the buccal mucosa and lips and often on the hands and feet also. Usually present in early childhood, the pigmentation may fade with age.

Intestinal polyps are most common in the upper small bowel but may also affect the stomach and colon. Malignant change is unusual but symptoms can arise from bleeding, obstruction, or intussusception. Large lesions causing symptoms

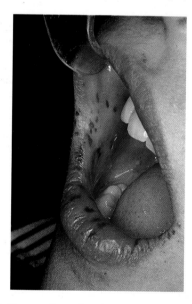

Fig. 4.3 Pigmented macules in the Peutz–Jeghers syndrome.

may have to be removed but repeated surgery can lead to problems with adhesions and the short-bowel syndrome [44]. A combined endoscopic and surgical approach can obtain a clear small bowel without resection [45]. Some doctors recommend regular screening by colonoscopy and gastroscopy every 2 years as an alternative to radiology [46,47]. Affected individuals are prone to malignancies of other organs, especially the ovaries and breasts.

Genetic aspects

This is an autosomal dominant trait with high penetrance and variable expressivity. No family history is known in about half of the cases. The gene has not yet been mapped.

Pathogenesis

This is not understood but skin fibroblasts from affected individuals are especially liable to malignant transformation by the murine sarcoma virus [46].

Multiple hamartoma syndrome (Cowden syndrome) (MIM 158350)

Clinical features

The presence of multiple facial tricholemmomas, extensive verrucous fibromas on the lips and inside the mouth, and warty acral keratoses, offers an early warning that tumours of other organs may occur later. Approximately 40–50% of affected females eventually develop carcinoma of the breast and some authorities recommend prophylactic bilateral total mastectomy by the third decade [48]. Thyroid adenomas and carcinomas, and hamartomata of many other organs may also be found [49].

Genetic aspects

This is an autosomal dominant trait with high penetrance. The gene itself has not yet been mapped [50].

Pathogenesis

This is not understood and raised levels of epidermal growth factor have not been found in body fluids [50]. Three of the most important genes currently being studied in relation to breast cancer were found to exist in an unamplified and unrearranged state in one patient with Cowden syndrome [48].

Muir–Torre syndrome (MIM 158320)

Clinical features

The association here is between sebaceous-gland tumours, usually adenomas, and visceral carcinomas. These are sometimes multiple but often have only a low degree of malignancy and most commonly are of the colon. Keratoacanthomas may be another feature of the syndrome. Some feel that even one sebaceous neoplasm should prompt a search for an internal tumour [51].

Genetic aspects

Inheritance is as an autosomal dominant trait [52]. The relationship with the cancer-family syndrome is not clear [53].

References

1 Evans DGR, Ladusans EJ, Rimmer S *et al.* Complications of the naevoid basal cell carcinoma syndrome: results of a population based study. *J. Med. Genet.* 1993; 30: 460–464.

2 Evans DGR, Farndon PA, Burnell LD, Rao GH, Birch JM. The incidence of Gorlin syndrome in 173 consecutive cases of medulloblastoma. *Br. J. Cancer* 1991; 64: 959–961.

3 Springate JE. The naevoid basal cell carcinoma syndrome. *J. Pediatr. Surg.* 1986; 21: 908–910.

4 Farndon PA, Del Mastro RG, Evans DGR, Kilpatrick MW. Location of gene for Gorlin syndrome. *Lancet* 1992; 339: 581–582.

5 Bale AT, Gailani MR, Leffel DJ *et al.* Naevoid basal cell carcinoma syndrome. *J. Invest Dermatol.* 1994; 103: 126S–130S.

6 Reis A, Kuster W, Linss G, Gebel E *et al.* Localisation of gene for the naevoid basal-cell carcinoma syndrome. *Lancet* 1992; 339: 617.

7 Gailani M, Leffell DJ, Bale AE. Evidence for a tumour suppressor gene on chromosome 9 in basal cell carcinoma of the skin. *Am. J. Hum. Genet.* 1991; 49 (Suppl): 454.

8 Ferguson-Smith J. A case of multiple primary squamous-celled carcinomata of the skin in a young man with spontaneous healing. *Br. J. Dermatol.* 1934; 46: 267–272.

9 Goudie DR, Yuille MAR, Leversha MA *et al.* Multiple self-healing squamous epitheliomata (ESSI) mapped to chromosome 9q22–q31 in families with common ancestry. *Nat. Genet.* 1993; 3: 165–169.

10 Ferguson-Smith MA, Wallace DC, James ZH, Renwick JH. Multiple self-healing squamous epithelioma. *Birth Defects* 1971; VII: 157–163.

11 Viksnins P, Berlin A. Follicular atrophoderma and basal cell carcinomas. *Arch. Dermatol.* 1977; 113: 948–951.

12 Gould DJ, Barker DJ. Follicular atrophoderma with multiple basal cell carcinomas (Basex). *Br. J. Dermatol.* 1978; 99: 431–435.

13 Scappatici S, Lambiase S, Orecchia G, Fraccaro M. Clonal chromosomal abnormalities with preferential involvement of chromosome 3 in patients with porokeratosis of Mibelli. *Cancer Genet. Cytogenet.* 1989; 43: 89–94.

14 Happle R. Somatic recombination may explain linear porokeratosis associated with disseminated superficial actinic porokeratosis. *Am. J. Med. Genet.* 1991; 39: 237.

15 Tucker MA, Fraser MC, Goldstein AM, Elder DE, Guerry D. Risk of melanoma and other cancers in melanoma-prone families. *J. Invest. Dermatol.* 1993; 100: 350S–355S.

16 Sigg C, Pelloni F, Schnyder UW. Increased incidence of multiple melanoma in sporadic and dysplastic nevus cell syndrome. *Hautarzt* 1989; 40: 548–552.

17 Kefford RF, Salmon J, Shaw MH, Donald JA, McCarthy WH. Hereditary melanoma in Australia: variable association with dysplastic naevi and absence of genetic linkage to chromosome 1p. *Cancer Genet. Cytogenet.* 1991; 51: 45–55.

18 Greene MH, Goldin LR, Clark WG *et al.* Familial cutaneous malignant melanoma: autosomal dominant trait possibly linked to the Rh locus. *Proc. Natl. Acad. Sci. USA* 1983; 80: 6071–6075.

19 Bale SJ, Dracopoli NC, Tucker MA *et al.* Mapping the gene for hereditary cutaneous malignant melanoma-dysplastic nevus to chromosome 1p. *N. Engl. J. Med.* 1989; 320: 1367–1372.

20 Dracopoli NC, Harnett P, Bale SJ *et al.* Loss of alleles from the distal short arm of chromosome 1 occurs late in melanoma tumor progression. *Proc. Natl. Acad. Sci. USA* 1989; 86: 4614–4618.

21 Goldstein AM, Dracopoli NC, Ho EC *et al.* Further evidence for a locus for cutaneous malignant melanoma-dysplastic naevus (CMM/DN) on chromosome 1p and

evidence for genetic heterogeneity. *Am. J. Hum. Genet.* 1993; 52: 537–550.

22 Cannon-Albrecht LA, Goldgar DE, Meyer LJ *et al.* Evidence against the reported linkage of the cutaneous melanoma–dysplastic nevus syndrome locus to chromosome 1p36. *Am. J. Hum. Genet.* 1990; 46: 912–918.

23 Meyer LJ, Zone JH. Genetics of cutaneous melanoma. *J. Invest. Dermatol.* 1994; 103: 112S–116S.

24 Nancarrow DJ, Palmer JM, Walters MK *et al.* Exclusion of the familial melanoma locus (M.L.M.) from the PND/D1S47 and MYCLI regions of chromosome arm 1p in 7 Australian pedigrees. *Genomics* 1992; 12: 18–25.

25 Copeman MC. The putative melanoma tumour-suppressor gene on human chromosome 6q. *Pathology* 1992; 24: 307–309.

26 Fountain JW, Karayiorgov M, Ernstoff MS, Kirkwood JM, Vlock DR. Homozygous deletions within human chromosome band 9p21 in melanoma. *Proc. Natl. Acad. Sci. USA* 1992; 89: 10557–10561.

27 Petty EM, Gibson LH, Fountain JW *et al.* Molecular definition of a chromosome 9p21 gene-line deletion in a woman with multiple melanomas and a plexiform neurofibroma: implications of 9p tumour suppressor gene. *Am. J. Hum. Genet.* 1993; 53: 96–104.

28 Cannon-Albrecht LA, Goldgar DE, Mayer LJ, Lewis CM, Bale AE. Assignment of a locus for familial melanoma, MLM, to chromosome 9p13–p22. *Science* 1992; 258: 1148–1152.

29 Battistutta D, Palmer J, Walters M *et al.* Incidence of familial melanoma and MLM 2 gene. *Lancet* 1994; 344: 1607–1608.

30 Sanchez MA, Zali MR, Khalil AA *et al.* Be aware of Gardner's syndrome: a review of the literature. *Am. J. Gastroenterol.* 1979; 71: 68–73.

31 Underwood MJ, Johnson VW. Familial colorectal cancer: discussion paper. *J. Roy. Soc. Med.* 1992; 85: 339–341.

32 Herrera L, Kakati S, Gibas L *et al.* Brief clinical report: Gardner syndrome in a man with an interstitial deletion of 5q. *Am. J. Med. Genet.* 1986; 25: 473–476.

33 Bodmer WF, Bailey CJ, Bodmer J *et al.* Localization of the gene for familial adenomatous polyposis on chromosome 5. *Nature* 1987; 328: 614–616.

34 Meera Khan P, Tops CM, Broek MVD *et al.* Close linkage of a highly polymorphic marker (D5S37) to familial adenomatous polyposis (FAP) and confirmation of FAP localization on chromosome 5q21–q22. *Hum. Genet.* 1988; 79: 183–185.

35 Groden J, Thliveris A, Samowitz W *et al.* Identification and characteristics of the familial adenomatous polyposis coli gene. *Cell* 1991; 66: 589–600.

36 Nishisho I, Nakamura Y, Miyoshi Y *et al.* Mutations of chromosome 5q21 genes in FAP and colorectal cancer patients. *Science* 1991; 253: 665–669.

37 Tops CM, Wijnen JT, Griffioen G *et al.* Presymptomatic diagnosis of familial adenomatous polyposis by bridging DNA markers. *Lancet* 1989; ii: 1361–1363.

38 Dunlop MG, Wylie AA, Steel CM, Piris J, Evans HJ. Linked DNA markers for presymptomatic diagnosis of familial adenomatous polyposis. *Lancet* 1991; 337: 313–316.

39 Kinzler KW. Personal communication quoted in *Mendelian Inheritance in Man*, vol. 1. (McKusick). Baltimore: John's Hopkins Press, 1992: 898.

40 Rasheed S, Rhim JS, Gardner EJ. Inherited susceptibility to retrovirus-induced transformation of Gardner syndrome cells. *Am. J. Hum. Genet.* 1983; 35: 919–931.

41 Chen S, Kazim D, Kraveka J, Pollack RE. Skin fibroblasts from individuals hemizygous for the familial adenopolyposis susceptibility gene show delayed crisis *in vitro*. *Proc. Natl. Acad. Sci. USA* 1989; 86: 2008–2012.

42 Hsui SH, Luk GD, Krush AJ, Hamilton SR, Hoover HH. Multiclonal origin of polyps in Gardner syndrome. *Science* 1983; 221: 951–953.

43 Ashton-Richardt PG, Dunlop ME, Makamura Y *et al.* High frequency of APC loss in sporadic colorectal carcinoma due to breaks clustered in 5q21–22. *Oncogene* 1989; 4: 1169–1174.

44 Mathus-Vliegen EMH, Tytgat GNJ. Peutz–Jeghers syndrome: Clinical presentation and new therapeutic strategy. *Endoscopy* 1985; 17: 102–104.

45 Eugene C, Tennenbaum R, Fingerhut A, Etienne JC. Treatment of tumours of the small intestine in Peutz–Jeghers syndrome: value of a combined endoscopic and surgical approach. *Gastroenterol. Clin. Biolog.* 1992; 16: 604–607.

46 Miyaki M, Akamatsu N, Rokutanda M *et al.* Increased sensitivity of fibroblasts of skin from patients with adenomatosis coli and Peutz–Jeghers syndrome to transformation by murine sarcoma virus. *Gann No Rinsho* 1980; 71: 797–803.

47 Williams CB, Goldblatt M, Delaney PV. 'Top and tail' endoscopy and follow-up in Peutz–Jeghers syndrome. *Endoscopy* 1982; 14: 82–84.

48 Williard W, Borgen P, Bol R, Tiwari R, Osborne M. Cowden's disease: a case report with analyses at the molecular level. *Cancer* 1992; 69: 2969–2974.

49 Starink TM, Van der Veen JPW, Awert F *et al.* The Cowden syndrome: a clinical and genetic study in 21 patients. *Clin. Genet.* 1986; 29: 222–233.

50 Carlson HE, Burns TW, Davenport SL *et al.* Cowden disease: gene marker studies and measurements of epidermal growth factor. *Am. J. Hum. Genet.* 1986; 38: 908–917.

48 Williard W, Borgen P, Bol R, Tiwari R, Osborne M. Cowden's disease: a case report with analyses at the molecular level. *Cancer* 1992; 69: 2969–2974.

51 Rothenburg J, Lambert WC, Vail JT, Nemlick AS, Schwartz RA. The Muir–Torre syndrome: the

significance of a solitary sebaceous tumour. *J. Am. Acad. Dermatol.* 1990; 23: 638–640.

52   Reiffers J, Laugier P, Hunziker N. Hyperplasies sebacées, keratoacanthomes, epitheliomas du visage et cancer du colon: une nouvelle entité? *Dermatologica* 1976; 153: 23–33.

53   Lynch HT, Fusaro RM, Roberts L, Voorhees G, Lynch JF. Muir–Torre syndrome in several members of a family with a variant of the cancer family syndrome. *Br. J. Dermatol.* 1985; 113: 295–301.

DNA repair and chromosome breakage disorders

Xeroderma pigmentosum (XP) (MIM 194400, 278700, 133510, 278720, 278730, 278740, 278760, 278780, 278750, 278800)

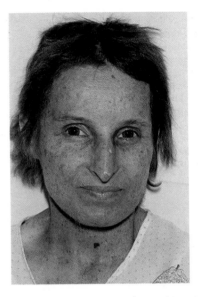

Fig. 4.4 Early photo-ageing in xeroderma pigmentosum.

Clinical features

XP is rare, affecting perhaps 5 per million in Europe and the USA, but rather more common in Japan. The many MIM numbers indicate its genetic heterogeneity but the following general description covers most of the shared clinical features.

The skin appears normal at birth but sun sensitivity becomes obvious within the first year or two. The changes seen on exposed skin at this early stage include dryness, atrophy, freckling, mottling and telangiectasia, but not elastosis. With this exception they are like those seen in elderly people with fair skins after many years of excessive sun exposure (Fig. 4.4).

Cutaneous malignancies soon occur against this background of damaged skin as excessive numbers of actinic keratoses, keratoacanthomas, squamous- and basal-cell carcinomas and malignant melanomas. These tumours show a significantly higher mutation frequency of the *ras* genes (50%) than do control tumours (22%) [1]. The same features affecting the eyes lead to photophobia, conjunctival inflammation and pigmentation, loss of eyelids and corneal clouding, sometimes resulting in blindness.

The disease advances unpredictably but life expectancy is much reduced. Many die before the age of 20; some as a consequence of their malig-

nancies but others from the severe neurological changes that together with XP make up the De Sanctis–Cacchione syndrome (MIM 278800) [2]. These are found most often in complementation group D (see below) and include progressive mental retardation, spasticity, sensorineural deafness, areflexia and ataxia.

Genetic aspects

XP is usually inherited as an autosomal recessive trait: most heterozygotes are normal but some show increased freckling. Genetic heterogeneity has been demonstrated by the cell fusion studies which are dealt with in the section on pathogenesis. XP has been subdivided on this basis into several complementation groups (A–H).

Pathogenesis

Ultraviolet (UV) light damages DNA by producing covalent linkages between adjacent pyrimidines. These distort the double helix and inhibit gene expression. In 1968, Cleaver showed that cells from XP patients lack the ability of normal cells to repair this damage [3]. All XP cells share this feature, which has been made the basis for prenatal diagnosis using amniotic fluid cells [4].

However, DNA repair is a complex process, using a large family of genes that encode a variety of interacting gene products. These coordinate, locate and prepare damaged sites for excision and replacement [5]. It is no surprise, therefore, that several genetic defects can lead to a similar clinical picture. Other abnormalities, including immunological ones, are needed to explain why XP patients develop skin malignancies while others with similar DNA repair defects, e.g. with trichothiodystrophy, do not [6].

XP has been divided into several complementation groups (Table 4.2) by studying the behaviour of cells obtained by fusing those from two different patients. The principle is simple enough. If the DNA repair defect is the same in both patients the fused cells will still show it: if the defect is different, then each cell will supply what the other lacks (i.e. complement it) and the fused cells will repair DNA normally.

The groups listed in Table 4.2 are still subject to debate and show much clinical heterogeneity within themselves. When 61 German XP cases were studied, three belonged to group A, 26 to group C, 16 to group D, three to group E and two to group F: 11 were of the XP variant type [7]. In contrast, 30 of 74 XP patients in Japan belonged to group A [8].

Some patients clinically indistinguishable from XP have normal DNA repair rates—sometimes this is referred to as the variant type of XP, or pigmentary xerodermoid (MIM 278750). Their cells are little more sensitive than normal to the cytotoxic effects of UV radiation but are more sensitive to its mutagenic effects [9] and replicate their DNA after UV irradiation in abnormally short fragments.

Complementation group A has been studied in most depth. The mouse DNA repair gene that complements the defect of group A has been cloned, and the human *XPAC* gene has been located to chromosome 9q34.1 by *in situ* hybridization [10]. The gene encodes a protein of 273 amino acids with a zinc-finger motif suggesting that it binds directly to DNA. Three mutations have been identified within the zinc-finger consensus sequence (nucleotides 313–387), which may be responsible for the loss of repair activity of the *XPAC* protein [11]: this may explain the clinical heterogeneity even within group A. In addition, another gene that partially complements group A has now been mapped to human chromosome 8 [12].

Most Japanese patients with XP group A are homozygous for the G to C transition mutation of the *XPAC* gene at the 3′ splice acceptor site of intron 3. This change can be detected by a combination of the polymerase chain reaction and AlwN1 restriction length polymorphism [13]. This technique has been used to confirm that a patient's parents were heterozygous for this mutation, and is likely to take over from the slower complementation tests, which cannot detect carriers. It may also become useful in prenatal diagnosis.

Complementation of the defect in group C has been achieved by the transfer of human chromosome 5, confirming the presence of a DNA repair

Table 4.2 Xeroderma pigmentosum complementation groups

Group (MIM*)	Mapping	Comment
A (278700)	9q34.1. Also gene on chromosome 8	Most common type in Japan
B (133510)	2q21 (*ERCC*-3 gene)	Rare. Association with Cockayne syndrome
C (278720)	Chromosome 5	Especially prone to develop melanomas
D (278730)	19q 13.2–13.3 (*ERCC*-2 gene)	Neurological abnormalities common
		May be linked to trichothiodystrophy
E (278740)	—	Mild type
F (278760)	?Chromosome 15	Mild type
G (278780)	—	Mild, rare
H	—	Associated with Cockayne syndrome

* First digit of MIM number indicates inheritance: 1 = autosomal dominant; 2 = autosomal recessive; 3 = X-linked.

gene there [14], and a DNA repair gene *(ERCC-2 on chromosome 19q13.2–13.3)* corrects the defective nucleotide excision repair in XP complementation group D cells [15]. Another DNA repair gene *(ERCC-3 on chromosome 2q21)* is the same as the XP complementation group B *(XPB)* gene. Rodent mutants deficient in this gene resemble human XP [16] and both genes had already been isolated by their ability to restore excision repair to the cells of UV-sensitive Chinese hamsters. Both possess sets of characteristic amino acid domains found in DNA 'helicases'— proteins that are able to unwind double-stranded nucleic acids. Other human DNA repair genes (e.g. *ERCC-1 on chromosome 19q13.2–13.3* and *ERCC-5 on 13q22–34)* are known but their role in human disease remains obscure.

A high level of UV-induced mutation, as is found in XP, trichothiodystrophy and Cockayne syndrome, does not always lead to being cancer-prone. Other factors such as catalase activity, immunosurveillance and perhaps linked cancer genes may also be important [17,18]. A topical liposomally delivered endonuclease repair enzyme is currently being tested in XP.

Cockayne syndrome (CS) (MIM 216400, 216410, 216411)

Clinical features

Affected children appear normal at birth but photosensitivity is soon obvious, followed within the first year or two by pigmentation and scarring, which simulate ageing. The facies becomes characteristic with sunken eyes, large ears and loss of subcutaneous fat. Other features include central and peripheral demyelination, optic atrophy, deafness, mental retardation, stunted growth and disproportionately large hands and feet. Unlike xeroderma pigmentosum, with which it may coexist, CS seems to carry no extra risk of carcinogenesis.

Genetic aspects

CS is inherited as an autosomal recessive trait. Three complementation groups exist [19]. The most common of these (group B) is due to mutations of the human DNA repair gene *ERCC-6* [20], which has been mapped to chromosome 10q11 [21]. The gene for the late-onset (group C) type may lie on the long arm of chromosome 10 [22].

Pathogenesis

In CS the defect lies in preferential nucleotide excision repair, a process that permits a quick resumption of transcription after UV exposure. It is concerned with repairing genes that are active. The human repair gene *ERCC-6*, important in group B, probably encodes a helicase that plays a part in unwinding the two strands of the double helix before DNA replication can begin [20]. Prenatal diagnosis can be based on the effect on RNA synthesis of the UV irradiation of cultured amniotic cells [23].

Trichothiodystrophy (TTD) (MIM 211390, 234050, 242170, 275550)

Clinical features

The name TTD [24] refers to the brittle, sulphur-deficient hairs that are a marker for a complex of clinically rather similar but genetically perhaps distinct disorders, the classification of which is still under debate.

The hairs themselves are sparse and unruly, and break off easily, cleanly and transversely (trichoschisis). Their flattened ribbon-like shafts show obvious weathering changes with loss of cuticle and exposure of the underlying cortex. Alternating dark and light bands can usually be seen under polarizing microscopy. The nails show similar biochemical abnormalities and may be hypoplastic and spooned with grooves and lamellar splitting.

The associated clinical features are conveniently listed as a series of overlapping acronyms. The BIDS syndrome [25] includes *b*rittle hair, *i*ntellectual impairment, *d*ecreased fertility and *s*hort stature. The Amish brittle hair syndrome (MIM 234050), the Sabinas brittle hair syndrome (MIM 211390) and the Pollitt syndrome (MIM

275550) are probably the same as BIDS. By extension the IBIDS syndrome also includes *ichthyosis*, and the PIBIDS syndrome *photosensitivity and ichthyosis.

Many sufferers from these syndromes have an unusual facies with protruding ears and a receding chin. Loss of subcutaneous fat may give them a prematurely aged look. Many other associated abnormalities have been reported [26].

Genetic aspects

The syndromes including TTD are inherited in an autosomal recessive manner. The three different patterns of cellular response to UV irradiation [27] point to genetic heterogeneity. An association between TTD and xeroderma pigmentosum in an inbred Italian kindred [28] may indicate possible genetic linkage between the two conditions.

Pathogenesis

The basis of the abnormality in sulphur metabolism is not understood but it has been suggested that an altered regulatory gene suppresses the synthesis of some high sulphur proteins [29] so that the levels of cystine/cysteine in the hairs may be reduced by 50%. The sulphur-rich proteins are also distributed abnormally within the shafts [30]. It is not known whether the CNS abnormalities are due to abnormal sulphur metabolism.

In addition, fibroblasts from patients with TTD vary in their response to UVB irradiation. Some behave quite normally, others show defects in excision repair similar to those in xeroderma pigmentosum (group D), and in a third category cells survive the irradiation normally but have a specific deficiency in their ability to repair pyrimidine (6–4) pyrimidone photodimers [27]. Patients in the last two groups usually have mutations in the XP group D *ERCC-2* gene [31]. It is still not clear why patients with TTD and Cockayne syndrome do not develop skin malignancies, whereas those with xeroderma pigmentosum do.

Abnormalities in colony-forming ability and of DNA repair have been found in UV-irradiated fetal fibroblasts, trophoblasts and amniotic fluid cells,

and formed the basis for the prenatal diagnosis of two cases of TTD [31].

Ataxia telangiectasia (Louis–Bar Syndrome) (MIM 208900)

Clinical features

Telangiectasia is often the least obvious feature, confined to the bulbar conjunctiva, or involving the face and ears. Other skin changes include pigmentation and eczema. More serious manifestations are progressive cerebellar ataxia and immunological abnormalities including thymic hypoplasia. Patients are exquisitely sensitive to X- and γ-irradiation. A more rapidly lethal form is accompanied by generalized skin pigmentation (MIM 208910). A syndrome has been reported with the same neurological features but no laboratory abnormalities (MIM 208920).

Carriers appear normal but have an increased incidence of malignancy, particularly breast cancer in women, possibly related to diagnostic or occupational exposure to ionizing radiation [32].

Genetic aspects

Inheritance is autosomal recessive but with a lower than expected rate of parental consanguinity and an incidence in sibs of index cases of only 1 in 7 [33]. Gatti *et al* [34] found linkage between ataxia telangiectasia (AT) and the gene *THY-1* at 11q22.3. Although *THY-1* codes for major cell-surface constituents of thymocytes and seemed a reasonable candidate gene for AT, recombinations between the two loci have been observed, excluding *THY-1* as the AT gene. AT has now been more precisely mapped to 11q23 [35].

Pathogenesis

The basic defect is unknown but appears to involve DNA processing, particularly in lymphoid tissue. AT cells fail to reduce their rate of replication after X-irradiation as normal cells do. There is defective excision repair of DNA damaged by γ- and X-rays—on the basis of this patients can be assigned to five different complementation groups [36]. AT patients have relatively more immature circulating lymphocytes and this may reflect an inability to switch expression of surface receptors from immature to mature type [37]. Chromosomal rearrangements are found much more frequently in lymphocytes than in fibroblasts [38]. Furthermore, T cells in AT patients particularly show breakpoints at loci implicated in immunological malignancy, including the gene for the α subunit of the T-cell antigen receptor (TCRA) at 14q11.2 and the T-cell lymphoma oncogene *TCL*-1 at 14q32.3 [39]. Characteristic rearrangements also occur at the loci for the T-cell receptor β and γ genes, immunoglobulin heavy-chain genes and other members of the immunoglobulin superfamily [40], and in fact the AT locus itself at 11q23 is adjacent to other members of this superfamily, namely CD3 and NCAM as well as *THY*-1. What causes these multiple specific breaks is, however, unknown.

Cells from a patient with the recently recognized Nijmegen breakage syndrome (MIM 251260), which resembles AT without skin manifestations, failed to complement one of the AT groups [41], demonstrating that these disorders overlap genetically as well as phenotypically.

Bloom syndrome (MIM 210900)

Clinical features

Growth retardation, a pinched face with a relatively large nose, patchy hyper- and hypopigmentation, cafe-au-lait macules, and telangiectasia of the light-exposed skin characterize this condition. Immune deficiency is common. Death may occur in early adulthood from infection, leucaemia or other malignancy.

Genetic aspects

Bloom syndrome is autosomal recessive. About one-third of patients have been of Jewish extraction. There are no consistent abnormalities in carriers.

Pathogenesis

The rate of DNA synthesis is reduced and there are increased spontaneous chromosomal anomalies. There are also frequent exchanges between pairs of chromosomes newly replicated from the same parent chromosome in mitosis ('sister chromatid exchange'): this phenomenon may be of no great pathogenetic importance as it entails no loss of genetic material, but is useful as a diagnostic test. It can also be used for antenatal diagnosis, but is normal in heterozygotes so it cannot be used to detect carriers. A consistent biochemical abnormality is defective activity of DNA ligase I, which functions during DNA replication, but no mutation has been found in the DNA ligase I gene, therefore the defect must be post-transcriptional [42]. Another enzyme, uracil DNA glycosylase may also be abnormal [43].

The chromosomal instability probably leads to increased hemizygosity and homozygosity (loss of heterozygosity) which are known to increase cancer risk.

Fanconi pancytopenia (MIM 227650)

Clinical features

This condition combines features of dyskeratosis congenita (pigmentation and marrow failure) and Rothmund–Thomson syndrome (radial ray aplasia). Diagnostic confusion may also occur with TAR syndrome (thrombocytopenia–absent radius, MIM 274000). The pigmentation is poorly defined but may be flexural. There may be renal and cardiac abnormalities. Death from pancytopenia usually occurs in childhood. The abnormalities in 370 patients enrolled in the International Fanconi Anaemia Registry have been summarized [44].

Genetic aspects

Inheritance is autosomal recessive. The condition has been mapped provisionally to 20q, but there is evidence of genetic heterogeneity [45].

Pathogenesis

The Fanconi mutation predisposes to multiple chromosome breaks. There are increased exchanges between non-homologous chromosomes (as opposed to between homologous chromosomes in Bloom syndrome). The chromosomal damage follows inability to remove DNA interstrand cross-links, probably caused by a deficiency, or an abnormal intracellular distribution of an enzyme such as DNA topoisomerase [46]. Complementation studies of the responses of various cell lines to DNA cross-linking agents such as mitomycin C suggest genetic heterogeneity [47] (as in xeroderma pigmentosum). The defect has been corrected in transfection experiments [48], perhaps opening the way to defining the gene. The mechanism of pigmentation in this disorder is unknown.

References

1 English JSC, Swerdlow AJ. The risk of malignant melanoma, internal malignancy and mortality in xeroderma pigmentosum patients. *Br. J. Dermatol.* 1987; 117: 457–461.

2 Daya-Grosjean L, Robert C, Drougard C, Sarasin A. High mutation frequency in ras genes of skin tumours isolated from DNA repair deficient xeroderma pigmentosum patients. *Cancer Res.* 1993; 53: 1625–1629.

3 Cleaver JE. Defective repair of DNA in xeroderma pigmentosum. *Nature* 1968; 218: 652–656.

4 Ramsay CA, Coltart TM, Blunts S *et al.* Prenatal diagnosis of xeroderma pigmentosum: report of the first successful case. *Lancet* 1974; ii: 1109–1112.

5 Cleaver JE. Do we know the cause of xeroderma pigmentosum? *Carcinogenesis* 1990; 11: 875–882.

6 Kraemer KH, Levy DD, Parris CN *et al.* Xeroderma pigmentosum and related disorders: examining the linkage between defective DNA repair and cancer. *J. Invest. Dermatol.* 1994; 103: 96S–101S.

7 Thielmann HW, Popanda U, Edler L, Jung EG. Clinical symptoms and DNA repair characteristics of xeroderma pigmentosum patients from Germany. *Cancer Res.* 1991; 51: 3456–3470.

8 Takebe H, Nishigori G, Satoh Y. Genetics and skin cancers of xeroderma pigmentosum in Japan. *Jap. J. Cancer Res.* 1987; 78: 1135–1143.

9 Wang Y-C, Maher VM, McCormick JJ. Xeroderma pigmentosum variant cells are less likely than normal cells to incorporate dAMP opposite photoproducts during replication of UV irradiated plasmids. *Proc. Natl. Acad. Sci. USA* 1991; 88: 7810–7814.

10 Tanaka K, Miura N, Satokata I *et al.* Analysis of a human DNA excision repair gene involved in group A xeroderma pigmentosum and containing a zinc-finger domain. *Nature* 1990; 348: 73–76.

11 Satokata I, Tanaka K, Okada Y. Molecular basis of group A xeroderma pigmentosum: a missense mutation and two deletions located in a zinc finger consensus sequence of the XPAC gene. *Hum. Genet.* 1992; 86: 603–607.

12 Kaur GP, Rinaldy A, Lloyd RS, Athwal RS. A gene that partially complements xeroderma pigmentosum group A cells maps to human chromosome 8. *Som. Cell Molec. Genet.* 1992; 18: 371–379.

13 Kore-Eda S, Tanaka T, Moriwaki S, Nishigori C, Imamura S. A case of xeroderma pigmentosum group A diagnosed with a polymerase chain reaction technique. *Arch. Dermatol.* 1992; 128: 941–971.

14 Kaur GP, Athwal RS. Complementation of the DNA repair defect in xeroderma pigmentosum cells of group C by transfer of human chromosome 5. *Som. Cell Molec. Genet.* 1993; 19: 83–93.

15 Flejter WL, McDaniel LD, Johns D, Freiberg EC and Schultz RA. Correction of xeroderma complementation group D mutant cell phenotypes by chromosome and gene transfer: involvement of the human ERCC2 DNA repair gene. *Proc. Natl. Acad. Sci. USA* 1992; 89: 261–265.

16 Weeda G, Wiegant J, VanDer Ploeg M *et al.* Localization of the xeroderma pigmentosum group B correcting gene ERCC3 to human chromosome 2q21. *Genomics* 1991; 10: 1035–1040.

17 Madzak C, Armier J, Stary A, Daya-Grosjean L, Sarasin A. UV induced mutations in a shuttle vector replicated in repair deficient trichothiodystrophy cells differ from those in genetically related cancer prone xeroderma pigmentosum. *Carcinogenesis* 1993; 14: 1255–1260.

18 Norris PG, Limb GA, Hamblin AS *et al.* Immune function, mutant frequency and cancer risk in DNA repair defective genodermatoses xeroderma pigmentosum, Cockayne's syndrome and trichothiodystrophy. *J. Invest. Dermatol.* 1990; 94: 94–100.

19 Lehman AR. Three complementation groups in Cockayne Syndrome. *Mutat. Res.* 1982; 106: 347–356.

20 Troelstra C, Hesen W, Hoeijmakers JH. Structure and expression of the excision repair gene ERCC6 involved in the human disorder Cockayne's syndrome group B. *Nucleic Acids Res.* 1993; 21: 419–426.

21 Hoeijmakers JHJ, Weeda G, Troelstra C *et al.* (Sub) chromosomal localization of the human excision repair genes ERCC-3 and -6 and identification of a gene (ASE-1) overlapping with ERCC-1. *Cytogenet. Cell. Genet.* 1989; 51: 1014.

22 Fryns JP, Bulcke J, Verdu P *et al.* Apparent late-onset Cockayne syndrome and interstitial deletion of the long arm of Chromosome 10. *Am. J. Med. Genet.* 1991; 40: 343–344.

23 Lehman AR, Francis AJ, Gianelli F. Prenatal diagnosis of Cockayne's syndrome. *Lancet* 1985; 1: 486–488.

24 Price VH. Trichothiodystrophy update. *Pediatr. Dermatol.* 1992; 9: 369–370.

25 Baden HP, Jackson CE, Weiss L *et al.* The physico-chemical properties of hairs in the BIDS syndrome. *Am. J. Hum. Genet.* 1976; 28: 514–521.

26 Chen T, Cleaver JT, Weber CA *et al.* Trichothiodystrophy: clinical spectrum, central nervous system imaging, and biochemical characterisation of two siblings. *J. Invest. Dermatol.* 1994; 103: 154S–158S.

27 Lehmann AR, Norris PG. DNA repair deficient photodermatoses. *Semin. Dermatol.* 1990; 9: 55–62.

28 Nuzzo F, Zei G, Stefanini M *et al.* Search for consanguinity within and among families of patients with trichothiodystrophy associated with xeroderma pigmentosum. *J. Med. Genet.* 1990; 27: 21–25.

29 Gillespie JM, Marshall RC. A comparison of the proteins of normal and trichothiodystrophic hair. *J. Invest. Dermatol.* 1983; 80: 195–202.

30 Gummer CL, Dawber RPR. Trichothiodystrophy: an ultra-structural study of the hair follicle. *Br. J. Dermatol.* 1985; 113: 273–280.

31 Sarasin A, Blanchet-Bardon C, Renault G *et al.* Prenatal diagnosis in a subset of trichothiodystrophy patients defective in DNA repair. *Br. J. Dermatol.* 1992; 127: 485–491.

32 Swift M, Morell D, Massey RB *et al.* Incidence of cancer in 161 families affected by ataxia-telangiectasia. *N. Engl. J. Med.* 1991; 325: 1831–1836.

33 Woods CG, Bundey SE, Taylor AMR. Unusual features in the inheritance of ataxia telangiectasia. *Hum. Genet.* 1990; 84: 555–562.

34 Gatti RA, Berkel I, Boder E *et al.* Localisation of an ataxia-telangiectasia gene to chromosome 11q22–23. *Nature* 1988; 336: 577–580.

35 Foroud T, Wei S, Ziv Y *et al.* Localization of an ataxia-telangiectasia locus to a 3cm interval on chromosome 11q23: linkage analysis of 111 families by an international consortium. *Am. J. Hum. Genet.* 1991; 49: 1263–1279.

36 Jaspers NGJ, Bootsma D. Genetic heterogeneity in ataxia-telangiectasia studied by cell fusion. *Proc. Natl. Acad. Sci. USA* 1982; 79: 2641–2644.

37 Peterson RDA, Funkhouser JD. Ataxia-telangiectasia: an important clue. *N. Engl. J. Med.* 1990; 322: 124–125.

38 Kojis TL, Schreck RR, Gatti RA, Sparkes RS. Tissue specificity of chromosomal rearrangements in ataxia-telangiectasia. *Hum. Genet.* 1989; 83: 347–352.

39 Croce CM, Isobe M, Palumbo A *et al.* Gene for the alpha-chain of human T-cell receptor: location on chromosome 14 region involved in T-cell neoplasms. *Science* 1985; 227: 1044–1047.

40 Aurias A, Dutrillaux B. Probable involvement of immunoglobulin superfamily genes in most recurrent chromosomal rearrangements from ataxia telangiectasia. *Hum. Genet.* 1986; 72: 210–214.

41 Curry CJR, Tsai J, Hutchinson HT *et al.* AT-Fresno: a phenotype linking ataxia-telangiectasia with the Nijmegen breakage syndrome. *Am. J. Hum. Genet.* 1989; 45: 270–275.

42 Petrini JHJ, Huwiler KJ, Weaver DT. A wild-type DNA ligase I gene is expressed in Bloom's syndrome cells. *Proc. Natl. Acad. Sci. USA* 1991; 88: 7615–7619.

43 Seal G, Brech K, Karp SJ *et al.* Immunological lesions in human uracil DNA glycosylase: association with Bloom syndrome. *Proc. Natl. Acad. Sci. USA* 1988; 85: 2339–2343.

44 Giampietro PF, Davis JD. Fanconi's anaemia. *N. Engl. J. Med.* 1994; 330: 720–721.

45 Mann WR, Venkatraj VS, Allen RG *et al.* Fanconi anaemia: evidence for linkage heterogeneity on chromosome 20q. *Genomics* 1991; 9: 329–337.

46 Wunder E. Further studies on compartmentalisation of DNA topoisomerase I in Fanconi anemia tissue. *Hum. Genet.* 1984; 68: 276–281.

47 Diatloff-Zito C, Papadopoulo D, Averbeck D, Moustacchi E. Abnormal response to DNA cross-linking agents of Fanconi anemia fibroblasts can be corrected by transfection with normal human DNA. *Proc. Natl. Acad. Sci. USA* 1986; 83: 7034–7038.

48 Shaham M, Adler B, Ganguly S. Transfection of normal human and Chinese hamster DNA corrects diepoxybutane-induced chromosomal hypersensitivity of Fanconi anemia fibroblasts. *Proc. Natl. Acad. Sci. USA* 1987; 84: 5853–5857.

Other degenerative disorders

Rothmund–Thomson syndrome (RTS) (MIM 268400)

Clinical features

Described independently by Rothmund, a German ophthalmologist, in 1868, and by Thomson, a British dermatologist, in 1923, there are now about 150 case reports in the world literature [1,2] many of them unwittingly duplicated [3].

Some patients have cataracts, but all have poikiloderma, diagnosed on the basis of atrophy, telangiectasia and pigmentation, often reticulate with round spared areas. The term poikiloderma congen-

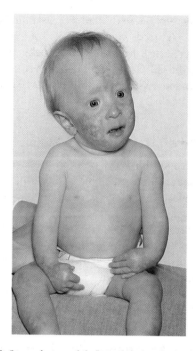

Fig. 4.5 Sparse hair, poikiloderma on the cheeks and hands and radial-ray defects in the Rothmund–Thomson syndrome. (A black and white version of this picture was published in Moss C, Bacon CJ, Mueller RF. Isolated radial ray defects may be due to Rothmund–Thomson syndrome. *Clin. Genet.* 1990; 38: 319.)

itale should be abandoned, as the skin changes do not appear until 6–9 months of age. Initially there are inflammatory papules, plaques and sometimes blisters on the cheeks, buttocks and extensor surfaces of hands, feet, forearms and legs (Fig. 4.5). There may be photosensitivity. The inflammation subsides within the first couple of years leaving atrophy. Later, warty keratoses may develop, particularly on the heels, elbows and knees. Intellect and life-span are normal. Sparse hair, atrophic nails and hypoplastic teeth have led some authors to classify this condition as an ectodermal dysplasia [4].

Associated skeletal abnormalities include short stature and defects of thumb and radius, which cause diagnostic confusion when they present before the characteristic skin changes [5]. Forty-two per cent of adult patients are hypogonadal and 40% of these can be recognized in childhood by their depressed nasal bridge ('saddle-nose'), a manifestation of mid-face hypoplasia, which presumably also affects the pituitary [1].

Patients with RTS are prone to two sorts of malignancy. Skin cancer has been overemphasized in the past—there have been only four reports of squamous carcinoma and two of dysplastic changes, usually in the warty lesions [1]. More significantly, osteosarcoma, first recognized as an association in 1990 [1], has now been reported in 11 patients, one of whom had multiple tumours. The lesions occur in the long bones, usually in areas of metaphyseal chondrodysplasia, which is a common radiological finding in RTS.

Genetic aspects

Inheritance is autosomal recessive. Early reviews suggested a 4 : 1 female predominance, but of the patients reported up to 1992 51% were female [2]. The gene has not been mapped. Two patients with cytogenetic abnormalities have been reported [6,7]. One had trisomy 15 and 22; his mother and maternal uncle who did not have RTS had trisomy 15 and the mother was also mosaic XX/XO. The other patient had trisomy 8 mosaicism.

Pathogenesis

Arguing that RTS was a cancer-prone disorder, Smith and Paterson [8] looked for, and found, reduced DNA repair of hypoxic γ-irradiation damage in fibroblasts from 2 out of 4 patients. This finding has not been confirmed by others. Abnormal karyotypes have been reported in cultured fibroblasts from poikilodermatous skin, suggesting chromosomal instability [9]. The fine skin and hyperextensibility of the fingers has led to the investigation of skin collagen, but no abnormalities have yet been found [1].

Dyskeratosis congenita (Zinsser–Cole–Engman syndrome) (MIM 305000, 224230, 127550)

Clinical features

A 'dirty neck' may be the first sign of the charac-

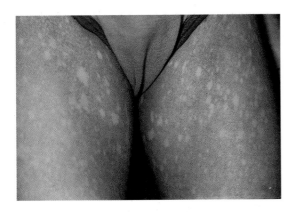

Fig. 4.6 Dyskeratosis congenita: typical flexural pigmentation with spared areas.

teristic flexural pigmentation that develops during early childhood, becoming poikilodermatous (Fig. 4.6). The nails grow poorly and mucous membranes show leucoplakia and sometimes develop squamous carcinomas. Other features are lachrymal-duct atresia, printless palms, plantar keratoderma and hypogonadism [10].

The most serious complication is bone-marrow aplasia, which develops during late childhood or teens. The disorder may be confused with Fanconi pancytopaenia, which is also associated with abnormal pigmentation that may be flexural.

The prognosis of this disorder is poor, with death due to infection or disseminated squamous-cell carcinoma usually occurring in the late teens.

Genetic aspects

Ninety-two of the 104 cases reviewed by Davidson and Connor [10] were male. Inheritance is usually X-linked with no clinical abnormalities found in the female carriers. However, autosomal dominant and recessive inheritance have also been reported [11].

Dyskeratosis congenita has been mapped to Xq28 by Connor *et al.* [12].

Pathogenesis

In some respects this condition shows premature ageing, with progressive atrophy of skin and nails,

together with marrow failure. De Bauche *et al.* found enhanced radiosensitivity of chromatids with increased frequency of breaks and gaps during the G2 phase [13]. Langlois *et al.* showed non-random X-inactivation in carrier females [14].

Premature ageing syndromes

These conditions share a progressive loss of subcutaneous fat and pigmentation of the skin. They differ in their age of onset, extent and associated features. Confusion can arise with the poikilodermatous conditions (especially Rothmund–Thomson) and collagen disorders (especially Ehlers–Danlos type IV). The three syndromes that are most clearly defined are described in full here, the rest are listed in Table 4.3. Their pathogeneses are unknown.

Progeria (Hutchinson–Gilford syndrome) (MIM 176670)

Clinical features

Senile degeneration begins in early childhood, and death from atherosclerosis occurs in the teens. The classical picture of proportionate dwarfism, thin taut skin, sparse hair and beaked nose is unmistakable.

Genetic aspects

Reports of progeria in siblings with normal parents were initially interpreted as meaning autosomal recessive inheritance. However, the low frequency of parental consanguinity and high paternal age has led to the current view that this is an autosomal dominant trait, most cases arising as new mutations [15]. Cytogenetic analysis in monozygotic twins with progeria showed an inverted insertion in the long arm of chromosome 1 in 70% of cells, suggesting a possible location on 1q [16].

Pathogenesis

Various metabolic abnormalities in fibroblasts

Table 4.3 Premature ageing syndromes

MIM*	Name	Onset	Distribution	Associated features
138920[1]	GRANDDAD syndrome	Infant	Face	Growth retardation, aged facies, normal development, decreased subcutaneous fat, autosomal dominant
176670	Progeria (Hutchinson–Gilford)	Infant	Generalized	Hair loss, atheroma contractures
176690[2]	Progeroid short stature with pigmented naevi (Baraitser)	Infant	Generalized	Multiple pigmented naevi, dwarfism, retardation
185069	Storm syndrome	Child	Face, hand feet	Calcific cardiac valve disease
201200	Acrogeria (Gottron)	Infant	Acral	None
219150[3]	Progeroid syndrome (de Barsy)	Infant	Generalized	Corneal clouding, mental retardation
231070[4]	Osteodysplastic geroderma (Walt Disney dwarfism)	Infant	Acral (lax skin, droopy jowls)	Multiple fractures, osteoporosis
233805	Werner-like syndrome	Birth	Generalized	Deficiency of IGF-1 and EGF
248010	—	Birth	Generalized	Short stature, osteoporosis, wrinkled skin
248370[5]	Mandibuloacral dysplasia	Child	Acral	Small jaw, acro-osteolysis
264090[6]	Neonatal pseudohydrocephalic progeroid syndrome (Wiedemann–Rautenstrauch)	Birth	Generalized	Growth and mental retardation
277700	Pangeria (Werner)	Teens	Generalized	Hair loss, cataract, atheroma, malignancy
278250[7]	Wrinkly skin syndrome	Birth	Acral	Hypotonia, retardation

* First digit of MIM number indicates inheritance: 1 = autosomal dominant; 2 = autosomal recessive; 3 = X-linked.
IGF-1, insulin-like growth factor 1; EGF, epidermal growth factor.
1 Marion RW, Goldberg RB, Young RS et al. The GRANDDAD syndrome: a disorder combining growth delay, "aged facies", normal development, and deficiency of subcutaneous fat. Am. J. Hum. Genet. 1989; 45: A53.
2 Baraitser M, Insley J, Winter RM. A recognisable short stature syndrome with premature aging and pigmented naevi. J. Med. Genet. 1988; 25: 53–56.
3 Karnes PS, Shamban AT, Olsen DR et al. De Barsy syndrome: report of a case, literature review, and elastin gene expression studies of the skin. Am. J. Med. Genet. 1992; 42: 29–34.
4 Hunter AGW. Is geroderma osteodysplastica underdiagnosed? J. Med. Genet. 1988; 25: 854–857.
5 Tenconi R, Miotti F, Miotti A et al. Another Italian family with mandibuloacral dysplasia: why does it seem more frequent in Italy? Am. J. Med. Genet. 1986; 24: 357–364.
6 Toriello HV. Wiedemann-Rautenstrauch syndrome. J. Med. Genet. 1990; 27: 256–257.
7 Casamassima AC, Wesson SK, Conlon CJ. Wrinkly skin syndrome: phenotype and additional manifestations. Am. J. Med. Genet. 1987; 27: 885–893.

have been reported, but the basis of the defect remains unknown.

Pangeria (Werner syndrome) (MIM 277700)

Clinical features

In this adult premature ageing syndrome, changes start after puberty with grey hair, sclerodactyly and keratoses. Diabetes, atherosclerosis, cataracts, leg ulcers and malignancies, particularly fibrosarcomas, may develop.

Genetic aspects

Inheritance is autosomal recessive. In a study of 21 families, Werner syndrome was mapped to the region 8p12–p11 [17]. Evidence from homozygosity mapping also supports this locus [18].

Pathogenesis

Numerous metabolic abnormalities have been described, including increased collagen synthesis [19] and decreased type VI collagen gene expression. There is also a high rate of spontaneous chromosome deletion. Skin fibroblast and lymphoblastoid cultures from patients with Werner syndrome show different clones, each characterized by a distinctive, apparently balanced chromosomal translocation, a phenomenon known as variegated translocational mosaicism [20]. One group studied the ability of cultured fibroblasts from Werner syndrome patients to join up (ligate) the ends of a linearized plasmid, restoring its circular shape. Werner cells are just as fast as normal cells at ligating the plasmid ends, but more often do it incorrectly, the errors usually being deletions [21]. Another relevant observation is that the lifespan of Werner syndrome fibroblast cultures is much shorter than normal, reaching only 20 rather than 60 population doublings, due to loss of replicative ability in more cells per generation than normal. Faragher *et al.* [22] have

postulated that a cell-division counting gene could explain this.

Acrogeria (Gottron syndrome) (MIM 201200)

Clinical features

Premature ageing confined to the extremities begins soon after birth. The skin on the hands and feet is atrophic, lacking subcutaneous fat. Hair and general health are normal. The appearance is similar to Ehlers–Danlos type IV, which is due to collagen III deficiency.

Genetic aspects

Inheritance is thought to be autosomal recessive, although cases in a mother and son have been reported [23].

References

1 Moss C. Rothmund–Thomson syndrome: a report of two patients and a review of the literature. *Br. J. Dermatol.* 1990; 122: 821–829.

2 Vennos EM, Collins M, James WD. Rothmund–Thomson syndrome: review of the world literature. *J. Am. Acad. Dermatol.* 1992; 27: 750–762.

3 Moss C. Duplicate reporting of patients with Rothmund–Thomson syndrome. *J. Am. Acad. Dermatol.* 1989; 21: 815–816.

4 Freire-Maia N, Pinheiro M. *Ectodermal Dysplasias: A Clinical and Genetic Study.* New York: Alan R Liss, 1984: 67–68.

5 Moss C, Bacon CJ, Mueller RF. "Isolated" radial ray defect may be due to Rothmund–Thomson syndrome. *Clin. Genet.* 1990; 38: 318–319.

6 Koch F, Santamouris C, Ulbrich F. D+G Trisomie bei einem Patienten mit Rothmund-Syndrom. *Zeitschr. Kinderheil.* 1967; 99: 1–13.

7 Ying KL, Oizumi J, Curry CJR. Rothmund–Thomson syndrome associated with trisomy 8 mosaicism. *J. Med. Genet.* 1990; 27: 258–260.

8 Smith PJ, Paterson MC. Enhanced radiosensitivity and defective DNA repair in cultured fibroblasts derived from Rothmund–Thomson syndrome patients. *Mutat. Res.* 1982; 94: 213–228.

9 Der Kaloustian, McGill VM, Vekemans JJ, Kopelman HR. Clonal lines of aneuploid cells in Rothmund–

Thomson syndrome. *Am. J. Med. Genet.* 1990; 37: 336–339.

10   Davidson HR, Connor JM. Dyskeratosis congenita. *J. Med. Genet.* 1988; 25: 843–846.

11   Pai GS, Morgan S, Whetsall C. Etiologic heterogeneity in dyskeratosis congenita. *Am. J. Med. Genet.* 1989; 32: 63–66.

12   Connor JM, Gathere D, Gray FC *et al.* Assignment of the gene for dyskeratosis congenita to Xq28. *Hum. Genet.* 1986; 72: 348–351.

13   De Bauche DM, Shashidar PG, Stanley WS. Enhanced G2 chromatid radiosensitivity in dyskeratosis congenita fibroblasts. *Am. J. Hum. Genet.* 1990; 46: 350–357.

14   Langlois S, Junker A, Yong SL *et al.* Carrier females for X-linked dyskeratosis congenita show non-random X-inactivation. *Am. J. Hum. Genet.* 1993; 53: 1188.

15   Jones KL, Smith DW, Harvey MAS *et al.* Older paternal age and fresh gene mutation: data on additional disorders. *J. Pediatr.* 1975; 86: 84–88.

16   Brown WT, Abdenur J, Goonewardena P *et al.* Hutchinson–Gilford progeria syndrome: clinical, chromosomal and metabolic abnormalities. *Am. J. Hum. Genet.* 1990; 47 (Suppl.): A50.

17   Goto M, Rubenstein M, Weber J *et al.* Genetic linkage of Werner's syndrome to five markers on chromosome 8. *Nature* 1992; 355: 735–738.

18   Schellenberg GD, Martin GM, Wijsman EM *et al.* Homozygosity mapping and Werner's syndrome. *Lancet* 1992; 339: 1002.

19   Bauer EA, Uitto J, Tan EM *et al.* Werner's syndrome. Evidence for preferential regional expression of a generalised mesenchymal cell defect. *Arch. Dermatol.* 1988; 124: 90–101.

20   Schonberg S, Niermeijer MF, Bootsma D *et al.* Werner's syndrome: proliferation in vitro of clones of cells bearing chromosome translocations. *Am. J. Hum. Genet.* 1984; 36: 387–397.

21   Runger TM, Bauer C, Dekant B *et al.* Hypermutable ligation of plasmid DNA ends in cells from patients with Werner syndrome. *J. Invest. Dermatol.* 1994; 102: 45–48.

22   Faragher RGA, Kill IR, Hunter JAA *et al.* The gene responsible for Werner syndrome may be a cell-division "counting" gene. *Proc. Natl. Acad. Sci. USA* 1993; 90: 12030–12034.

23   De Groot WP, Tafelkruyer J, Woerdeman MJ. Familial acrogeria (Gottron). *Br. J. Dermatol.* 1980; 103: 213–223.

5
GENETICALLY DETERMINED
BENIGN TUMOURS

Heritable benign tumours

All skin tumours probably result from mutations in genes responsible for normal controlled cell growth, and therefore embody clues to normal development. However, very little is known about the mutations responsible for benign skin tumours. As with naevi, the mutations must occur after conception (somatic or postzygotic mutations). The earlier the mutation, particularly if it is in the epidermis, the more likely it is to produce a linear lesion, because the orientation of the abnormal clone will correspond to the direction of embryonic cell migration (see section on Blaschko's lines, p. 8). Later mutations such as those responsible for the benign tumours discussed here, tend to produce round lesions in no particular pattern.

If acquired tumours arise from mutations occurring after conception, it is hard to understand how they can be inherited from one generation to the next, as indeed they are (Table 5.1). The explanation must be a 'two-hit hypothesis' as in familial cancer syndromes: a 'susceptibility mutation' is present in all cells and is heritable, but the development of tumours requires a second event, perhaps another mutation, loss of heterozygosity, or some environmental factor.

Familial, multiple, benign skin tumours sometimes occur as part of a syndrome, the best known of which are referred to as the phakomatoses (from the Greek *phakus*, a lens or lentil). In these conditions the heritable susceptibility mutation is presumably also responsible for the associated non-cutaneous developmental defects.

Tricho-epithelioma (epithelioma adenoides cysticum) (MIM 132700)

Clinical features

The multiple small, pink, translucent tumours arise at puberty and are most common around

Table 5.1 Heritable benign tumours. For most of these tumours a positive family history is the exception rather than the rule

MIM*	Condition
125600	Dermatosis papulosa nigra
132700	Trichoepitheliomas
190340	Trichodiscomas
190345	Desmoplastic trichoepitheliomas
182000	Seborrhoeic warts
167900	Familial cutaneous papillomatosis
185069	Syringomas
123850	Multiple cylindromas
313100	Multiple cylindromas
132600	Calcifying epitheliomas
157400	Multiple milia
184500	Steatocystoma multiplex
184510	Steatocystoma multiplex
162900	Multiple melanocytic naevi
137550	Giant pigmented hairy naevus with multiple smaller melanocytic naevi
151900	Multiple lipomatosis
206550	Angiolipomas
156610	Michelin-tyre baby syndrome (extensive lipomas)
103060	Adiposis dolorosa (Dercum disease)
154800	Mastocytomas
138000	Multiple glomus tumours
150800	Familial leiomyomas
115250	Familial cutaneous collagenomas
148100	Keloids
149100	Knuckle pads

First digit of MIM number indicates inheritance: 1 = autosomal dominant; 2 = autosomal recessive; 3 = X-linked.

the eyes, on the cheeks and in the nasolabial folds. Malignant change is rare. In some families scalp cylindromas also occur [1].

Genetic aspects

Inheritance is as an autosomal dominant trait but the gene has not yet been mapped. The condition seems distinct from multiple desmoplastic trichoepitheliomas (MIM 190345), although this too is an autosomal dominant trait.

Pathogenesis

This is not understood. The tumours, which are

multicellular in origin [2], show differentiation towards hair follicles.

Multiple cylindromas (MIM 123850, 313100)

Clinical features

Firm, domed, smooth, pink to red tumours arise in early adult life and grow slowly, a few up to 5 cm in diameter. Lesions are most common on the scalp, where they are hairless, and less common on the face and neck (Fig. 5.1). Some 10% of cases have lesions on the trunk and limbs also. Occasionally, extensive scalp involvement may justify the term turban tumour. The condition is probably distinct from hereditary benign cystic trichoepithelioma, although the two conditions coexist in some families [3]. Malignant change seldom occurs.

Genetic aspects

The disorder is more commonly seen in females than males but is probably inherited as an autosomal dominant with stronger expression in the female rather than as an X-linked dominant.

Multiple lipomatosis (MIM 151900)

Clinical features

Multiple soft lobulated lipomas appear in the subcutaneous tissues. The condition is usually asymptomatic.

Genetic aspects

Inheritance is as an autosomal dominant trait. Studies of chromosome abnormalities in solitary lipomas have demonstrated balanced rearrangements and ring chromosomes involving chromosome 12, with breakpoints at either 12q13 or 12q14 [4]. It is not yet known whether familial multiple cases show linkage to markers on 12q.

Urticaria pigmentosa (MIM 154800)

The term refers to a variety of skin eruptions characterized by an excess of mast cells (Fig. 5.2): systemic involvement occurs in a minority. Most cases are sporadic but 50 affected families have been documented [5]; in two the condition ran through three generations [6]. Concordantly

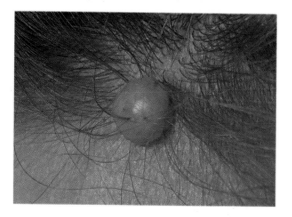

Fig. 5.1 Cylindroma: sometimes these cover the scalp, hence the name of turban tumour.

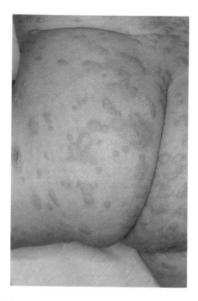

Fig. 5.2 Mastocytomas in infantile urticaria pigmentosa.

affected monozygotic twins and even triplets have been recorded [7] but clinical and genetic heterogeneity is likely.

Hereditary multiple leiomyomas (MIM 150800)

Clinical features

These small pink skin tumours of smooth muscle are thought to arise from the arrector pilorum muscles, which may explain the characteristic discomfort felt in the cold. In some families cutaneous leiomyomas have been associated with uterine myomas [8].

Genetic aspects

Inheritance of this trait is dominant with incomplete penetrance. A patient has been described in whom mental retardation and multiple cutaneous leiomyomas were associated with trisomy of the short arm of chromosome 9 and monosomy of the end of the short arm of chromosome 18 [9].

Familial cutaneous collagenoma (MIM 115250)

Several families have been described in which the presence of multiple dermal nodules has been inherited as an autosomal dominant trait [10]. An association with testicular failure and cardiomyopathy in some affected individuals argues that the skin changes are part of a systemic disorder. Enhanced transcriptional activity of collagen genes has been suggested as a possible mechanism.

Keloids (MIM 148100)

A racial and familial predisposition has long been noted [11]; in one family the tendency passed through five generations [12]. Keloid formation is a notable feature of the Rubinstein–Taybi syndrome, the gene for which has been tentatively assigned to chromosome 16p13.3 [13]. An occasional association with Ehlers–Danlos syndrome is

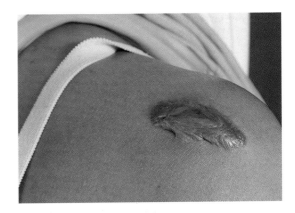

Fig. 5.3 A keloid on one shoulder.

also of interest in view of the activation of type I and VI collagen gene expression known to occur in keloids [14].

References

1 Autio-Harmainen H, Pakko P, Alavaikko M, Karvonen J, Leisti J. Familial occurrence of malignant lymphoepithelial lesion of the parotid gland in a Finnish family with dominantly inherited trichoepithelioma. *Cancer* 1988; 61: 161–166.

2 Gartler SM, Ziprkowski L, Krakowski A *et al.* Glucose-6-phosphate dehydrogenase mosaicism as a tracer in the study of hereditary multiple trichoepithelioma. *Am. J. Hum. Genet.* 1966; 18: 282–287.

3 Welch JP, Wells RS, Kerr CB. Ancell-Spiegler cylindromas (turban tumours) and Brooke–Fordyce trichoepitheliomas: evidence for a single genetic entity. *J. Med. Genet.* 1968; 5: 29–35.

4 Turc-Carel C, Dal Cin P, Boghosian L, Leong SPL, Sandberg AA. Breakpoints in benign lipoma may be at 12q13 or 12q14. *Cancer Genet. Cytogenet.* 1988; 36: 131–135.

5 Anstey A, Lowe DG, Kirby JD, Horton MA. Familial mastocytosis: a clinical, immunophenotypic, light and electron microscopic study. *Br. J. Dermatol.* 1991; 125: 583–587.

6 Clark DP, Buescher L, Havey A. Familial urticaria pigmentosa. *Arch. Intern. Med.* 1990; 150: 1742–1744.

7 Rockoff AS. Urticaria pigmentosa in identical twins. *Arch. Dermatol.* 1978; 114: 1227–1228.

8 Reed WB, Walker R, Horowitz R. Cutaneous leiomyomata with uterine leiomyomata. *Acta Derm. Venereol.* 1973; 53: 409–416.

9 Fryns JP, Haspeslagh M, de Muelenaere A, van den Berghe H. 9p trisomy/18p distal monosomy and

multiple cutaneous leiomyomata: another specific chromosomal site (18pter) in dominantly inherited multiple tumours? *Hum. Genet.* 1985; 70: 284–286.

10 Uitto J, Santa-Cruz DJ, Eisen AZ. Familial cutaneous collagenoma: genetic studies on a family. *Br. J. Dermatol.* 1979; 101: 185–195.

11 Murray JC, Pollack SV, Pinnell SR. Keloids: a review. *J. Am. Acad. Dermatol.* 1981; 4: 461–470.

12 Bloom D. Heredity of keloids: review of the literature and report of a family with multiple keloids in five generations. *NY J. Med.* 1956; 56: 511–519.

13 Tommerup N, Van der Hagen CB, Heiberg A. Tentative assignment of a locus for Rubinstein–Taybi syndrome to 16p13.3 by a *de novo* reciprocal translocation. *Cytogenet. Cell Genet.* 1991; 58: 2002–2003.

14 Peltonen J, Hsiao LL, Jaakkola *et al.* Activation of collagen gene expression in keloids: colocalization of type I and VI collagen and transforming growth factor-B1 mRNA, *J. Invest. Dermatol.* 1991; 97: 240–248.

Syndromes featuring benign tumours

There are many syndromes in which multiple benign skin tumours are a diagnostic feature. Usually the cutaneous lesions are pigmentary or dermal. Syndromes featuring multiple epidermal or appendage-derived tumours are remarkably rare: they include epidermal naevus syndrome and acanthosis nigricans, which are discussed elsewhere (pp. 22 and 61).

Syndromes with multiple pigmented lesions

These are listed in Table 5.2. Moles, or naevocytic naevi are melanocytic hamartomas; lentigines are brown macules composed of increased numbers of melanocytes without evidence of focal proliferation; while ephelides (freckles) simply show an overproduction of melanin by a normal number of melanocytes. A blue naevus is composed of a group of functioning melanocytes in the dermis. A clue to the pathogenesis of melanocytic naevi may be provided by the development of multiple moles following chemotherapy.

Syndromes featuring multiple benign dermal tumours (Table 5.3)

This section includes the phakomatoses—a poorly defined group of disorders featuring hamartomas in the skin. Several of these are discussed in detail because considerable advances have been made in understanding their pathogenesis.

Buschke–Ollendorf syndrome (MIM 166700)

Clinical features

Yellow papules develop in childhood, particularly on the limbs and buttocks [1]. Radiologically there is osteopoikilosis due to uneven bone formation.

Genetic aspects

This is an autosomal dominant trait.

Pathogenesis

There is abnormal accumulation of elastin in the dermis. *In vitro*, there is increased elastin production by fibroblasts, with elevated elastin mRNA [2].

Tuberous sclerosis (TSC, tuberous sclerosis complex) (MIM 191100) [3,4] (Figs 5.4–5.6)

Clinical features

Tuberous sclerosis is a complex multisystem disorder renowned for its variable expression within and between families, and for the trouble that this causes in genetic and epidemiological studies.

It is now known that the full classical triad of features (epilepsy, low intelligence and adenoma sebaceum) is shown by less than 1 in 3 of those with the disease. Modern imaging technology can now detect cerebral and extracerebral lesions in asymptomatic subjects. Past estimates of the prevalence of the disease have inevitably been too low because minimally affected individuals do not come to medical attention. The frequency of TSC at birth could be as high as one in 10 000, prevalence falling thereafter, as life expectancy is less than for the general population [5].

Table 5.2 Syndromes with pigmented naevi

MIM*	Name	Associated features
(a) Moles (naevocytic naevi)		
—	Turner syndrome	Multiple moles may occur with XO phenotype
163200 165630	Epidermal naevus syndrome	Multiple moles may occur with epidermal naevi and neurological defects
137550[1]	Giant pigmented hairy naevus	Multiple small naevi in relatives
249400[2]	Neurocutaneous melanosis	Giant hairy naevi, meningeal pigmentation, melanoma
(b) Ephelides and lentigines, +/− naevocytic naevi, blue naevi		
137270[3]	Gastrocutaneous syndrome	Peptic ulcer/hiatus hernia, multiple lentigines, hyperteleorism/myopia
150900[4]	Lentiginosis	Generalized lentigines with no associations
151000[5]	Touraine lentiginosis	Centrofacial lentigines with retardation
151001[6]	Inherited patterned lentiginosis	Small lentigines on extremities and buttocks
151100	LEOPARD syndrome	Lentigines, ECG abnormalities, ocular hyperteleorism, pulmonary stenosis, abnormal genitalia, retardation of growth, deafness
157800[7]	—	Mitral regurgitation, conductive deafness, fusion of cervical vertebrae and of carpal/tarsal bones, short stature, freckling of face and iris
160980[8]	NAME syndrome	Naevi, atrial myxoma, myxoid neurofibromas, ephelides
160980[9]	LAMB syndrome	Lentigines, atrial myxoma, mucocutaneous myxoma, blue naevi
160980[10]	Carney syndrome	Spotty cutaneous pigmentation, myxomas, endocrine adenomatosis
175200	Peutz–Jeghers	Periorificial lentiginosis with small intestinal polyposis
140900[11]	—	Peutz–Jeghers type lentiginosis with haemangiomas of small intestine
—	Laugier–Hunziker[12]	Peutz–Jeghers type lentiginosis with black streaks in nails and no systemic features
175500[13]	Cronkhite–Canada	Polyposis, pigmentation, alopecia, nail dystrophy

* First digit of MIM number indicates inheritance: 1 = autosomal dominant; 2 = autosomal recessive; 3 = X-linked.

1 Goodman RM, Caren J, Ziprkowski M *et al.* Genetic considerations in giant pigmented hairy naevus. *Br. J. Dermatol.* 1971; 85: 150–157.
2 Kaplan AM, Itabashi HH, Hanelin LG, Lu AT. Neurocutaneous melanosis with malignant leptomeningeal melanoma. *Arch. Neurol.* 1975; 32: 669–671.
3 Halal F, Gervais MH, Baillargeon J, Lesage R. Gastrocutaneous syndrome: peptic ulcer-hiatal hernia, multiple lentigines–cafe-au-lait spots, hypterolism and myopia. *Am. J. Med. Genet.* 1982; 11: 161–176.
4 Pipkin AC, Pipkin SB. A pedigree of generalised lentigo. *J. Hered.* 1950; 41: 79–82.
5 Dociu I, Galaction-Nitelea O, Sirjita N, Murgu V. Centrofacial lentiginosis. *Br. J. Dermatol.* 1976; 94 : 39–43.
6 O'Neill JF, James WD. Inherited patterned lentiginosis in blacks. *Arch. Dermatol.* 1989; 125: 1231–1235.
7 Forney WR, Robinson SJ, Pascoe DJ. Congenital heart disease, deafness, and skeletal malformations: a new syndrome? *J. Pediatr.* 1966; 68: 14–26.
8 Atherton DJ, Pitcher DW, Wells RS, MacDonald DM. A syndrome of various pigmented cutaneous lesions, myxoid neurofibromata and atrial myxoma: the NAME syndrome. *Brit. J. Dermatol.* 1980; 103: 421–429.
9 Rhodes AR, Silverman RA, Harrist TJ, Perez-Atayde AR. Mucocutaneous lentigines, cardiomucocutaneous myxomas, and multiple blue nevi: the LAMB syndrome. *J. Am. Acad. Dermatol.* 1984; 10: 72–82.
10 Carney JA, Headington JT, Su WPD. Cutaneous myxomas: a major component of the complex of myxomas, spotty pigmentation, and endocrine overactivity. *Arch. Dermatol.* 1986; 122: 790–798.
11 Bandler M. Haemangiomas of the small intestine associated with mucocutaneous pigmentation. *Gastroenterology* 1960; 38: 641–645.
12 Koch SE, LeBoit PE, Odom RB. Laugier-Hunziker syndrome. *J. Am. Acad. Dermatol.* 1987; 16: 431–434.
13 Daniel ES, Lugwig S, Lewin KJ *et al.* The Cronkhite–Canada syndrome. *Medicine* 1982; 61: 293–309.

Table 5.3 Syndromes featuring multiple benign dermal tumours

MIM*	Name	Naevi/hamartomas present
191100	Tuberous sclerosis	Sacral collagenoma (shagreen patch), subungual fibromas, facial angiofibromas
166700[1]	Buschke–Ollendorf	Elastomas (with osteopoikilosis)
115250[2]	Familial cutaneous collagenomas	Collagenomas on trunk, cardiomyopathy, hypogonadism
158350	Cowden syndrome	Facial trichilemmomas and other hamartomas of skin, mucous membranes, breast and thyroid
—	Encephalocranio cutaneous lipomatosis[3]	Multiple lipomas of head, neck and brain
162200	Neurofibromatosis I	
101000	Neurofibromatosis II	Neurofibromas
162260	Neurofibromatosis III	
162270	Neurofibromatosis IV	
167730	Coloboma–lipoma syndrome	Lipomas

* First digit of MIM number indicates inheritance: 1 = autosomal dominant; 2 = autosomal recessive; 3 = X-linked.
1 Verbov J, Graham R. Buschke–Ollendorf syndrome: disseminated dermatofibrosis with osteopoikilosis. *Clin. Exp. Dermatol.* 1986; 11: 17–26.
2 Sacks HN, Crawley IS, Ward JA, Fine RM. Familial cardiomyopathy, hypogonadism, and collagenoma. *Ann. Intern. Med.* 1980; 93: 813–817.
3 Sanchez NP, Rhodes AR, Mandell F *et al.* Encephalocraniocutaneous lipomatosis: a new neurocutaneous syndrome. *Br. J. Dermatol.* 1981; 104: 89–96.

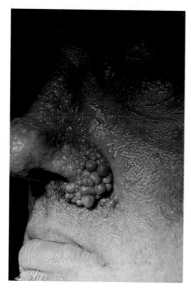

Fig. 5.4 Angiofibromas in tuberous sclerosis.

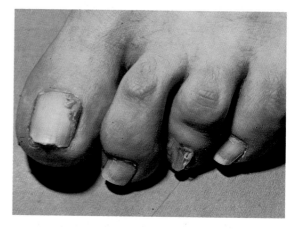

Fig. 5.5 Periungual fibromas may be the only manifestation of tuberous sclerosis.

These problems have led to the evolution of a strict set of diagnostic criteria that have now been widely adopted [6] (Table 5.4) and are especially useful in the investigation of families that include an apparently sporadic case of TSC. In up to 30% of such cases, a battery of non-invasive tests (e.g. Wood's light examination, cranial CT scan, specialist ophthalmic and dental assessments, skeletal survey and echocardiography) will reveal that one of the parents has unsuspected disease. Correct genetic counselling can then be given [7].

Those who screen families for TSC have to appreciate that its manifestations are age dependent. The

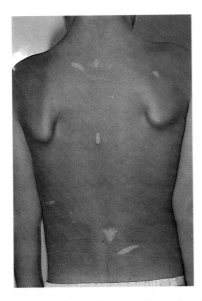

Fig. 5.6 The orientation of the ash-leaf macules of tuberous sclerosis often corresponds to hair lines.

skin lesions are a good example of this. Depigmented macules (Fig. 5.6) are the most important and earliest indicator and are usually present at birth. Wood's light should be used to detect them. Facial angiofibromas (Fig. 5.4) develop after the third year of life; periungual fibromas (Fig. 5.5) do not appear until the second decade.

Genetic aspects

TSC is inherited as an autosomal dominant trait with high penetrance and great variability of expression. Approximately 60–70% of cases still seem to be genuinely new mutations even after careful screening of their parents.

The genetics of TSC has advanced rapidly over the last few years. In 1987, a linkage was reported between the TSC gene and the ABO locus on the distal long arm of chromosome 9 (TSC-I, MIM 191100) [8]. This has now been confirmed and the locus lies on chromosome 9q34, close to the Albelson oncogene and the gene for prostaglandin D_2 synthetase. Linkage to 9q34 is found in only 40% of TSC families, being more common in British than American studies.

More recently, a second important gene (TSC-2, MIM 191090) has been mapped to a locus on chromosome 16p13.3 [9]. The protein product of this gene, tuberin, has a region of homology to the GTPase activity protein GAP3 [10]. Between them the genes on chromosomes 9 and 16 account for most cases of TSC. A small minority of cases may be due to an abnormality of genes lying on other chromosomes: claims, so far unconfirmed, have been put forward for genes on 11q22–23 [11], and on 12q22–24.1 [12].

Table 5.4 Hierarchy of features for the diagnosis of TSC [6]. (The presence of a direct relative with TSC should change a patient's diagnostic class from suspect to presumptive or from provisional to definitive. Two 'presumptive' features also make the diagnosis definitive)

Definitive	Presumptive	Suspect
Cortical tuber	Single retinal hamartoma	Infantile spasms
Subependymal nodules	Confetti-like spots on skin	Generalized or partial seizures
Giant-cell astrocytoma	Single angiomyolipoma of kidney	Hypomelanotic macules of skin
Hamartomas of retina	Multiple rhabdomyomas of heart	Kidney cysts
Facial angiofibromas	Lymphangiomyomatosis	Single cardiac rhabdomyoma
Ungual fibromas	of lungs	Spontaneous pneumothorax
Fibrous forehead plaque	Rectal polyps	Chylothorax
Multiple angiomyolipomas	Shagreen patches	Honeycomb image of lungs
of kidneys		Enamel pits of teeth
		Gingival fibromas
		Thyroid adenoma
		Angiomyolipoma of adrenal, gonads or liver
		Bone cysts
		Periosteal new bone

Changes in more than one gene can lead to an identical clinical picture, perhaps by affecting any of several components of a multimeric protein, or any of a series of enzymes on a sequential pathway. It is not yet known whether a clinical distinction can be made between families manifesting mutations at these different loci. Some have claimed that 'chromosome 9 families' are less prone to mental retardation, and one TSC family, not linked to chromosome 9, had an unusual pattern of depigmentation, and curious nuchal skin tags [13]. In one large study [14], chromosome-9-linked families had a higher incidence of ungual fibromas but no other clinical differences were found.

Pathogenesis

Ideas on this have run ahead of the facts. However, the curious cells consistently grown from TSC lesions in tissue culture seem to be neuronal precursors [15]. A two-stage pathogenesis has been suggested in which these cells first spread widely throughout the body and then interact with surrounding cells to induce hamartomas and tumours. The primary mutation in TSC may therefore involve a molecule important for the migration of neuronal precursor cells. In this context it is of interest that a gene for a neural cell adhesion molecule (N-CAM), has been mapped to chromosome 11q and is a possible candidate gene for the putative TSC loci there.

Neurofibromatosis

There are two genetically distinct types (NF-1 and NF-2) together with several other variants of uncertain status designated NF-III–NF-VIII by Riccardi [16]. Eighty-five per cent of patients with neurofibromatosis have NF-1.

Von Recklinghausen's neurofibromatosis: NF-1 (MIM 162200)

Clinical features

This disorder affects 1 in 3–5000 people. The diagnosis may be difficult in early childhood because of the delayed appearance of some of the characteristic signs. Some cafe-au-lait macules (CALs) may be present at birth; flexural freckling appears during childhood, and neurofibromas are unusual before adolescence (Fig. 5.7). Lisch nodules (pigmented iris hamartomas best seen with the slit lamp) appear during childhood and increase with age; however, a study claiming to show that all adults with NF-1 have Lisch nodules [17] was flawed by a circular argument: one of the diagnostic criteria used to distinguish affected and unaffected individuals for the study was the presence of Lisch nodules. Juvenile xanthogranulomas [18] are more common in children with NF-1 than in healthy children. The combination of NF-1 and xanthogranuloma may be a predictor for juvenile chronic myeloid leucaemia [19]. Naevus anaemicus [20] also appears to be associated with NF-1, as are certain other vascular phenomena. The non-cutaneous features of NF-1 are shown below in Table 5.5, and the diagnostic criteria in Table 5.6.

Genetic aspects

NF-1 is an autosomal dominant trait. Patients born of affected mothers have more severe disease

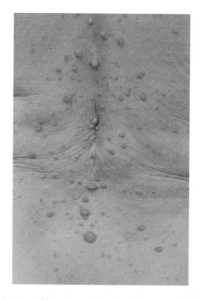

Fig. 5.7 Neurofibromas and scoliosis in neurofibromatosis type 1.

Table 5.5 Non-cutaneous features of NF-1

Ophthalmic	Lisch nodules
	Retinoblastoma
	Optic glioma
	Congenital glaucoma
Central nervous system	Plexiform neuroma
	Neurofibrosarcoma
	Meningioma
	Acoustic neuroma
	Hypothalamic hamartoma
	Learning disability
Skeletal system	Short stature
	Scoliosis
	Macrocephaly
	Sphenoid dysplasia
	Pseudarthrosis
Other tumours	Phaeochromocytoma
	Carcinoid tumour
	Wilms tumour
	Fibrosarcoma
	Leucaemia, especially juvenile chronic myeloid leucaemia
Vascular	Renovascular hypertension
	Large-vessel aneurysm
	Arterial fibrodysplasia
Other	Fibrosing alveolitis

Table 5.6 Minimal diagnostic criteria for NF-1 [21]

Two or more of the following
Six or more cafe-au-lait macules over 5 mm diameter
(prepuberty), or over 15 mm (adult)
Two or more neurofibromas or one plexiform neuroma
Axillary or inguinal freckling
Optic glioma
Two or more Lisch nodules
A distinctive bone lesion, e.g. sphenoid dysplasia, cortical
thinning, with or without pseudarthrosis
A first-degree relative with NF-1 by these criteria

than those born of affected fathers, an example of genetic imprinting so far unexplained. One-third to a half of index cases have no preceding family history: the mutation rate of 1 in 10 000 gametes is one of the highest for a human disorder. Interestingly, new mutations usually occur on the paternally derived chromosome 17 [22]. Furthermore, there is a striking distinction between expression of NF-1 in descendants and predecessors: once classical NF-1 has appeared in a family it is passed on with 100% penetrance, while atypical incomplete forms are limited to patients with no antecedent family history [23]. This can be explained by NF-1 arising as a somatic mutation, with cutaneous and gonadal mosaicism. Segmental NF probably falls into this category, and is further discussed in the section on Blaschko's lines (p. 8).

The hunt for the NF-1 gene has been well summarized [24]. Attempts to map NF-1 were frustrated for years by the absence of linkage to any of the known biochemical or haematological polymorphisms. There were no clues until, at an international meeting in 1987, investigators pooled their negative findings and constructed an exclusion map. Workers were then able to concentrate their efforts on the few remaining candidate sites, and within months NF-1 was localized to chromosome 17. Subsequent work on patients with translocations involving the NF-1 gene defined the locus as 17q11.2. The NF-1 gene is very large (300 kb), which may explain the high mutation rate, and has now been cloned and sequenced [25].

It is not yet possible to identify the molecular defect in all affected individuals: several different mutations have now been identified [26,27], but there is no technique to scan the whole gene for mutations. Several closely linked and intragenic markers have been developed, and these can be used for diagnosis and genetic counselling in informative families [28,29].

Pathogenesis

Nerve growth factor was at one stage considered the most likely candidate gene, especially when it was mapped to the same area of 17q as NF-1. In fact, the two genes are now known to be quite distinct. The NF-1 gene encodes a 2818 amino acid, 250 kDa protein, which has been found in all tissues and all vertebrates so far studied [30]. Within this polypeptide is a 48 kDa domain identical to mammalian GAP (guanosine triphosphate (GTP) activating protein), which can convert the active GTP-bound form of the *ras* p21 oncogene to the inactive guanosine diphosphate (GDP)-bound form. An inability to inactivate *ras* could explain the susceptibility of NF-1 patients to tumour formation [31]. The function of the rest of the gene product is unknown but may be responsible for the non-tumorous manifestations of NF-1, including CALs.

Bilateral acoustic neurofibromatosis: NF-2 (MIM 101000)

Clinical features

This condition is characterized by tumours of the eighth cranial nerve, meningiomas, Schwannomas and cataracts, and usually presents with raised intracranial pressure and deafness. There are few, if any, neurofibromas, and CALs if present at all are larger and paler than in NF-1.

Genetic aspects

Inheritance is autosomal dominant. The observation of cytogenetic change in chromosome 22 in meningioma, a tumour characteristic of NF-2, prompted a search for the NF-2 gene on chromosomes 22. It has now been mapped to 22q11.21–13.1 [29] and the gene cloned. It encodes a novel tumour-suppressor protein 'Merlin', which is ubiquitously expressed.

Mixed central and peripheral neurofibromatosis: NF-III (MIM 162260)

This combines the cutaneous signs of NF-1 with a tendency to multiple tumours of the central nervous system. It has not been mapped.

Variant NF: NF-IV (MIM 162270)

This heterogeneous category is for patients who do not fit into any of the other groups.

Segmental NF: NF-V (Fig. 5.8)

This probably represents somatic mutation for the NF-1 gene: the patient is genetically mosaic for NF-1, and this is reflected in the skin and possibly in the gametes. This is the likely explanation for

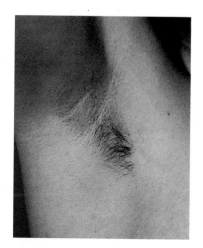

a

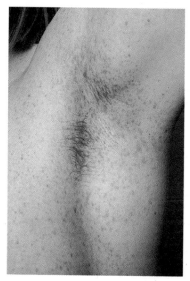

b

Fig. 5.8 Asymmetric axillary freckling (a, b), in a patient with segmental neurofibromatosis who has a daughter with full blown neurofibromatosis type 1 (von Recklinghausen's). (Black and white versions of these pictures appeared in [32].

patients with cutaneous lesions of NF-1 following Blaschko's lines (see p. 8), and offspring with classical NF-1 [32]. The dermatological entities zosteriform lentiginous naevus and segmental naevus spilus may be segmental NF. Whether patients with just a small cluster of neurofibromas or a few CALs also have segmental NF with a risk of full-blown NF-1 in offspring is not yet known.

Watson syndrome (MIM 193520)

This condition combines the skin lesions of NF-1 with the 'male-Turner'-like phenotype of Noonan syndrome, and pulmonary stenosis. Linkage studies suggest that this may be an allelic variant of NF-1 [33]. However, classical Noonan syndrome is not linked to the NF-1 gene [34].

CALs with no associated abnormalities

Some families have CALs only. This may be another allelic variant of NF-1.

References

1 Verbov J, Graham R. Buschke–Ollendorf syndrome: disseminated dermatofibrosis with osteopoikilosis. *Clin. Exp. Dermatol.* 1986; 11: 17–26.
2 Giro MG, Duvic M, Smith LT *et al.* Buschke–Ollendorf syndrome associated with elevated elastin production by affected skin fibroblasts in culture. *J. Invest. Dermatol.* 1992; 99: 129–137.
3 Stefansson K. Tuberous sclerosis. *Mayo Clin. Proc.* 1991; 66: 868–872.
4 Webb DW, Osborne JP. New research in tuberous sclerosis. *BMJ* 1992; 304: 1647–1648.
5 Sampson JR, Scahill SJ, Stephenson JBR, Mann L, Connor JM. Genetic aspects of tuberous sclerosis in the West of Scotland. *J. Med. Genet.* 1989; 26: 28–31.
6 Gomez MR. Phenotypes of the tuberous sclerosis complex with a revision of diagnostic criteria. *Ann. NY Acad. Sci.* 1991; 615: 1–7.
7 Al-Gazali LI, Arthur RJ, Lamb JT *et al.* Diagnostic and counselling difficulties using a fully comprehensive screening protocol for families at risk of tuberous sclerosis. *J. Med. Genet.* 1989; 26: 694–703.
8 Fryer AE, Chalmers A, Connor JM *et al.* Evidence that the gene for tuberous sclerosis is on chromosome 9. *Lancet* 1987; 1: 659–661.
9 Kandt RS, Haines JL, Smith M *et al.* Linkage of an important gene locus for tuberous sclerosis to a chromosome 16 marker for polycystic kidney disease. *Nat. Genet.* 1992; 2: 37–41.
10 The European Chromosome 16 Tuberous Sclerosis Consortium. Identification and characterization of the tuberous sclerosis gene on chromosome 16. *Cell* 1993; 75: 1305–1315.
11 Smith M, Yoshiyama K, Wagner C, Flodman P, Smith B. Genetic heterogeneity in tuberous sclerosis. Map position of the TSC2 locus on chromosome 11q and future prospects. *Ann. NY Acad. Sci.* 1991; 615: 274–283.
12 Fahsold T, Rott HD & Lorenz P. A third gene locus for tuberous sclerosis is closely linked to the phenylalanine hydroxylase gene locus. *Hum. Genet.* 1991; 88: 85–90.
13 Winship IM, Connor JM, Beighton PH. Genetic heterogeneity in tuberous sclerosis: phenotypic correlations. *J. Med. Genet.* 1990; 27: 418–421.
14 Northrup H, Kwiatowski DJ, Roach ES *et al.* Evidence for genetic heterogeneity in tuberous sclerosis: one locus on chromosome 9 and at least one locus elsewhere. *Am. J. Hum. Genet.* 1992; 51: 709–720.
15 Davidson M, Yoshidome H, Stenroos E, Johnson WG. Neuron-like cells in culture of tuberous sclerosis tissue. *Ann. NY Acad. Sci.* 1991; 615: 196–210.
16 Riccardi VM, Eichner JE. *Neurofibromatosis: Phenotype, Natural History and Pathogenesis.* Baltimore: Johns Hopkins University Press, 1986.
17 Lubs M-LE, Bauer S, Formas ME, Djokic B. Lisch nodules in neurofibromatosis type 1. *N. Eng. J. Med.* 1991; 324: 1264–1266.
18 Jensen NE, Sabharwal S, Walker AE. Naevoxanthoendothelioma and neurofibromatosis. *Br. J. Dermatol.* 1971; 85: 326–330.
19 Morier P, Merot Y, Paccaud D *et al.* Juvenile chronic granulocytic leukaemia, juvenile xanthogranulomas, and neurofibromatosis: case report and review of the literature. *J. Am. Acad. Dermatol.* 1990; 22: 962–965.
20 Piorkowski FO. Nevus anemicus (Voerner). *Arch. Dermatol.* 1944; 50: 374–377.
21 National Institutes of Health Consensus Development Conference. Neurofibromatosis: conference statement. *Arch. Neurol.* 1988; 45: 575–578.
22 Stephens K, Kayes L, Riccardi VM *et al.* Preferential mutation of the neurofibromatosis type 1 (NF1) gene in paternally derived chromosomes. *Hum. Genet.* 1992; 88: 279–282.
23 Riccardi VM, Lewis RA. Penetrance of von Recklinghausen neurofibromatosis: a distinction between predecessors and descendants. *Am. J. Hum. Genet.* 1988; 42: 284–289.
24 Goldberg NS, Collins FS. The hunt for the neurofibromatosis gene. *Arch. Dermatol.* 1991; 127: 1705–1707.
25 Marchuk DA, Saulino AM, Tavvakol R *et al.* cDNA cloning of the type 1 neurofibromatosis gene: complete sequence of the NF1 gene product. *Genomics* 1991; 11: 931–940.
26 Horiuchi T, Hatta N, Matsumoto M *et al.* Nonsense mutations at ARG-1947 in two cases of familial neurofibromatosis type 1 in Japanese. *Hum. Genet.* 1994; 93: 81–83.
27 Shen MH, Upadhyaya M. A de-novo nonsense mutation in exon 28 of the neurofibromatosis type 1 gene. *Hum. Genet.* 1993; 92: 410–412.
28 Upadhyaya M, Fryer A, MacMillan J *et al.* Prenatal diagnosis and presymptomatic detection of neurofibromatosis type 1. *J. Med. Genet.* 1992; 29: 180–183.

29 Wertelecki W, Rouleau GA, Superneau DW *et al.* Neurofibromatosis 2: clinical and DNA linkage studies of a large kindred. *N. Engl. J. Med.* 1988; 319: 278–283.

30 Gutmann DH, Wood DL. Identification of the neurofibromatosis type 1 gene product. *Proc. Natl. Acad. Sci. USA* 1991; 88: 9658–9662.

31 Basu TN, Gutmann DH, Fletcher JA. Aberrant regulation of ras proteins in malignant tumour cells from type 1 neurofibromatosis patients. *Nature* 1992; 356 (6371): 713–715.

32 Moss C, Green SH. What is segmental neurofibromatosis? *Br. J. Dermatol.* 1994; 130: 106–110.

33 Stern HJ, Saal HM, Lee JS *et al.* Clinical variability of type 1 neurofibromatosis: is there a neurofibromatosis–Noonan syndrome? *J. Med. Genet.* 1992; 29: 184–187.

34 Sharland M, Taylor R, Patton MA *et al.* Absence of linkage of Noonan syndrome to the neurofibromatosis type 1 locus. *J. Med. Genet.* 1992; 29: 188–190.

6
GENETIC INFLAMMATORY SKIN DISORDERS

The numerous mediators of inflammation, their sources, targets, actions and interactions are beyond the scope of this book. However, the genes for many inflammatory substances, as well as for their receptors and inhibitors, are now known and no doubt have a role in the multitude of hereditary inflammatory dermatoses (Table 6.1).

Psoriasiform conditions

Psoriasis (MIM 177900)

Clinical features

These are too well known to need detailed description here. The disease is characterized by sharply marginated, red, scaly plaques (Figs 6.1) but many clinical patterns exist with or without arthritis; for example, flexural, guttate, small and large plaque, erythrodermic, and localized and generalized types of pustular psoriasis.

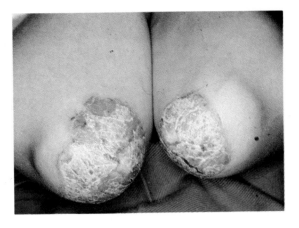

Fig. 6.1 Chronic and typical psoriatic plaques on the elbows.

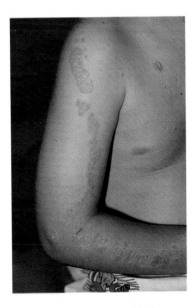

Fig. 6.2 Linear psoriasis is presumably due to mosaicism for the mutant gene.

Table 6.1 Familial inflammatory dermatoses

MIM*	Name
177900	Psoriasis
173200	Pityriasis rubra pilaris
151620	Lichen planus
147050	Atopy
221700	Atopic dermatitis and deafness
106100	Hereditary angioedema
191950	Heat urticaria
120100	Cold urticaria
191850	Aquagenic urticaria
125630	Dermodistortive urticaria (vibratory angioedema)
125635	Dermographism
147540	Hypersensitivity to stings
191900	Urticaria, amyloidosis and deafness
106500	Annular erythema
132990	Erythema nodosum
109650	Behçet syndrome
150590	Leg ulcers
192310	Vasculitis with nodules
Several	Porphyrias
219095	Photosensitivity and colitis
236300	Hooft disease
139000	Granulosis rubra nasi
—	Acne
142690	Hidradenitis suppurativa

* First digit of MIM number indicates inheritance: 1 = autosomal dominant; 2 = autosomal recessive; 3 = X-linked.

Genetic aspects [1]

Psoriasis undoubtedly has a strong genetic component (Fig. 6.2) and Table 6.2 supplies useful information for parents who have one psoriatic child about the risk of other children developing the disease. However, the mode of inheritance is uncertain for the following reasons.

1 Psoriasis may not be a single disease. The different clinical types may represent distinct genetic subpopulations. Early-onset psoriasis is more strongly associated with human leucocyte antigen

Table 6.2 Proportion of siblings of psoriatic probands also affected by psoriasis [2]

Neither parent affected	One parent affected	Both parents affected
8%	16%	50%

(HLA)-CW6 and with a family history of the disease [3] than late-onset disease. The genetic associations of psoriasis also vary strikingly from country to country and from family to family [4].
2 The ascertainment of cases, especially if based on questionnaires [5], is often incomplete. Expression may be minimal and psoriatics do not always advertise their disease.
3 Environmental as well as genetic factors affect psoriasis. This is reflected in the concordance rate of monozygotic twins, which in one study was 72%, although still much higher than the 17% of dizygotics [6]. In another study [7], the concordance rate for monozygotic twins was 35% while that for dizygotic twins was only 12%.

Lomholt's studies and their interpretation. Lomholt's famous and laboriously compiled pedigrees from the Faroe Islands, published in 1963, illustrate many of the difficulties of understanding the inheritance of psoriasis. The findings may even be unrepresentative of less isolated populations but illustrate clearly how the same information can be reworked to provide different answers. Lomholt himself [8] had felt that his data would fit either an autosomal dominant mode of inheritance with incomplete penetrance or with inheritance based on two pairs of autosomal recessive genes. Kimberling and Dobson [9] reassessed Lomholt's families, selecting only those in which at least one child over the age of 21 had psoriasis, and leaving out all subjects, affected or unaffected, who had not been examined by Lomholt. They came down heavily on the side of an autosomal dominant inheritance. Ten years later Iselius and Williams [10] returned to Lomholt's data and used complex segregation analysis, concluding that the pattern of inheritance differed from family to family, being monogenic in some and multifactorial in others.

Finally, Traupe *et al.* [11] have found evidence of genomic imprinting in Lomholt's data as the children of fathers with psoriasis seem to have developed the disease far more often than those with psoriatic mothers. They have also shown that the children of psoriatic fathers are heavier at birth than those of psoriatic mothers.

The precise mode of inheritance is still *sub judice*. The finding of HLA associations (see below) and one large study based on questionnaires [12] support the idea of polygenic inheritance. Further evidence for this is the decrease in risk ratio by a factor of 7 going from the first to the second generation [1]. Other workers prefer the idea of autosomal dominant inheritance with a 60% penetrance, doubting if a polygenic disorder would manifest itself through six generations of one family as has been recorded in psoriasis. The idea of an autosomal recessive mode of inheritance is still favoured by some [13].

Genetic linkages. Studies on genetic markers in psoriasis have shown an over-representation of blood group A (chromosome 9q), the Lewis blood group Le (a-b-) (chromosome 19), the SS type of the MNSs blood group (chromosome 4q28–32) [14] and possibility of slow acetylator status [15].

HLA-associations. The relative risks of the above associations, however, are small (less than three times) compared with those of bearing HLA-CW6 (up to 15) and HLA-DR7 on the human major histocompatibility complex on the short arm of chromosome 6 [16].

Recent analyses using restriction fragment length polymorphisms [17] and pulsed field gel electrophoresis [18] show tight linkage between the HLA-C locus and a gene controlling susceptibility to psoriasis. In Japan a new high-risk haplotype has been found with specific and extensive DNA deletions near HLA-DR genes [19]. In addition, alanine at position 73 of HLA-C molecules seems to be a good marker for psoriasis [20].

Nationality differences are particularly striking in the associations between psoriasis and arthritis, although an increase in HLA-B27 expression is usually found. In English patients, the use of a

DNA probe for the switch region of immunoglobulin heavy-chain genes (on chromosome 14q32), together with a restriction endonuclease, demonstrated a particular polymorphic pattern in 60.7% of patients with psoriatic arthritis but only in 12.2% of patients with psoriasis alone [21]. The same group found no association between arthritis and IgH gene polymorphisms in Italian patients, but a strong association was seen between psoriasis itself and a genotype 5′ of the JH region, giving a relative risk of 27 [22]. These differences are difficult to interpret.

Localized pustular psoriasis does not share the same HLA associations as psoriasis vulgaris, and this supports the argument that it is a different disease. Generalized pustular psoriasis, on the other hand, associates strongly with HLA-B27 and with arthritis.

A psoriasis susceptibility gene on chromosome 17q [4]. Eight multiply affected families with plaque psoriasis have been tested for DNA markers cosegregating with the condition, using a set of polymorphic microsatellites spanning the genome. Linkage to markers at the distal end of chromosome 17q was found when psoriasis was treated as a dominant trait. The maximum LOD score (see Glossary) was obtained when a penetrance of 80% was assumed in the calculations. In families with linkage to 17q, no association between psoriasis susceptibility and HLA-CW6 was found. However, weak associations with HLA-CW6 were found in two families lacking the 17q linkage, but not in two others. This suggests that there may be at least one additional psoriasis susceptibility locus. One possible candidate gene lying within the same region of chromosome 17q is that coding for interleukin enhancer binding factor (ILF).

Pathogenesis

The time has not yet come when the genetic associations mentioned above can be linked in detail to what is known about the pathogenesis of psoriasis. However, the associations with the major histocompatibility complex, and with the heavy-chain gene cluster on chromosome 14, are of great interest now that psoriasis is being thought of as an immunological disease. It has been argued [1] that the relatively high prevalence (about 10%) of psoriasis in CW6-positive individuals reflects the participation of only one major non-HLA predisposing gene.

Psoriasis is a disease of keratinocyte proliferation and inflammation, which follow infiltration by activated T-helper cells and mononuclear cells, and the release of pro-inflammatory cytokines [4,5]. It is possible that, in families showing linkage to 17q, affected members harbour alterations in ILF that alter regulation of interleukin (IL) 2 transcription in such a way that it is expressed inappropriately, thereby triggering the inflammatory and proliferative events characteristic of psoriasis [4].

In addition, monoclonal antibodies raised to streptococcal antigens will bind to keratinocyte products [22]. It has been suggested that memory T cells specific for streptococci may later recognize keratinocytes carrying these antigens and cause them to proliferate. The high prevalence of psoriasis in some northern countries may even relate to a selective advantage conferred against streptococcal infections [23].

Finally, the IL-1 receptor antagonist gene has been put forward as a possible candidate gene, and the HLA gene cluster contains several other genes whose products may be involved in psoriasis such as complement components, tumour necrosis factor α and β and newly discovered peptide transporters [1].

Pityriasis rubra pilaris (PRP) (MIM 173200)

Clinical features

These include varying degrees of hyperkeratosis of the palms and soles, follicular plugging, perifollicular erythema and a red scaly eruption showing characteristic areas of sparing. At least five types have been recognized [25,26]. Inherited PRP tends to be more limited in extent than the acquired type but, in contrast to the ichthyosiform erythrodermas, is not present at birth.

Genetic aspects

PRP occasionally affects several generations of a single family and then an autosomal dominant inheritance seems likely. However, genetic heterogeneity is obvious and relatives are not affected in Griffiths types I and III, and seldom in types II, IV and V [24].

References

1 Elder JT, Nair RP, Guo S *et al.* The genetics of psoriasis. *Arch. Dermatol.* 1994; 130: 216–224.
2 Watson W, Cann HM, Faber EM, Nall ML. The genetics of psoriasis. *Arch. Dermatol.* 1972; 105: 197–207.
3 Henseler T, Christophers E. Psoriasis of early and late onset: characterisation of two types of psoriasis vulgaris. *J. Am. Acad. Dermatol.* 1985; 13: 450–456.
4 Tomfohrde J, Silverman A, Barnes R *et al.* Gene for familial psoriasis susceptibility mapped to the distal end of human chromosome 17q. *Science* 1994; 264: 1141–1145.
5 Valdimarsson H, Baker BS, Jonsdittir I, Fry L. Psoriasis: a disease of abnormal keratinocyte proliferation induced by T lymphocytes. *Immunol. Today* 1986; 7: 256–259.
6 Brandrup F, Hauge M, Hennigsen K, Eriksen B. Psoriasis in an unselected series of twins. *Arch. Dermatol.* 1978; 114: 874–878.
7 Duffy DL, Spelman LS, Martin NG. Psoriasis in Australian twins. *J. Am. Acad. Dermatol.* 1993; 29: 428–434.
8 Lomholt G. *Psoriasis, Prevalence, Spontaneous Course and Genetics.* Copenhagen: GEC GAD, 1963.
9 Kimberling W, Dobson RL. The inheritance of psoriasis. *J. Invest. Dermatol.* 1973; 60: 538–540.
10 Iselius L, Williams WR. The mode of inheritance of psoriasis: evidence for a major gene as well as a multifactorial component and its implication for genetic counselling. *Hum. Genet.* 1984; 68: 73–76.
11 Traupe H, Van Gurp P, Happle R, Boezeman J, Van de Kerkhof P. Psoriasis vulgaris, fetal growth and genomic imprinting. *Am. J. Med. Genet.* 1992; 42: 649–654.
12 Barker JNWN. The pathophysiology of psoriasis. *Lancet* 1991; 338: 227–230.
13 Swanbeck G, Inerot A, Martinsson T, Wahlstrom J. A population genetic study of psoriasis. *Acta Dermato-Venereolog.* 1994; 186 (Suppl.): 7–8.
14 Beckman L, Bergdahl K, Cedergren B, Liden S. Genetic markers in psoriasis. *Acta Dermatov.* (Stockholm) 1977; 57: 247–251.
15 Jimenez-Nieto LC, Ladero JM, Fernandez-Gundin MJ, Robledo A. Acetylator phenotype in psoriasis. *Dermatologica* 1989; 178: 136–137.
16 Elder JT, Henseler T, Christophers E *et al.* Of genes and antigens: the inheritance of psoriasis. *J. Invest. Dermatol.* 1994; 103: 150S–153S.
17 Ozawa A, Ohkido M, Inoko H, Ando A, Tsuji K. Specific restriction fragment length polymorphism on the HLA-C region and susceptibility to psoriasis. *J. Invest. Dermatol.* 1988; 90: 402–405.
18 Nakagawa H, Akazaki S, Tokunaga K *et al.* Major histocompatibility complex markers in Japanese patients with psoriasis vulgaris. *J. Invest Dermatol.* 1990; 94: 558.
19 Nakagawa H, Akazaki S, Asahina A *et al.* Study of HLA class I, class II and complement genes (C2, C4A, C4B and BF) in Japanese psoriatics and analysis of a newly found high-risk haplotype by pulse field gel electrophoresis. *Arch. Dermatol. Res.* 1991; 283: 281–284.
20 Asahina A, Akazaki S, Nakagawa H *et al.* Specific nucleotide sequence of HLA-C is strongly associated with psoriasis vulgaris. *J. Invest. Dermatol.* 1991; 97: 254–258.
21 Sakkas LI, Dermaine AG, Panayi GS, Welsh KI. Arthritis in patients with psoriasis is associated with an immunoglobulin gene polymorphism. *Arthritis Rheum.* 1988; 31: 276–178.
22 Sakkas LI, Marchesoni A, Kerr LA *et al.* Immunoglobulin heavy chain gene polymorphism in Italian patients with psoriasis and psoriatic arthritis. *Br. J. Rheumatol.* 1991; 30: 449–450.
23 Swerlick RA, Cunningham MW, Hall NK. Monoclonal antibodies cross-reactive with group A streptococci and normal and psoriatic human skin. *J. Invest. Dermatol.* 1986; 87: 367–371.
24 McFadden JP. Hypothesis—the natural selection of psoriasis. *Clin. Exp. Dermatol.* 1990; 15: 39–43.
25 Griffiths WAD. Pityriasis rubra pilaris. *Clin. Exp. Dermatol.* 1980; 5: 105–112.
26 Piamphongsant T, Akarphant R. Pityriasis rubra pilaris: a new proposed classification. *Clin. Exp. Dermatol.* 1994; 19: 134–138.

Eczema

Atopy (MIM 147050) [1]

Clinical features

Atopy is a state in which an exuberant production of IgE occurs as a response to common environmental allergens, and atopic subjects may or may not develop one or more of the atopic diseases such as asthma, hayfever and eczema (Fig. 6.3). All of these disorders can usually be

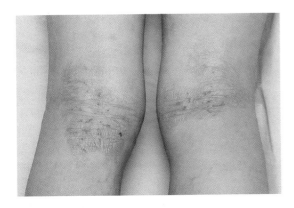

Fig. 6.3 Typical flexural atopic eczema.

recognized on clinical grounds but precise diagnostic criteria have been hard to establish. Those suggested several years ago for atopic eczema [2], for example, are still in the process of being validated [3]. The subject has an extra significance now as epidemiological studies confirm that the preval-ence of atopic disease has risen significantly over the last 30 years [4].

Genetic aspects

A strong genetic component has always been obvious; but so too has a contribution from the environment. For example, exposure to house-dust-mite antigen in the first year of life increases the chance of asthma developing later [5].

Workers investigating the genetics of atopy have had two options: to study IgE levels or to look for the atopic diseases themselves, and of course the two do not always correspond. Up to 30% of those with undoubted atopic eczema, for example, have normal IgE levels.

In 1988, an important paper was published by a multidisciplinary group in Oxford interested in respiratory allergy and defining atopy, not on the basis of clinical disease but as a positive prick test, a positive specific IgE, a high total concentration of IgE or any combination of these [6]. An autosomal dominant mode of inheritance was proposed and a gene important in atopy was mapped to chromosome 11q13 [7]. Inheritance via this locus was found to occur only through the female line [8]. Despite this, atopy can of course be inherited

paternally and the authors felt that the proportion attributable to the locus on chromosome 11 was only about 60%.

Several other groups have failed to confirm linkage to chromosome 11q13 either in the families of those with atopic eczema [9] or with respiratory allergy [10–12]. The reasons for this are still not clear [13,14]. Atopy is a complex condition: genetic heterogeneity and differences in definition, in selection and in race may all have played some part.

Such contradictions have often been seen in earlier clinical studies. Atopic eczema, for example, with a reported concordance rate of 0.86 in monozygotic and 0.21 in dizygotic twins [15], has in its time been said to follow autosomal dominant, recessive and polygenic modes of inheritance. Confusion remains, but recent studies using more precise clinical definitions have demonstrated two interesting phenomena. First, atopic diseases tend to run true to type within each family (intrafamilial organ constancy). In some families most of the affected members will have eczema while in others asthma or hayfever will predominate [16,17]. This has still to be explained. Second, some clinical studies confirm that atopic diseases, whether respiratory or eczematous [18,19] are inherited more often from the mother than from the father.

This echoes the findings of the Oxford group who have now put forward a candidate gene that looks all the more plausible because of their IgE-based definition of atopy. The gene coding for the β subunit of the high-affinity IgE receptor lies on chromosome 11q13 and is closely linked to the suspected gene for atopy [20].

Pathogenesis

These strands of information have still to be woven into a coherent theory and it remains likely that many genes and environmental factors play a part in the pathogenesis of atopic diseases. However, the high affinity IgE receptor is found both on mast cells, important in immediate sensitivity, and on Langerhans cells, important as antigen-presenting cells within the skin. The latter are the only cells in the epidermis to express it [21] and do so especially in atopic eczema [22] in which IgE may be involved in antigen presentation [23]. At last a link may be emerging between the immediate hypersensitivity components of atopy, such as asthma and hayfever, and the delayed ones such as eczema. The well-established associations of atopic eczema with phenyl-ketonuria, Wiskott–Aldrich syndrome, Dubovitz syndrome and hypohidrotic ectodermal dysplasia may also provide clues to pathogenesis.

Contact dermatitis [24]

Allergic (Fig. 6.4)

Animal breeding experiments have shown that the ability to become sensitized to contact allergens is under genetic control [25], sometimes being inherited as an autosomal dominant trait [26]. The genes controlling these reactions have been mapped to the major histocompatibility complex [27].

In humans the picture is less clear-cut. Nevertheless, there are differences between individuals in the ease with which they can be sensitized, and this does seem to be familial. For example, if both parents in a family can be sensitized to dinitrochlorobenzene (DNCB), about 90% of their children can be sensitized too. If only one parent can be sensitized, the corresponding figure for their children is about 50% [28].

Twin studies also confirm the idea of genetic control. In one Danish study the concordance rate of nickel allergy in female monozygotic twins was 0.32, significantly different from that in dizygotic twins (0.14) [29]. The study had the double merit of using unselected twins, entering the register independently of disease, and dealing with only one allergen, as it is known that the ability to become sensitized to one allergen does not automatically imply ease of sensitization to others [30]. Perhaps for this reason, some twin studies using multiple allergens [31] have not confirmed the importance of genetic factors.

There may be human leucocyte-associated antigen (HLA) associations too, in view of those with the major histocompatibility complex in animals. Most studies have been negative but an increase in the HLA class II polymorphism BFF has been found in a group of nickel-sensitive patients [32]. A significant association has also been found between nickel allergy and a *Taq*-1 HLA-DQA allelic restriction fragment [33].

Irritant

The genetics of irritant dermatitis has largely escaped attention. However, a higher degree of concordance has been found in 54 monozygotic than 46 dizygotic pairs with respect to reactions to three well-known irritants (benzalkonium chlor-ide, sodium lauryl sulphate and potash soap) [34]. The skin of atopic subjects is particularly easy to irritate.

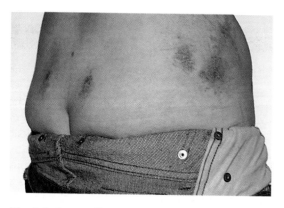

Fig. 6.4 Contact allergy to nickel in jean studs.

References

1 Savin JA. Atopy and its inheritance. *BMJ* 1993; 307: 1019–1020.
2 Hanifin JM, Rajka G. Diagnostic factors of atopic dermatitis. *Acta Dermato-Venereol.* 1980; 92 (Suppl.) 44–47
3 Williams HC, Burney P, Hay RH. The UK diagnostic criteria for atopic dermatitis. *Br. J. Dermatol.* 1922; 127 (Suppl. 40): 75–77.
4 Williams HC. Is the prevalence of atopic dermatitis increasing? *Clin. Exp. Dermatol.* 1992; 17: 385–391.
5 Sporik R, Holgate ST, Platts-Mills TAE, Cogswell JJ. Exposure to house dust mite allergen (Derpl) and the development of asthma in childhood—a prospective study. *N. Engl. J. Med.* 1990; 323: 502–507.

6 Cookson WOCM, Hopkin JM. Dominant inheritance of atopic immunoglobulin-E responsiveness. *Lancet* 1988; 1: 86–88.

7 Cookson WOCM, Sharp F, Faux JA, Hopkin JM. Linkage between immunoglobulin-E responses underlying asthma and rhinitis and chromosome 11q. *Lancet* 1989; 1: 1292–1295.

8 Cookson WOCM, Young RP, Sandford AJ *et al.* Maternal inheritance of atopic IgE responsiveness on chromosome 11q. *Lancet* 1992; 340; 381–384.

9 Coleman R, Trembath RC, Harper JI. Chromosome 11q13 and atopy underlying atopic eczema. *Lancet* 1993; 341: 1121–1122.

10 Amelung PJ, Panhuysen CIM, Postma DS *et al.* Atopic and bronchial hyperresponsiveness: exclusion of linkage to markers on chromosomes 11q and 6p. *Clin. Exp. Allergy* 1992; 22: 1077–1084.

11 Hizawa N, Yamaguchi O, Ohe M *et al.* Lack of linkage between atopy and locus 11q13. *Clin. Exp. Allergy* 1992; 22: 1065–1069.

12 Lympany P, Welsh K, Maccochrane G, Kemeny DM, Tak HL. Genetic analysis using DNA pleomorphism of the linkage between chromosome 11q13 and atopy and bronchial hyper-responsiveness to methacholine. *J. Allergy Clin. Immunol.* 1992; 89; 619–628.

13 Moffatt MF, Sharp PA, Faux JA *et al.* Factors confounding genetic linkage between atopy and chromosome 11q. *Clin. Exp. Allergy* 1992; 22: 1046–1051.

14 Morton NE. Major loci for atopy? *Clin. Exp. Allergy* 1992; 22: 1041–1043.

15 Larsen FS, Holm NV, Henningsen K. Atopic dermatitis. A genetic-epidemiological study in a population-based twin sample. *J. Am. Acad. Dermatol.* 1986; 15: 487–494.

16 Diepgen TL, Fartasch M. Recent epidemiological and genetic studies in atopic dermatitis. *Acta Dermato-Venereol.* 1993; 176 (Suppl.): 13–18.

17 Dold S, Wjst M, Von Mitius E, Retimeir P, Stiepel E. Genetic risk for asthma, allergic rhinitis and atopic dermatitis. *Arch. Dis. Child.* 1992; 67: 1018–1022.

18 Ruiz RG, Kemeny DM, Price JF. Higher risk of infantile atopic dermatitis from maternal atopy than from paternal atopy. *Clin. Exp. Allergy* 1992; 22: 762–766.

19 Kuster W, Petersen M, Christophers E. A family study of atopic dermatitis. Clinical and genetic characteristics of 188 patients and 2151 family members. *Arch. Dermatol. Res.* 1990; 282: 98–102.

20 Sandford AJ, Shirakawa T, Moffat MF *et al.* Localisation of atopy and β subunit of high-affinity IgE receptor (FCERI) on chromosome 11q. *Lancet* 1993; 341: 332–334.

21 Reiger A, Wang B, Kilgus O, *et al.* FceR1 mediates IgE binding to human epidermal Langerhans cells. *J. Invest. Dermatol.* 1992; 9: 305–325.

22 Barker JNWN, Alegre CA, MacDonald DM. Surface-bound immunoglobulin-E on antigen presenting cells in cutaneous tissue of atopic dermatitis. *J. Invest. Dermatol.* 1988; 90: 117–21.

23 Mudde GC, Van Reijsen FC, Bruijnzeel-Koomen CAFM. IgE-positive Langerhans cells and TH2 allergen specific T cells in atopic dermatitis. *J. Invest. Dermatol.* 1992; 99: 1035.

24 Menné T, Holm NV. Genetic susceptibility in human allergic contact sensitisation. *Semin. Dermatol.* 1986; 5: 301–306.

25 Chase M. Inheritance in guinea pigs of the susceptibility to skin sensitisation with simple chemical compounds. *J. Exp. Med.* 1941; 73: 711–726.

26 Polak L, Barnes JM, Turk JL. The genetic control of contact sensitisation to inorganic metal compounds in guinea pigs. *Immunology* 1968; 14: 707–711.

27 Ishii N, Ishii H, Ono H *et al.* Genetic control of nickel sulfate delayed-type hypersensitivity. *J. Invest. Dermatol.* 1990; 94: 673–676.

28 Walker FB, Smith PD, Maibach HI. Genetic factors in human allergic contact dermatitis. *Int. Arch. Allergy* 1967; 32: 453–462.

29 Menné T, Holm NV. Nickel allergy in a female twin population. *Int. J. Dermatol.* 1983; 22: 22–28.

30 Landsteiner K, Rostenberg A, Sulzberger MB. Individual differences in susceptibility to eczematous sensitisation with simple chemical substances. *J. Invest. Dermatol.* 1939; 2: 25–29.

31 Forsbeck M, Skog E, Ytterborn KH. Delayed type of allergy and atopic disease among twins. *Acta Dermato-Venereol.* 1968; 48: 192–197.

32 Orecchia G, Perfetti L, Finco O, Dondi E, Cuccia M. Polymorphisms of HLA class III genes in allergic contact dermatitis. *Dermatology* 1992; 184: 254–259.

33 Olerup O, Emtestam L. Allergic contact dermatitis to nickel is associated with a Taq 1 HLA-DQA allelic restriction fragment. *Immunogenetics* 1988; 28: 310–313.

34 Holst R, Müller H. One hundred twin pairs patch tested with primary irritants. *Br. J. Dermatol.* 1975; 93: 145–149.

The porphyrias

The porphyrias are due to deficiencies in the enzymes involved in haem synthesis (Table 6.3). The abnormal metabolism usually occurs in the liver, although in two varieties (erythropoietic protoporphyria and congenital erythropoietic porphyria) it affects haemopoietic tissue. Accumulated precursors damage the skin, nervous system or both. In general, enzyme defects higher up the pathway cause neurological problems while those further down are most likely to cause skin problems (see Table 6.3). To some extent this corre-lates with the biochemistry and metabolism of the accumulated precursor: earlier metabolites are more water soluble and can be excreted in the urine, whereas the later, water-insoluble metabolites are excreted in the faeces and deposited in the skin.

Some porphyrias are characterized by acute attacks of neurophyschiatric disorder with red porphyrin-laden urine.

Porphyrins in the skin are photoactivated by ultraviolet light of wavelength 400 nm, emitting red fluorescence and generating free radicals [1]. Membrane lipids are particular targets for the activated oxygen, and in the skin this causes inflammation, pain and blistering.

Congenital erythropoietic porphyria (CEP) (Gunther disease) MIM 263700

Clinical features

This is the classical 'werewolf' picture of severe photosensitive blistering with mutilating scars, hypertrichosis and red fluorescence of teeth and urine. Haemolytic anaemia may be due to photohaemolysis in superficial blood vessels.

Table 6.3 The enzymes involved in haem synthesis, and their deficiency disorders

MIM*	Metabolite (*enzyme*)	Disorder		
	Glycine + succinyl CoA			
	↓ *ALA synthase*			
	Aminolaevulinic acid (ALA)			
125270	↓ *ALA dehydratase*	Acute hepatic porphyria		
	Porphobilinogen (PBG)			
176000	↓ *Porphobilinogen deaminase*	Acute intermittent porphyria		
	Hydroxymethylbilane			
263700	↓ *Uroporphyrinogen III cosynthase*	Congenital erythropoietic porphyria	Neurological features (except PCT and CEP) and urinary porphyrins	
	Uroporphyrinogen III			Photosensitivity and faecal porphyrins
176090 176100	↓ *Uroporphyrinogen decarboxylase*	Porphyria cutanea tarda/hepatoerythropoietic porphyria		
	Coproporphyrinogen III			
121300	↓ *Coproporphyrinogen oxidase*	Hereditary coproporphyria		
	Protoporphyrinogen IX			
176200	↓ *Protoporphyrinogen oxidase*	Variegate porphyria		
	Protoporphyrin IX			
177000	↓ *Ferrochelatase*	Erythropoietic protoporphyria		
	Haem			

* First digit of MIM number indicates inheritance: 1 = autosomal dominant; 2 = autosomal recessive; 3 = X-linked.
CEP, congenital erythropoietic porphyria; PCT, porphyria cutanea tarda.

Genetic aspects and pathogenesis

Inheritance is autosomal recessive. This condition is due to mutations in the uroporphyrinogen III cosynthase gene. Damage is caused by an accumulation not of the precursors aminolaevulinic acid (ALA) and porphobilinogen (PBG), but of the abnormal products uroporphyrin I and coproporphyrin I synthesized in haemopoietic tissue. In homozygotes, the enzyme level is less than 20% of normal; in heterozygotes, who are usually asymptomatic, the level is approximately 50%. A cDNA encoding this enzyme was cloned in 1987 [2], and the gene was mapped to 10q25.2–26.3 in 1991 [3]. Mutations have so far been characterized in three patients [4,5]: one was a compound heterozygote with a codon 73 mutation on one allele and a codon 53 mutation on the other (MIM 263700.0001); a second was homozygous for the codon 53 mutation (MIM 263700.0002); a third was heterozygous for mutations in codons 73 and 66 (MIM 263700.0003).

Treatment

Therapy has been attempted with sunscreens, β-carotene, splenectomy, transfusion and charcoal. Theoretically, bone-marrow transplantation should cure the condition but has not been reported. A more radical approach would be autologous marrow transplantation using normoblasts into which the missing gene had been inserted.

Porphyria cutanea tarda (PCT)

This is the most common form of porphyria (Fig. 6.5). Eighty per cent of cases are sporadic (MIM 176090) and 20% are familial (MIM 176100). There is evidence for heterogeneity, even between families with inherited PCT.

Clinical features

Photosensitive blistering appears at any age in patients with the familial form, but usually in middle age in sporadic cases. Fragility, scarring, pigmentary changes and hypertrichosis are also seen on exposed skin. Sporadic PCT may be precipitated by alcohol, oestrogens, iron and polyhalogenated cyclic hydrocarbons as in the epidemic in Turkey caused by wheat contaminated with the fungicide hexachlorobenzene. Iron overload is usually present. Venesection improves the condition.

Genetic aspects

The familial cases show autosomal dominant inheritance.

Pathogenesis

Both forms are due to reduced uroporphyrinogen decarboxylase activity, which in the sporadic form only develops in the presence of certain acquired stresses. Enzyme levels are reduced to 50% in the liver in sporadic PCT, and in liver and extrahepatic tissues in familial PCT. Excessive amounts of uroporphyrin III are excreted in urine and faeces. The gene for uroporphyrinogen decarboxylase has been cloned and mapped to 1q34, and two different mutations have been found in familial PCT. In 1990, Garey *et al.* [6] identified the same mutation in 5 of 22 unrelated families with PCT (MIM 176100.0003): the product of this mutant gene was shorter than the normal protein, lacked catalytic activity and was rapidly degraded. They had previously found a different mutation in the

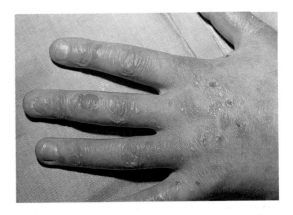

Fig. 6.5 Blistering and milia in porphyria cutanea tarda.

same gene in another patient with familial PCT (176100.0001) [7]. In sporadic PCT, uroporphyrinogen decarboxylase appears to be inhibited by abnormal oxidation products of uroporphyrinogen possibly involving cytochrome P-450 enzymes and iron chelates.

Hepatoerythropoietic porphyria (MIM 176100.0002)

This condition appears to be a homozygous form of PCT. Inheritance is recessive and a specific mutation has been identified in the uroporphyrinogen decarboxylase gene in two unrelated families [8]. It differs from the mutation found in PCT families, which presumably is more severe as it behaves in a dominant manner.

Hereditary coproporphyria (MIM 121300)

Clinical features

This is characterized by both blistering photosensitivity and acute neuropsychiatric attacks.

Genetic aspects

Inheritance is autosomal dominant. Severely affected homozygous individuals have been described [9].

Pathogenesis

The activity of coproporphyrinogen oxidase is 50% in heterozygotes and less than 10% in homozygotes. The gene for this enzyme has been mapped to chromosome 9 [10]. So far there have not been any reports of gene mutations in this disorder.

Variegate porphyria (MIM 176200)

Clinical features

This disorder usually presents in early adult life with photosensitive blistering. Acute neurovisceral attacks may also occur, generally precipitated by drugs.

Genetic aspects

This rare disorder is relatively common in South Africans of Dutch descent. Dean [11] suggested that the 8000 South Africans affected are all descended from the same original settler. The trait is inherited in an autosomal dominant manner but the biochemical abnormality is present without symptoms in about 50% of affected adults. It has been suggested that King George III had variegate porphyria. Several patients have been described who were apparently homozygous for variegate porphyria, protoporphyrinogen oxidase levels being very low in the patients and half normal in both parents [12].

This disorder has not been mapped precisely, but is closely linked to the α_1-antitrypsin locus on chromosome 14 [13].

Pathogenesis

This condition is probably due to deficiency of protoporphyrinogen oxidase. Faecal protoporphyrin and coproporphyrin are elevated during and between attacks.

Erythropoietic protoporphyria (EPP) (MIM 177000)

Clinical features

This disorder classically presents in early childhood with burning pain after exposure to sunlight. Small scars are seen on the face and backs of hands but there is no blistering. Symptoms improve during adolescence. Later, gallstones and liver failure occur due to deposition of protoporphyrin.

Genetic aspects and pathogenesis

EPP is due to mutations in the gene for ferrochelatase, which controls the final step in the synthesis of haem. There is accumulation of the precursor of haem, protoporphyrin, in erythrocytes, bile and faeces. Protoporphyrin is insoluble in water and therefore not excreted in the urine.

Inheritance was initially thought to be autosomal dominant. However, the level of the enzyme is reduced to 10–25% in affected individuals, rather than 50% as expected for a dominant trait [14]. Subsequent studies have suggested that the disorder is either recessive or that inheritance of more than one gene may be required for disease expression [15,16].

Mutations have now been identified in two patients: one (MIM 177000.0001,0002), was a compound heterozygote for two different mutations of the ferrochelatase gene [17], while the other (177000.0003), who had 50% ferrochelatase activity, had a point mutation in only one allele [18]. Thus, the disorder was recessive in the first and dominant in the second.

The ferrochelatase gene has been cloned [19] and mapped to 18q21.3 [20].

Management

Patients benefit from sun avoidance, β-carotene and cholestyramine, which decreases hepatic protoporphyrin content.

References

1 Carraro C, Pathak MA. Studies on the nature of *in vitro* and *in vivo* photosensitisation reactions by psoralens and porphyrins. *J. Invest. Dermatol.* 1988; 90: 267–275.

2 Tsai S-F, Bishop DF, Desnick RJ. Human uroporphyrinogen III synthase: molecular cloning, nucleotide sequence, and expression of a full length cDNA. *Proc. Natl. Acad. Sci. USA* 1988; 85: 7049–7053.

3 Astrin KH, Warner CA, Yoo HW *et al.* Regional assignment of the human uroporphyrinogen III synthase (UROS) gene to chromosome 10q25.2–26.3. *Hum. Genet.* 1991; 87: 18–22.

4 Deybach J-C, de Verneuil H, Boulechfar S *et al.* Point mutations in the uroporphyrinogen III synthase gene in congenital erythropoietic porphyria (Gunther's disease). *Blood* 1990; 75: 1763–1765.

5 Warner CA, Yoo HW, Tsai SF *et al.* Congenital erythropoietic porphyria: characterisation of the genomic structure and identification of mutations in the uroporphyrinogen III synthase gene. *Am. J. Hum. Genet.* 1990; 47 (Suppl.): A83.

6 Garey JR, Hansen JL, Franklin KF *et al.* Uroporphyrinogen decarboxylase: a splice site mutation causes the deletion of exon 6 in multiple families with porphyria cutanea tarda. *J. Clin. Invest.* 1990; 86: 1416–1422.

7 Garey JR, Hansen JL, Harrison LM *et al.* A point mutation in the coding region of uroporphyrinogen decarboxylase associated with familial porphyria cutanea tarda. *Blood* 1989; 73: 892–895.

8 de Verneuil H, Hansen J, Picat C *et al.* Prevalence of the 281 (gly-to-glu) mutation in hepatoerythropoietic porphyria and porphyria cutanea tarda. *Hum. Genet.* 1988; 78: 101–102.

9 Grandchamp B, Phung N, Nordman Y. Homozygous case of hereditary coproporphyria (Letter). *Lancet* 1977; ii: 1348–1349.

10 Grandchamp B, Weil D, Nordman Y *et al.* Assignment of the human coproporphyrinogen oxidase gene to chromosome 9. *Hum. Genet.* 1983; 64: 180–183.

11 Dean G. *The Porphyrias: A Story of Inheritance and Environment*, 2nd edn. Philadelphia: JB Lippincott, 1972.

12 Norris PG, Elder GH, Hawk JLM. Homozygous variegate porphyria: a case report. *Br. J. Dermatol.* 1990; 122: 253–257.

13 Bissbort S, Hitzeroth HW, du Wentzel DP *et al.* Linkage between the variegate porphyria (VP) and the alpha-1-antitrypsin (PI) genes on human chromosome 14. *Hum. Genet.* 1988; 79: 289–290.

14 Bloomer JR. Characterisation of deficient heme synthase activity in protoporphyria with cultured skin fibroblasts. *J. Clin. Invest.* 1980; 65: 321–328.

15 Norris PG, Nunn AV, Hawk JLM, Cox TM. Genetic heterogeneity in erythropoietic protoporphyria: a study of the enzymatic defect in nine affected families. *J. Invest. Dermatol.* 1990; 95: 260–263.

16 Went LN, Klasen EC. Genetic aspects of erythropoietic protoporphyria. *Ann. Hum. Genet.* 1984; 48: 105–117.

17 Lamoril J, Boulechfar S, de Verneuil H *et al.* Human erythropoietic protoporphyria: two point mutations in the ferrochelatase gene. *Biochem. Biophys. Res. Commun.* 1991; 181: 594–599.

18 Nakahashi Y, Fujita H, Taketani S *et al.* The molecular defect of ferrochelatase in a patient with erythropoietic protoporphyria. *Proc. Natl. Acad. Sci. USA* 1992; 89: 281–285.

19 Nakahashi YN, Taketani ST, Okuda MO *et al.* Molecular cloning and sequence analysis of cDNA encoding human ferrochelatase. *Biochem. Biophys. Res. Commun.* 1990; 173: 748–755.

20 Inazawa J, Taketani S, Nakagawa H *et al.* Assignment of the human ferrochelatase gene (FCE) to chromosome 18 at region q21.3 (Abstract). *Cytogenet. Cell Genet.* 1991; 58: 2014.

Other inflammatory conditions

Hereditary angioedema (HAE) (MIM 106100)

Clinical features

The condition is rare but important, as up to 35%

of sufferers die from laryngeal obstruction. Urticaria does not occur, but only about 5% of patients with angiodema without urticaria have the hereditary type.

Attacks usually begin in childhood. The non-itching swellings affect the skin and mucous membranes including the larynx and the intestine, spreading for several hours and lasting for several days. They often seem to be triggered by trauma, notably dental extractions and surgery. A reticulated erythema may be seen as a prodromal eruption [1].

Genetic aspects

HAE is inherited as an autosomal dominant trait. There are two main types, clinically indistinguishable, and both are due to abnormalities in the gene coding for C1 esterase inhibitor, lying on chromosome 11q11–13.1 [2].

HAE Type I is found in 85% of patients, who have abnormally low levels of an apparently normal C1 esterase-inhibitor protein. Type II HAE is characterized by the presence of a dysfunctional mutant protein—levels measured immunologically may appear normal or even high. Several genetic abnormalities have now been described. Patients with type I have either a deleted gene or a truncated transcript due to a stop-codon: patients with type II tend to have a single base substitution.

Pathogenesis

Defective hepatic synthesis of the C1 inhibitor is the basis for its deficiency in the plasma [3]. It regulates the first component of complement (C1) by inhibition of the proteolytic activity of its subcomponents C1R and C1S. This prevents activation of C4 and C2 by C15. During acute attacks, plasma levels of complexes of C1 and C1 inhibitor rise, and the fibrinolytic system is activated [4].

C1 esterase-inhibitor concentrate, if available, is useful for acute episodes and can also be used prophylactically before dental extractions, etc.

Sufferers should avoid angiotensin-converting enzyme inhibitors [5]. Long-term treatments include attenuated androgens such as danazol, which increase synthesis of the C1 inhibitor, and tranexamic acid, which suppresses esterase enzymes. Acute episodes can be helped by esterase inhibitors such as trasylol and ε-amino caproic acid, but resuscitation may be needed.

Acne

Clinical features

Acne is an inflammatory disorder of pilosebaceous follicles, common in adolescence and characterized by comedones, papules, pustules and cysts.

Genetic aspects

A genetic influence is suggested by the fact that a history of acne is more common in parents of children with acne than in parents of children without acne [6], and by the almost complete concordance between monozygotic twins [7]. Cunliffe's group had earlier concluded that monozygotic twins were discordant for acne grade [8] in a study flawed by the fact that few of the subjects studied actually had significant levels of acne [9].

Moderate to severe acne, extending to the forearms, is a feature of Apert syndrome (acrocephalosyndactyly) [10].

Pathogenesis

Acne lesions result from increased sebum excretion, infection and inflammation of the pilosebaceous duct, and hyperkeratosis of the follicular duct.

Of these, the first is certainly under genetic control [7,8]. Sebaceous activity depends on androgens: free hormone levels as well as androgen-receptor activity may be genetically determined. Sebum excretion is greater in males than females and XYY males may have severe acne [11]. A patient with worse acne and greater sebum excretion on one side of the back than the other was presumably genetically mosaic [12]. Another possibly mosaic situation is Becker's naevus, which arises on the upper trunk at puberty in males more often than females, and may show more acne lesions as well as more pigment than the surrounding skin.

Duct hyperkeratosis may also be genetically determined: hidradenitis suppurativa (MIM 142690), another follicular occlusion disorder, appears to be dominantly inherited [13]. Similarly, steatocystoma multiplex is sometimes dominantly inherited (MIM 184500) and, judging from its association with pachyonychia congenita, may be due to a keratin disorder.

Fixed drug eruptions

These occur in the same areas of skin whenever the responsible drug is taken (Fig. 6.6). In one family [14] a genetic predisposition was found to be linked to HLA-B22.

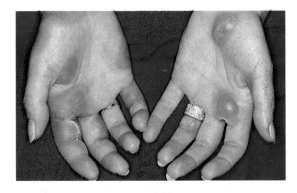

Fig. 6.6 Bullous fixed drug eruption due to barbiturates.

References

1 Williamson DM. Reticulate erythema—a prodrome in hereditary angio-oedema. *Br. J. Dermatol.* 1979; 101: 548–552.

2 Theriault A, Whaley K, McPhadden AR, Boyd E, Connor JM. Regional assignment of the human C1-inhibitor gene to 11q11–q13.1. *Hum. Genet.* 1990; 84; 477–479.

3 Johnson AM, Alper CA, Rosen FS, Craig JM. C-prime-1-inhibitor: evidence for decreased hepatic synthesis in hereditary angioneurotic edema. *Science* 1971; 173: 553–554.

4 Cugno M, Hack CE, de Boer JP *et al.* Generation of plasmin during acute attacks of hereditary angioedema. *J. Lab. Clin. Med.* 1993; 121: 38–43.

5 Megerian CA, Arnold JE, Berger M. Angioedema: 5 years experience with a review of the disorder's presentation and treatment. *Laryngoscope* 1992; 102: 256–260.

6 Liddell K. *Genetic study of acne vulgaris.* MD thesis. Leeds University, 1980.

7 Ebling FJG, Cunliffe WJ. Disorders of the sebaceous glands. In *Textbook of Dermatology*, 15th edn (Champion RH, Burton JL, Ebling FJG eds). Oxford: Blackwell, Scientific Publications 1992: 1717.

8 Walton S, Wyatt EH, Cunliffe WJ. Genetic control of sebum excretion and acne—a twin study. *Br. J. Dermatol.* 1988; 118: 393–396.

9 Moss C. Genetic control of sebum excretion and acne—a twin study (Letter). *Br. J. Dermatol.* 1989; 121: 144.

10 Solomon LM, Fretzin D. Pilosebaceous abnormalities in Apert's syndrome. *Arch. Dermatol.* 1970; 102: 381–385.

11 Vorhees JJ, Wilkins JW Jr, Hayes E *et al.* Nodulocystic acne as a phenotypic feature of the XYY genotype. Report of five cases, review of all known XYY subjects with severe acne, and discussion of XYY cytodiagnosis. *Br. J. Dermatol.* 1972; 105: 913–919.

12 Shuster S. In *Androgens and Anti-androgen Therapy* (Jeffcote SL ed.) Chichester: John Wiley and Sons, 1982: 1.

13 Fitzsimmons JS, Guilbert PR, Fitzsimmons EM. Evidence of genetic factors in hidradenitis suppurativa. *Br. J. Dermatol.* 1985; 113: 1–8.

14 Pellicano R, Ciavarelli G, Lomuto M, Di Giorgio G. Genetic susceptibility to fixed drug eruption. *J. Am. Acad. Dermatol.* 1994; 30: 52–54.

7
IMMUNOLOGICAL
DISORDERS

Autoimmunity

Autoimmune disorders are said to affect up to 4% of most populations [1] and include several conditions, both with and without organ specificity, of importance to dermatologists. They follow complex modes of inheritance in which the effects of multiple genes are entangled with those of the environment.

Autoimmune disorders are presumably due to mutations in genes that play a role in the selective censoring of self-reactive T or B cells. Sometimes their autoimmune aetiology can be proved directly, as when IgG from pemphigus patients causes similar lesions to appear in newborn mice [2]. But proof is less easy when the disease is caused by autoantigen-specific T cells rather than by antibody. Indirect evidence is then needed from animal models.

Further circumstantial evidence includes a lymphocytic infiltration of the target organ, an association with other autoimmune disorders in the same individual or the same family and a statistical association with a particular human leucocyte antigen (HLA) haplotype [3]. Indeed, in humans the HLA complex remains the most firmly established susceptibility region for the breaking of self-tolerance, although animal studies have shown that many other genes of importance in this context are not related to the MHC cluster [4].

The HLA complex

In humans the major histocompatibility complex (MHC) lies on chromosome 6q21.3 and is usually referred to as the HLA complex. Its genes are conventionally divided into three classes but only classes I and II, which encode cell-surface glycoprotein antigens, will be discussed further here. Class III genes are responsible for several components of the complement system.

The overall function of MHC molecules is to collect peptides inside the cell and transport them to the cell surface where they can be surveyed by T cells [5]. Class I antigens, coded by HLA-A, B

and C genes, are found on the surface of all nucleated cells. They are composed of a polymorphic heavy (H) chain and an invariant light chain (B_2 microglobulin). The heavy chain has three extracellular domains that form a peptide-accommodating groove. In addition, three new 'non-classical' class IB genes (HLA-E, F and G) have been discovered [6]. Their roles have yet to be defined.

The class II genes (HLA-DR, DQ and DP) also have many alleles. They code for antigens with two chains (α and β) both of which may be polymorphic. They are expressed on the surface of lymphocytes and antigen-presenting cells.

Despite its complexity, the HLA gene cluster covers a relatively short stretch of DNA and so cross-overs between its components are rare. This results in extended haplotypes that tend to be inherited as discrete units, one from each parent. The number of possible haplotypes is enormous given the large number of alleles at each gene within the HLA complex. However, their distribution in any population is not random as certain combinations of alleles are more common than one would expect by chance. This is an example of linkage disequilibrium.

On the clinical side, two generalizations can be made. First, the inheritance pattern of diseases with strong HLA associations tends to be polygenic; secondly, autoimmunity is often a prominent feature.

Systemic lupus erythematosus (SLE) [7] (MIM 152700)

Clinical features

Many subsets have been defined and it is clear that SLE is both clinically and genetically heterogeneous. Prominent skin features include photosensitivity, facial erythema and nail-fold telangiectasia.

Genetic aspects

SLE is not inherited as a simple Mendelian trait. The difference in concordance rates between monozygotic (24%) and dizygotic human twins (2%) reflects contributions from both heredity and environment [8]. The latter seems to be larger than estimated in earlier twin studies [9]. Concordant twins show similar autoantibody titres and specificities but so do twins discordant for the disease. Discordance is therefore greater in disease expression than in autoantibody production [10].

Pathogenesis

SLE is characterized by an excessive and spontaneous production of antibodies to DNA: it is therefore not organ specific. Several murine models exist in which the development of SLE is clearly genetic and related to the MHC region. In humans, the production of particular autoantibodies seems linked to polymorphisms in the class II HLA-DQ loci [11]; for example, the combination of HLA-DQW2.1/DQW6 is found in many patients with autoantibodies to Ro and La [12]. Other genetic associations in SLE include those leading to deficiency of complement component C4 [13].

Other autoimmune disorders

Familial aggregations of autoimmune skin diseases have often been seen without a clear-cut mode of inheritance being established. Indeed, little light has so far been shed on the general question of whether an autoimmune trait *per se*, defined by the presence of autoantibodies and autoimmune disorders of various types, has itself a specific mode of inheritance. In one large study [14] such an autoimmune trait was found to be inherited in an autosomal dominant manner with a penetrance of 92% for females and 49% for males. The particular type of autoimmunity which developed in each case was thought to depend on the actions of other genes including those of the HLA complex.

Vitiligo (MIM 193200) (Fig. 7.1)

Up to 40% of patients with vitiligo have a family history of the condition [15]. The relative risk for

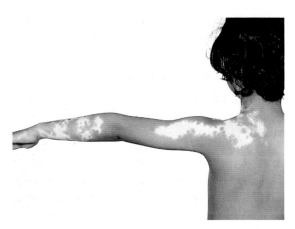

Fig. 7.1 Segmental vitiligo.

relations of affected individuals has been estimated to be 12 for siblings and 36 for offspring [16]. In one large Japanese study, 22% of patients with non-segmental vitiligo were classified as familial: they developed their vitiligo younger than non-familial cases (mean age of onset 24.8 years vs. 42.2 years). Both groups had a similar increased prevalence of circulating autoantibodies to the thyroid and other organs but differed in their HLA associations (familial cases—HLA-BW6; non-familial ones—HLA-A31 and CW4) [17]. The inheritance of familial vitiligo has variously been interpreted as an autosomal dominant trait [18] and along the lines of a multiple recessive homozygous model [19]. Abnormalities have also been recorded in the genes coding for the fourth component of complement [20].

An interesting murine model for vitiligo has been developed [21]: the gene has been mapped to mouse chromosome 6 and is inherited as an autosomal recessive.

Alopecia areata (MIM 104000)

A study of the families of 348 severely affected patients showed that in 7% one of their parents had also been affected. The lifetime risk of a child of an affected parent developing the disease was estimated to be about 6% [22]. The HLA associations of the disorder are still not defined [23,24] but a possible linkage has been suggested with a chromosome 2 gene coding for the immunoglobulin κ light-chain determinant Kml [25].

Pemphigus vulgaris (MIM 169610)

Blisters arise when interkeratinocyte adhesion is reduced by autoantibodies reacting with desmoglein adhesion molecules on their surface. The gene coding for this pemphigus vulgaris antigen has been mapped to chromosome 18 [26].

Familial examples of pemphigus are uncommon but 25 families have now been recorded including 53 affected individuals [27,28]. Their HLA associations have often appeared contradictory and clearly vary with the race of the patient [29]. In one interesting study [30] low levels of pemphigus vulgaris antibody were found in 48% of 120 asymptomatic relatives of 31 patients, exhibiting an apparently dominant mode of inheritance. This inheritance was linked to the MHC (LOD score (see Glossary) of 9.07), usually to a DR4 or DR6 haplotype. The conclusion drawn was that pemphigus occurs in susceptible individuals who already have low levels of antibody after another factor, perhaps environmental, has induced levels high enough to produce blisters.

Lichen planus (MIM 151620)

An autoimmune basis for lichen planus has not been firmly established, nor are its HLA associations clear-cut. Familial examples have occasionally been recorded [31]. Its occasional occurrence in a linear (clonal) distribution strongly suggests an epidermal gene conferring susceptibility to lichen planus.

Systemic sclerosis (MIM 181750)

Familial examples of localized scleroderma and systemic sclerosis have been described. However, it is not clear that the clinical subsets of these disorders share a common genetic background. Certainly their HLA associations are not the same [32].

Several intriguing genetic clues exist but have still to be followed up. Chromosome fragility is a recognized feature of systemic sclerosis with the most common fragile site being at 3p14 [33]. A mutant fibronectin gene was identified in fibroblasts from Japanese but not Dutch patients with systemic sclerosis [34]. Finally, antibodies to topoisomerase I are often found in systemic sclerosis and it has been suggested that this could form a link with collagen gene expression if the DNA flanking these genes were particularly susceptible to the action of topoisomerase I [35].

References

1 Todd JA, Steinman L. Genetic dissection of tolerance. *Curr. Opin. Immunol.* 1992; 4: 699–702.

2 Anhalt GJ, Labib RS, Voorhees JJ, Beals TF, Diaz LA. Induction of pemphigus in neonatal mice by passive transfer of IgG from patients with the disease. *N. Engl. J. Med.* 1982; 306: 1189–1196.

3 Rose NR, Bona C. Defining criteria for autoimmune diseases. *Immunol. Today* 1993; 14: 426–430.

4 Garchon HJ. Non-MHC-linked genes in autoimmune diseases. *Curr. Opin. Immunol.* 1992; 4: 716–722.

5 Rammensee H, Falk K, Rötzschke O. MHC molecules as peptide receptors. *Curr. Opin. Immunol.* 1993; 5: 35–44.

6 Geraghty DE. Structure of the HLA class I region and expression of its resident genes. *Curr. Opin. Immunol.* 1993; 5: 3–7.

7 Harley JB, Sheldon P, Neas B *et al.* Systemic lupus erythematosus: considerations for a genetic approach. *J. Invest Dermatol.* 1994; 103: 144S–149S.

8 Deapen D, Escalante A, Weinrib L *et al.* Revised estimate of twin concordance in systemic lupus erythematosus. *Arth. Rheum.* 1992; 35: 311–318.

9 Block SR, Winfield JB, Lockshin MD, D'Angelo WA, Christian CL. Studies of twins with systemic lupus erythematosus. *Am. J. Med.* 1975; 59: 533–552.

10 Reichlin M, Harley JB, Lockshin MD. Serologic studies of monozygotic twins with systemic lupus erythematosus. *Arth. Rheum.* 1992; 35: 457–464.

11 Arnett FC. Genetic aspects of human lupus erythematosus. *Clin. Immunopathol.* 1992; 63: 4–6.

12 Reveille JD, MacLeod MJ, Whittington K, Arnett FC. Specific amino acid residues in the second hypervariable region of HLA-DQA1 and DQB1 chain genes promote the Ro (SS-A)/La (SS-B) autoantibody responses. *J. Immunol.* 1991; 146: 3871–3876.

13 Fan Q, Uring-Lambert B, Weill B *et al.* Complement component C4 deficiencies and gene alterations in patients with systemic lupus erythematosus. *Eur. J. Immunogenet.* 1993; 20: 11–21.

14 Bias WB, Reveille JD, Beaty TH, Meyers DA, Arnett FC. Evidence that autoimmunity in man is a mendelian

dominant trait. *Am. J. Hum. Genet.* 1986; 39: 584–602.

15 Lerner AB. On the etiology of vitiligo and grey hair. *Am. J. Med.* 1971; 51: 141–147.

16 Majunder PP, Nordlund JJ, Nath SK. Pattern of familial aggregation of vitiligo. *Arch. Dermatol.* 1993; 129: 994–998.

17 Ando I, Chi H, Nakagawa H, Otsuka F. Difference in clinical features and HLA antigens between familial and non-familial vitiligo of non-segmental type. *Br. J. Dermatol.* 1993; 129: 408–410.

18 Lerner AB. Vitiligo. *J. Invest. Dermatol.* 1959; 32: 285–310.

19 Majunder PP, Das SK, Li CC. A genetical model for vitiligo. *Am. J. Hum. Genet.* 1988; 43: 119–125.

20 Venneker GT, Westerhof W, De Vries IJ *et al.* Molecular heterogeneity of the fourth component of complement and its genes in vitiligo. *J. Invest.Dermatol.* 1992; 99: 853–858

21 Lamoreux ML, Boissy RE, Womack JE, Norlund JJ. The vit gene maps to the mi (microphthalmia) locus of the laboratory mouse. *J. Hered.* 1992; 83: 435–439.

22 Van der Steen P, Traupe H, Happle R *et al.* The genetic risk for alopecia areata in first degree relatives of severely affected patients. An estimate. *Acta Dermato-Venereol.* 1992; 72: 373–375.

23. Morling N, Frentz G, Fugger L *et al.* DNA polymorphism of the HLA class II genes in alopecia areata. *Dis. Markers* 1991; 9: 35–42.

24 Zlotogorski A, Weintrauch L, Brautbar C. Familial alopecia areata: no linkage with HLA. *Tiss. Anti.* 1990; 35: 40–41.

25 Galbraith GM, Panday JP. Kml allotype association with one sub-group of alopecia areata. *Am. J. Hum. Genet.* 1989; 44: 426–428.

26 Arnemann J, Spurr NK, Buxton RS. The human gene (DSG3) coding for the pemphigus vulgaris antigen is, like the genes coding for the other two known desmogleins, assigned to chromosome 18. *Hum. Genet.* 1992; 89: 347–350.

27 Feinstein A, Yorav S, Movshovitz M, Schewach-Millet M. Pemphigus in families. *Int. J. Dermatol.* 1991; 30: 347–351.

28 Laskaris G, Sklavounou A, Stavrou A, Stavropoulou K. Familial pemphigus vulgaris with oral manifestations affecting two Greek families. *Oral Pathol.* 1989; 18: 1–53.

29 Ahmed AR, Yunis EL, Alper CA. Complotypes in pemphigus vulgaris: differences between Jewish and non-Jewish patients. *Hum. Immunol.* 1990; 27: 298–304.

30 Ahmed AR, Mohimen A, Yunis EJ *et al.* Linkage of pemphigus vulgaris antibody to the major histocompatibility complex of healthy relatives of patients. *J. Exp. Med.* 1993; 177: 419–424.

31 Katzenelson V, Lotem M, Sandbank M. Familial lichen planus. *Dermatologica* 1990; 180: 166–168.

32 Holzmann H, Sollberg S, Kuhni P. Scleroderma and HLA antigens. *Hautarzt* 1989; 40: 134–140.

33 Tsay GJ, Lan JL, Li SY. Chromosome studies in systemic sclerosis with consideration of antibodies to topoisomerase I. *Ann. Rheum. Dis.* 1992; 51: 624–626.

34 Verheijen R, Oberye EH, Van den Hoogen FH, Van Venrooij WJ. The mutations in the fibronectin gene described in Japanese patients with systemic sclerosis are not present in Dutch patients. *Arth. Rheum.* 1991; 34: 490–492.

35 Briggs D, Welsh KI. Major histocompatibility complex class II genes and systemic sclerosis. *Ann. Rheum. Dis.* 1991; 50 (Suppl. 4): 862–865.

Immunodeficiency

The complex components of a normal immune system act in concert to protect against infection. They are controlled genetically and, inevitably, inherited conditions exist in which these defence mechanisms are abnormal. Several are of particular interest to dermatologists: good examples of this include ataxia telangiectasia (p. 116), Wiskott–Aldrich syndrome (p. 146) and cartilage hair hypoplasia (p. 67). Dermatologists also see patients whose defect lies in resistance to a particular pathogen; for example, epidermodysplasia verruciformis (p. 164), chronic mucocutaneous candidiasis (p. 163) and susceptibility to the herpes simplex virus (MIM 142450).

Sometimes the defect is a general one of humoral or cellular immunity, or both. Although these conditions are more likely to be seen by paediatricians than dermatologists, some are described briefly here after a short discussion of the genetics underlying immunity.

Humoral immunity

This is mediated by antibodies synthesized by stimulated B lymphocytes (plasma cells). Each antibody has to recognize the stereochemical shape of a particular antigen, and as there are a huge number of antigens that may be encountered, the immune system has to be able to make a corresponding number of antibodies. The mystery has always been how so few genes can code for so many different antibodies.

Antibodies are immunoglobulins that share a basic Y-shaped structure made up of two identical heavy (H) chains and two identical light (L) chains held together by disulphide bridges. Both H and L chains have constant (C) regions, variable (V) regions and junctional (J) regions. In addition, the heavy chains have a short diversity (D) region between V and J. Finally, L chains are of two types (κ and λ), and each class of immunoglobulin (IgA, IgD, IgE, IgG and IgM) has its own characteristic H-chain constant region.

The three main gene clusters controlling the κ and λ L chains and the H chains lie on different chromosomes, 2, 22 and 14 respectively. The H-chain gene cluster consists of about 200 variable genes, about 50 diversity genes, six junctional genes, and one or more genes for the constant region of each class of immunoglobulin. The L-chain gene clusters have about 200 variable genes, four junctional genes, a single constant gene and no diversity genes.

A process of gene shuffling (somatic recombination) allows for a huge number of combinations of these different regions in the H and L chains to be created, so that each clone of cells can make its own antibodies with unique binding sites.

The cellular immune system

T lymphocytes which have become differentiated in the thymus recognize foreign antigens using antigen-specific cell-surface receptors with α and β polypeptide chains that have many features in common with immunoglobulins. The gene families responsible for regulating these chains lie on chromosomes 14 and 7 respectively. Their numerous V and J region genes can be rearranged to produce a variety of α and β chains by the same sort of shuffling process that occurs with immunoglobulins. However, for an antigen to be recognized, accessory cells have to present it to T cells in association with the accessory cell's own human leucocyte antigen (HLA) glycoprotein molecules. Cytotoxic T cells recognizing antigen in association with HLA class I molecules, will then kill cells bearing foreign antigens or virus infected cells.

Helper T cells recognize antigen with HLA class II molecules and will then, amongst other things, help B cells to complete their differentiation.

X-linked agammaglobulinaemia (types I and II) (MIM 300300, 300310)

Clinical features

This is the classic example of a disorder of humoral immunity. Affected boys begin to suffer from repeated bacterial infections, often of the ears, lungs and sinuses, from the age of 5 months onwards. Associated features include eczema and pyogenic skin infections.

Genetic aspects

The gene for type I lies on chromosome Xq21.3–22 [1]. It has now been cloned and this means that once a mutation has been defined in an affected individual precise carrier detection and prenatal diagnosis become possible for that particular family [2]. The gene seems similar to the *src* family of proto-oncogenes [3], which mediate cellular signalling pathways regulating proliferation and differentiation.

Pathogenesis

Circulating B lymphocytes are absent whereas B-cell precursors are present in normal numbers in the bone marrow. This lack of B-cell maturation is due to a failure of immunoglobulin H-chain variable region rearrangement [4].

Injections of replacement immunoglobulins can reduce morbidity.

Severe combined immunodeficiencies (SCID)

Clinical features

Affected infants fail to thrive and may have extensive candidiasis. They are highly vulnerable to viral, bacterial and fungal infections. The risk of graft vs. host disease developing after blood transfusions can be lessened by prior irradiation of blood products. Few sufferers survive longer than 2 years without bone marrow transplantation.

Genetic aspects

Several forms exist, most of which are genetically determined. Approximately half of the patients with SCID inherit it as an X-linked recessive trait (MIM 300400; gene mapped to Xq13.1–21.1 [5]) and some 20% as an autosomal recessive trait (MIM 202500) with the relevant gene perhaps lying on chromosome 8 [6].

Some of the remaining patients are examples either of adenosine deaminase (ADA) deficiency (MIM 102700; gene mapped to chromosome 20q12–13.11 [7]) or of nucleoside phosphorylase deficiency (MIM 164050; gene mapped to chromosome 14q11.2). Both enzymes are part of the breakdown pathway of inosine to hypoxanthine.

ADA deficiency and nucleoside phosphorylase deficiency are both good candidate diseases for gene therapy. Little enzyme activity is required to correct the clinical defect completely. Normal ADA genes have already been transfected into haematopoietic progenitors and transplanted back into the patient with apparently good results in the USA [10], and permission has been given for similar work to go ahead in the UK [11].

Two uncommon causes of SCID are also worth mentioning. In the bare lymphocyte syndrome, class II HLA antigens are poorly expressed on lymphocytes. Finally, cartilage hair hypoplasia (p. 67) may be associated with SCID.

Pathogenesis

In the more common types, the thymus, lymph nodes and spleen are poorly developed and levels of circulating B and T cells are low. Little immunoglobulin is formed [8] and cell-mediated immunity is impaired also. The lymphoid precursor cells may fail to differentiate because of a primary defect in the thymus. X-linked SCID is due to mutations in the gene encoding the γ polypeptide chain of the interleukin (IL)2 receptor. This reduces the receptor's affinity for IL-2 and so interferes with T-cell activation and differentiation [9].

Chronic granulomatous disease (CGD)

Clinical features [12]

CGD is rare but much more common in males than females. Infected eczematous lesions of the scalp and face in the first year of life are often the first manifestation, to be followed by furuncles and subcutaneous abscesses that heal slowly leaving draining fistulae. Lymph nodes enlarge and suppurate, and chronic granulomatous infections may involve the lungs, liver and gut. The infecting organism is usually *Staphylococcus aureus* but may be an unusual pathogen such as *Serratia marescens*. Laboratory abnormalities include a neutrophil leucocytosis, anaemia and raised serum levels of IgM, IgG and IgA.

Carriers are not especially susceptible to infection but may have discoid lupus erythematosus and oral ulcers.

Genetic aspects

At least four genetically distinct types of CGD are now recognized. The most common (MIM 306400) is inherited as an X-linked recessive trait. The gene has been mapped to a locus on chromosome Xp21 [13] which encodes the heavy (β) subunit of cytochrome b-245, and so this type is cytochrome b negative. Another cytochrome b-negative type is inherited as an autosomal recessive trait (MIM 233690) and is due to an abnormality in the gene on chromosome 16q24 [14,15], which encodes the light (α) subunit of cytochrome b-245. Two further autosomal recessive types (MIM 233700, mapped to chromosome 7q11.23 [16]; and 233710, mapped to chromosome 1q25 [16]) are cytochrome b positive, being due to a lack of neutrophil cytosol factors I and II, which are necessary to activate nicotinamide-adenine dinucleotide phosphate (NADPH) oxidase.

Pathogenesis

Normal phagocytes kill engulfed bacteria by generating oxidative metabolites such as superoxide and hydrogen peroxide. In CGD, phagocytosis is normal but the cells are unable to deliver activated oxygen into their phagocytic vacuoles. Those pathogens which themselves generate hydrogen peroxide, such as streptococci, may still be killed normally, but others, such as *Staphylococcus aureus*, are not.

The chain of reactions required for this 'metabolic burst' involves NADPH, a flavoprotein and cytochrome b-425. The section on genetic aspects explains how defects at various points in this chain can result in the same phenotype.

The nitroblue tetrazolium (NBT) test depends on the ability of normal phagocytes, but not those in CGD, to reduce this colourless soluble dye to an insoluble blue component. It can be used to detect carriers, only 50% of whose phagocytes will show blue inclusions. It can also be used to make a prenatal diagnosis if performed on fetal blood samples [17]. Bone marrow transplantation has also been tried therapeutically [18] and gene therapy is under consideration [19].

Chediak–Higashi syndrome (CHS) (MIM 214500)

Clinical features

This condition is rare but unmistakable. The skin is pale and the hair has a curious silvery grey sheen. Abnormal susceptibility to infection, particularly of the skin and respiratory tract, leads to death in the first decade. Lymphomatous transformation may be provoked by infection with the Epstein–Barr virus or other viruses.

Genetic aspects

CHS is inherited as an autosomal recessive trait. Similar disorders have been identified in 10 species [20]—the Aleutian blue mink and the 'beige' mouse being the best-known examples. Using the mouse model it has been predicted that the human CHS gene lies on chromosome 1q [21].

Pathogenesis

There is a generalized defect in cytoplasmic granules. Lysosomes fuse to form the pathognomonic giant granules found in circulating neutrophils, renal tubular cells and neurones. Neutrophils show decreased chemotaxis and abnormal degranulation. Melanocytes contain giant melanosomes and the pigmentary dilution is due to a failure to transfer melanin to keratinocytes. The clinically similar Griscelli syndrome (MIM 214450) lacks the characteristic giant granules.

Chronic mucocutaneous candidiasis (CMC)

Clinical features (Fig. 7.2)

The inherited types tend to start in early childhood with persistent oral candidiasis, which is sometimes hypertrophic, chronic paronychia with nail plate involvement, and lesions in the flexures.

CMC has a variety of causes [22]. It may be just one component of the mixture of infections seen in patients with severe combined immunodeficiency disease (p. 161). It may also be part of the autoimmune polyendocrinopathy–candidiasis–ectodermal dystrophy syndrome (MIM 240300), often evident several years before any other manifestation [23]. Finally, CMC may exist in patients in good general health who otherwise have no more than a slight excess of dermatophyte OP human papilloma virus infection.

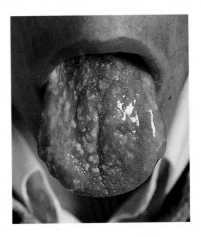

Fig. 7.2 Chronic mucocutaneous candidiasis.

Genetic aspects

Just as CMC has many causes, so it has a matching variety of inheritance patterns. Autosomal recessive [22] (MIM 212050) and dominant [24] (MIM 114580) types exist. Polyendocrinopathy-associated CMC is inherited as an autosomal recessive trait [25]. The relevant genes have not yet been mapped.

Pathogenesis

No consistent pattern of abnormalities in cellular immunity have been found. Iron deficiency is often present but its cause and effects remain obscure.

Epidermodysplasia verruciformis (MIM 303350, 226400)

Clinical features

Skin lesions appear during childhood and persist. On exposed parts they look like plane warts but may fuse on the trunk into plaques resembling pityriasis versicolor. Malignant change may eventually occur, usually into squamous carcinomas on exposed skin. Etretinate may improve the condition.

Genetic aspects

Autosomal dominant [26], recessive and X-linked [27] patterns of inheritance have been described.

Pathogenesis

The immunological defects underlying this heavy and persistent human papillomavirus infection have not yet been classified. HPV types 3 and 10, which cause ordinary plane warts, and many other HPV types specific to epidermodysplasia verruciformis, may be involved. HPV types 5 and 8 are most commonly associated with malignant change, in which ultraviolet light plays an important part as do defects in anti-oncogenes and HLA associations [28].

References

1 Mensink EJBM, Thompson A, Schot JDL *et al.* Genetic heterogeneity in X-linked agammaglobulinemia complicates carrier detection and prenatal diagnosis. *Clin. Genet.* 1987; 31: 91–96.
2 Flinter FA, Vetrie D, Bobrow M. The implications of cloning the XLA gene. *J. Roy. Coll. Phys. Lond.* 1993; 27: 233–235.
3 Vetrie D, Vorechovsky I, Sideras P *et al.* The gene involved in X-linked agammaglobulinaemia is a member of the src family of protein-tyrosine kinases. *Nature* 1993; 361: 226–233.
4 Schwaber J, Chen RH. Premature termination of variable gene rearrangement in B lymphocytes from X-linked agammaglobulinemia. *J. Clin. Invest.* 1988; 81: 2004–2009.
5 Puck JM, Conley ME, Bailey LC. Refinement of linkage of human severe combined immunodeficiency (SCDX1) to polymorphic markers in Xq13. *Am. J. Hum. Genet.* 1993; 53: 176–184.
6 Itoh M, Hamatani K, Komatsu K *et al.* Human chromosome 8 (p12–q22) complements radiosensitivity in the severe combined immunodeficiency (SCID) mouse. *Radiation Res.* 1993; 134: 364–368.
7 Jhanwar SC, Berkvens TM, Breukel C *et al.* Localisation of human adenosine deaminase (ADA) gene sequences to the q12–q13.11 region of chromosome 20 by *in situ* hybridisation. *Cytogenet. Cell Genet.* 1989; 50: 168–171.
8 Lever AML. Gene therapy for genetic, malignant, metabolic and infectious disease. *Proc. of the Roy. Coll. Phys. Edin.* 1993; 23: 424–427.
9 Beecham L. Green light for gene therapy. *Br. Med. J.* 1993; 306: 658.
10 Hendrickson EA, Schatz DG, Weaver DT. The SCID gene encodes a trans-acting factor that mediates the rejoining event of Ig gene rearrangement. *Genes Dev.* 1988; 2: 817–829.
11 Noguchi M, Yi H, Rosenblatt HM, *et al.* Interleukin-2 receptor gamma chain mutation results in X-linked severe combined immuno-deficiency in humans. *Cell* 1993; 73: 147–157.
12 Johnston RB, Newman SL. Chronic granulomatous disease. *Pediat. Clin. North Am.* 1977; 24: 365–376.
13 Baehner RL, Kunkel LM, Monaco AP *et al.* DNA linkage analysis of X chromosome-linked chronic granulomatous disease. *Proc. Natl. Acad. Sci. USA* 1986; 83: 3398–3401.
14 De Boer M, Der Klein A, Hossile JP *et al.* Cytochrome b 558-negative, autosomal recessive chronic granulomatous disease: two new mutations in the cytochrome b 558 light chain of the NADPH oxidase (p22-phox). *Am. J. Hum. Genet.* 1992; 51: 1127–1135.
15 Dinauer MC, Pierce EA, Bruns GAP, Curnutte JT, Orkin SH. Human neutrophil cytochrome b light

chain (p22-phox): gene structure, chromosomal location, and mutations in cytochrome-negative autosomal recessive chronic granulomatous disease. *J. Clin. Invest.* 1990; 86: 1729–1737.

16 Francke U, Hsieh CL, Foellmer BE, Lomax KJ, Malech HL, Leto TL. Genes for two autosomal recessive forms of chronic granulomatous disease assigned to 1q25 (NCF2) and 7q11.23 (NCF1). *Am. J. Hum. Genet.* 1990; 47: 483–492.

17 Gallin JI, Buescher ES, Seligmann BE. Recent advances in chronic granulomatous disease. *Ann. Inter. Med.* 1983; 99: 657–674.

18 Kamani N, August CS, Douglas SD. Bone marrow transplantation in chronic granulomatous disease. *J. Paediatr.* 1984; 105: 42–46.

19 Sekhsaria S, Gallin JI, Linton GF *et al.* Peripheral blood progenitors as a target for genetic correction of p47 phox-deficient chronic granulomatous disease. *Proc. Nat. Acad. Sci. USA* 1993; 90: 7446–7450.

20 Kahraman MM, Prieur DJ. Chediak–Higashi syndrome in the cat: prenatal diagnosis by evaluation of amniotic fluid cells. *Am. J. Med. Genet.* 1990; 36: 321–327.

21 Jenkins NA, Justice MJ, Gilbert DJ, Chu ML, Copeland NG. Nidogen/entactin (Nid) maps to the proximal end of mouse chromosome 13 linked to beige (bg) and identifies a new region of homology between mouse and human chromosomes. *Genomics* 1991; 9: 401–403.

22 Wells RS, Higgs JM, Valdimarsson H, Holt PJL. Familial chronic muco-cutaneous candidiasis. *J. Med. Genet.* 1972; 9: 302–310.

23 Ahonen P, Myllarniemi S, Sipila I, Perheentupa J. Clinical variation of autoimmune polyendocrinopathy–candidiasis–ectodermal dystrophy (APECED) in a series of 68 patients. *N. Engl. J. Med.* 1990; 322: 1829–1836.

24 Sams WM, Jorizzo JL, Snyderman R *et al.* Chronic mucocutaneous candidiasis: immunologic studies of three generations of a single family. *Am. J. Med.* 1979; 67: 948–959.

25 Ahonen P. Autoimmune polyendocrinopathy–candidosis–ectodermal dystrophy (APECED): autosomal recessive inheritance. *Clin. Genet.* 1985; 27: 535–542.

26 Jablonska S, Orth G, Jarzabek-Chorzelska M *et al.* Twenty-one years of follow-up studies of familial epidermodysplasia verruciformis. *Dermatologica* 1979; 158: 309–327.

27 Androphy EJ, Dvoretzky I, Lowy DR. X-linked inheritance of epidermodysplasia verruciformis: genetic and virologic studies of a kindred. *Arch. Dermatol.* 1985; 121: 864–868.

28 Majewski S, Jablonska S. Epidermodysplasia verruciformis as a model of human papillomavirus-induced genetic cancers: the role of local immunosurveillance. *Am. J. Med. Sci.* 1992; 304: 174–179.

8
CHROMOSOMAL
DISORDERS

Chromosomal aberrations have to be large (more than 4 million base pairs) before they can be seen with the light microscope. They are found in 6–7% of all conceptions, but most of these miscarry leaving a live birth frequency of 0.6%. Of these about one-third have abnormalities in the number of sex chromosomes, one-third in the number of autosomal chromosomes and the remainder have chromosomal rearrangements.

Trisomy, the presence of an extra chromosome, is the most common numerical abnormality in those who survive. It arises when homologous pairs of chromosomes fail to separate (non-dysjunction) during meiosis. Gametes are therefore formed with either an extra or a missing chromosome. Non-dysjunction becomes more frequent with increasing maternal age.

Structural aberrations occur if chromosomes break and are rejoined in a faulty position. Such breaks are usually random but some especially 'fragile' sites are recognized. The terminology of chromosomal aberrations is as follows.

Loss of part of a chromosome is a 'deletion'. High-resolution cytogenetic techniques can now detect microdeletions that are responsible for contiguous gene disorders in which associations occur between uncommon disorders, such as X-linked ichthyosis and Kallman syndrome.

Reciprocal translocation occurs when two chromosomes break and exchange their broken-off segments. In a 'balanced' reciprocal translocation there is no loss of DNA and the individual is usually normal although capable of producing 'unbalanced' gametes and therefore chromosomally unbalanced offspring. If both arms of a chromosome break, and their ends fuse, a 'ring' chromosome is formed. An 'inversion' occurs when two breaks in a single chromosome allow a segment to rotate through 180° before the chromosome is reconstituted. Sections of chromosomes may also be duplicated.

One obvious feature of these chromosome abnormalities is that large numbers of genes are involved: the disorders are therefore often serious

Table 8.1 Some chromosomal abnormalities with associated skin features

Disorder	Chromosomal abnormality	Birth frequency	Skin features
Down syndrome	Usually trisomy 21	1/700	See text
Edwards syndrome	Trisomy 18	1/3000	Redundant neck skin; flexed hands with overlapping fingers, single palm creases, hypoplastic nails, abnormal fingerprints; capillary haemangiomas; hypertrichosis
Patau syndrome	Trisomy 13	1/5000	Scalp defects; capillary haemangioma; narrow hyperconvex nails; single palmar crease; redundant neck skin; scrotal penile skin
Supermale	XYY	1/1000 males	Tall with severe acne
Klinefelter syndrome	XXY	1/600	Poor beard and trunk hair; association with systemic lupus erythematosus; risk of leg ulcers
Turner syndrome	XO	1/5000 females	Low posterior hairline; redundant neck skin; multiple pigmented naevi; hypoplastic nails; lymphoedema; keloids
Fragile X-associated mental retardation	Fragile site on X chromosome	1/1000	Hyperelastic skin
Wolf–Hirschhorn syndrome	Deletion of short arm of chromosome 4		Pre-auricular skin tags; sacral dimples; mid-line scalp defects

and tend to involve many systems. Dysmorphic features and mental retardation are common. If a generalization is possible it is that deletions tend to be more harmful than duplications.

Some of the more common chromosomal disorders that have associated skin abnormalities are listed in Table 8.1. Only Down syndrome will be dealt with in detail in the text.

Down's syndrome

Clinical features

These are too well known to need much elaboration here. The condition is found in 1 in 700 live births and a clinical diagnosis can usually be made with confidence on the basis of mental retardation and a variable constellation of abnormalities which include a characteristic facies (medial epicanthic folds, a short nose and an open mouth displaying a large scrotal tongue), irides with areas of decreased pigmentation (Brushfield spots), a single mid-palmar tranverse (simian) crease and incurved little fingers.

The skin is spongy and soft at birth, often with loose folds around the neck. With age, it becomes generally dry and often shows lichenified patches, particularly on the extremities, which are acrocyanotic. A distinctive chronic erythematous follicular eruption may appear on the upper trunk [1]. Syringomas [2] and elastosis perforans serpiginosa [3], are more common than in the rest of the population. So too are alopecia areata [4] and vitiligo, reflecting an increased prevalence of autoimmune disorders. Sweat osmolality is consistently raised [5]. Skin infections are common in institutionalized patients.

Genetic aspects

Trisomy 21 accounts for about 95% of cases, with non-dysjunction arising usually, but not invariably, at the first maternal meiotic division. About 1% of affected individuals are mosaics of normal and trisomy 21 cell lines, and their clinical abnormalities are often less striking. The remaining 4% have a chromosomal rearrange-

ment involving extra chromosome 21 material introduced by one parent who has a balanced translocation. Maternal age is not a risk factor for this sometimes familial type, although it is important in trisomy 21 itself. Screening and prenatal diagnosis [6,7] are not discussed here.

Pathogenesis

This is still not clear. Studies of reciprocal translocations suggest that the errors of gene dosage responsible for the Down's phenotype may relate particularly to the 21q–22 band [8]. It is of interest that several genes important in brain function (e.g. those coding for the amyloid β precursor protein, and for the β subunit of the S-100 protein) lie in this area. Genes encoding collagen VI are also located at the end of the long arm of chromosome 21 and may account for the hypermobile joints and doughy skin of Down syndrome. Chromosome 21, one of the smallest chromosomes, has now been completely sequenced.

References

1 Finn OA, Grant PW, McCallum DI, Raffle E. A singular dermatosis of mongols. *Arch. Dermatol.* 1978; 114: 1943–1944.

2 Butterworth T, Strean LP, Beerman H, Wood MA. Syringoma and mongolism. *Arch. Dermatol.* 1964; 90: 483–487.

3 Rasmussen JE. Disseminated elastosis perforans serpiginosa in four mongoloids. *Br. J. Dermatol.* 1972; 86: 9–13.

4 Du Vivier A, Munro DD. Alopecia areata, autoimmunity and Down's syndrome. *BMJ* 1975; 1: 191–192.

5 Geetha H, Shetty KT. Sweat osmolality in Down's syndrome and cystic fibrosis in an Indian population. *BMJ* 1987; 294: 156.

6 Connor M. Biochemical screening of Down's syndrome. *BMJ* 1993; 306: 1705–1706.

7 Mutton DE, Ide R, Alberman E, Bobrow M. Analysis of national register of Down's syndrome in England and Wales: trends in prenatal diagnosis 1989–91. *BMJ* 1993; 306: 431–432.

8 Williams JD, Summit RL, Martens PR. Familial Down's syndrome due to t (10; 21) translocation: evidence that the Down phenotype is related to trisomy of a specific segment of chromosome 21. *Am. J. Hum. Genet.* 1975; 27: 478–485.

9
ANTENATAL DIAGNOSIS AND GENE THERAPY

Antenatal diagnosis

Most genodermatoses can easily be lived with; a few rare ones cannot. Families at high risk of the latter will want to ensure that no more of their members are affected and will require prenatal diagnoses at as early a stage as possible, so that selective termination is easy and safe.

Before undertaking prenatal diagnosis with any of these methods, several questions have to be asked.

1 Is the family diagnosis certain? This has to be confirmed by reassessment of the family history and medical records, and perhaps by a re-examination of affected members.

2 Is the condition severe enough to justify the risks of the procedure? The couple concerned are the best judges of this and their informed consent is needed. Estimates of fetal loss rates are 2% for chorionic villus sampling, 0.5% for amniocentesis and 5% for fetal biopsy.

3 Are the parents prepared to act on the results? Some may be opposed to selective termination.

4 Is an accurate radiological or *in vitro* test available for this condition?

5 What is the most suitable procedure?

Several techniques [1] are available but those based on DNA analyses score over fetoscopy and fetal skin biopsy.

(a) *Ultrasonography* and perhaps radiography will detect major deformities but are not helpful for most skin disorders.

(b) *Fetoscopy and fetal skin biopsy* [2]: these are usually performed at 18–20 weeks to allow the skin to develop sufficiently for a diagnostic pathology to be recognized with confidence. A fibreoptic fetoscope can be introduced into the amniotic cavity via an abdominal puncture. Biopsies are obtained under direct vision using special biopsy forceps. Alternatively, skin samples can be obtained using ultrasound to position the forceps. The full-thickness skin samples can be examined with the light and electron microscopes and in other ways for diagnostic abnormalities. Table 9.1 lists the skin conditions in which this technique has been found useful [3]

(c) *Amniocentesis* is seldom performed before the 14th week, and the few cells derived from the fetus have to be cultured, sometimes for several weeks, until there are enough for testing. Amplification with the polymerase chain reaction (PCR) can overcome problems with a low yield of cells [4]. This technique can be used for chromosome and DNA analysis, and to study inherited metabolic disorders and abnormalities of DNA repair, but not for disorders only diagnosable on the basis of skin structure.

(d) *Chorionic villus sampling* can be performed as early as 8–11 weeks of gestation. The specimen is obtained via a small flexible catheter guided through the cervix or transabdominally. The latter seems to carry the lower risk of infection. The samples can be used for the same studies as amniocentesis. It supplies more DNA and can be performed earlier than amniocentesis but its fetal loss rate is higher (2% vs. 0.5%). Success has been achieved in the prenatal diagnosis of recessive dystrophic epidermolysis bullosa [5].

(e) *Preimplantation diagnosis* lies in the future [5]. A single cell could be removed from the eight-cell blastocyst stage of *in vitro* fertilized embryos. The DNA in this cell could be amplified using the PCR and then checked for mutations in the candidate gene. Only blastocysts not containing the mutation would be implanted in the uterus using routine *in vitro* fertilization procedures, thereby ensuring that only unaffected children will be conceived.

Gene therapy [6]

Current treatments for genetic disease are exercises in damage limitation that aim only to minimize the biological consequences of gene mutation. Too often they are not effective. One study of 351 major single gene disorders showed that a normal lifespan was achieved in only 15% and a normal social life in 6%. Treatment was ineffective in 48% [7]. The general argument applies equally to inherited skin disorders even though mortality is lower.

Gene therapy has now been recognized officially as a logical alternative. A government committee

Table 9.1 Conditions in which fetal skin biopsy has been useful [3]

Epidermolysis bullosa	Junctional, recessive and dominant dystrophic, and simplex types
Disorders of keratinization	Bullous and non-bullous congenital ichthyosiform erythrodermas, harlequin ichthyosis, Sjögren–Larsson syndrome
Disorders of pigmentation	Tyrosinase-negative albinism, incontinentia pigmenti
Ectodermal dysplasias	X-linked hypohidrotic and autosomal recessive anhidrotic types
Others	Tay syndrome, Chediak–Higashi syndrome, Griscelli disease, restrictive dermopathy

[8] concluded that it 'offers for the first time the prospect of effective treatment and cure in many genetic diseases'. The committee did not give blanket approval for all types of gene therapy. It did not sanction genes being introduced into germ cells so that they could be passed on to future generations. Major ethical issues would then come into play. Nor did it condone attempts to tamper with personality, intelligence or physique. In contrast, somatic gene therapy for specific genetic diseases, introducing a normal gene into an appropriate tissue but not into the germ line, seems to raise no greater ethical problems than well-established procedures such as blood transfusion.

Gene therapy and the skin

The rules governing gene therapy apply here as to other organs. Candidate diseases are likely to be those controlled by single genes and inherited in a recessive manner. Their prognosis with and without treatment must be known. The gene must have been isolated and its major regulatory regions defined. Appropriate target cells must be available and safe vectors are needed to introduce the gene into them. Preliminary animal work must have shown that genes inserted in this way will work effectively and long term.

The skin has a number of advantages that make it a particularly attractive target for somatic gene therapy [9,10]. Access to skin cells presents no problem. Keratinocytes, melanocytes and fibroblasts can be obtained, cultured and to some extent replaced. However, most of them are already likely to be terminally differentiated. Only if a gene is inserted into skin stem cells will it persist long term *in vivo*; much work is still needed on how to recognize and isolate these cells.

Easy access carries two other advantages. First, should the transgene have deleterious effects, the cells carrying it can be removed. Secondly, it may be possible to modify the expression of transgenes by topical means. For example, if a steroid-sensitive promoter had also been inserted into the target cells, local steroid applications could perhaps be used to regulate gene expression [9].

The future

The potential dangers of gene therapy have to be taken seriously. Can engineered vector viruses themselves ever cause disease? Where do the inserted genes go in the genome? Can they ever interfere with genes critical for cell survival or activate oncogenes and so cause neoplastic change?

If questions of this sort can be answered, two obvious lines of progress lie ahead. In the first, genes inserted into fibroblasts or keratinocytes can be used to create substances that pass into the circulation and restore deficiencies in inherited metabolic diseases. Animal models already exist in which human growth hormone [11] and factor IX [12] genes have remained active in human keratinocytes grafted subcutaneously into nude mice.

The second approach must be to look at gene therapy for skin diseases that are themselves due to inherited abnormalities of keratinocytes or fibroblasts. Already, steroid sulphatase deficiency has been corrected by gene transfer in cultured keratinocytes from patients with X-linked ichthyosis [13]. Attempts are being made to use a topical liposomally delivered endonuclease repair enzyme in xeroderma pigmentosum: an obvious alternative would be to insert the normal gene for the repair enzyme into keratinocytes. Similarly, in recessive epidermolysis bullosa, inserting a normal type VII collagen gene into keratinocytes might be helpful even if the treatment could be used only in skin areas where the disease is most severe.

Gene therapy clearly has immense potential, but it is not for the immediate future [14]. The appropriate attitude is one of guarded optimism.

References

1 Anton-Lamprecht I. Prenatal diagnosis of genodermatoses. *Analysis* 1992; 7 (Suppl.); 131–155.

2 Eady RAJ. Fetoscopy and fetal skin biopsy for prenatal diagnosis of genetic skin disorders. *Semin. Dermatol.* 1988; 7: 2–8.

3 Holbrook KA, Smith LT, Elias S. Prenatal diagnosis of genetic skin disease using fetal skin biopsy samples. *Arch. Dermatol.* 1993; 129: 1437–1454.

4 Fisk NM, Bower S. Fetal blood sampling in retreat. *BMJ* 1993; 307: 143–144.

5 Christiano AM, Uitto J. DNA-based prenatal diagnosis of heritable skin diseases. *Arch. Dermatol.* 1993; 129: 1455–1459.

6 Davies K, Williamson B. Gene therapy begins. *BMJ* 1993; 306: 1625–1626.

7 Lever AML. Gene therapy for genetic, malignant, metabolic and infectious disease. *Proc. Roy. Coll. Phys. Edin.* 1993; 23: 424–427.

8 Clothier C. *Report of the Committee on the Ethics of Gene Therapy.* London: HMSO, 1992.

9 Vogel JC. Keratinocyte gene therapy. *Arch. Dermatol.* 1993; 129: 1478–1483.

10 Greenhalgh DA, Rothnagel JA, Roop DR. Epidermis: an attractive target tissue for gene therapy. *J. Invest. Dermatol.* 1994; 103: 63S–69S.

11 Morgan JR, Barrandon Y, Green H, Mulligan RC. Expression of an exogenous growth hormone gene by transplantable human epidermal cells. *Science* 1987; 237: 1476–1479.

12 Gerrard AJ, Hudson DL, Brownlee GG, Watt FM. Towards gene therapy for hemophilia B using primary human keratinocytes. *Nat. Genet.* 1993; 3: 180–183.

13 Jensen TG, Jensen UB, Ibsen HH *et al.* Correction of steroid sulfatase deficiency by gene transfer into basal cells of tissue cultured epidermis from patients with recessive X-linked ichthyosis. *Exp. Cell Res.* 1993; 209: 392–397.

14 Krueger GG, Morgan JR, Jorgensen CM *et al.* Genetically modified skin to treat disease: potential and limitations. *J. Invest. Dermatol.* 1994; 103: 76S–84S.

APPENDICES

A: LOCALIZATION OF DERMATOLOGICAL GENES

In the following table, chromosomes are listed in numerical order. Chromosome regions are numbered outwards from the centromere (cen) along the short (p) and long (q) arms. Status indicates whether the localization is tentative (t), provisional (p) or confirmed (c). There are many more genes of possible relevance, particularly immune-related genes, in addition to these listed here.

Chromosome region	MIM	Locus name (deficiency disease)	Status
1 p36	155600	Dysplastic naevus syndrome	t
1 p34	176100	Uroporphyrinogen decarboxylase (porphyria cutanea tarda)	c
1 cen–q32	233710	Neutrophil cytosolic factor 2 (chronic granulomatous disease autosomal 2)	p
1 q21	135940	Profilaggrin/filaggrin	p
1 q21–q22	147360	Involucrin	p
1 q22–q25	131210	Endothelial adhesion molecule	c
1 q23	147139/40	Receptors for Fc fragments of IgE	c
1 q23	146740/90	Receptors for Fc fragments of IgG	c
1 q23–q25	153240	Lymphocyte adhesion molecule 1	p
1 q25	233710	Chronic granulomatous disease (cytochrome b +ve)	p
1 q31	150290	Laminin β_2 polypeptide	c
1 q32	120830/1	Complement binding proteins	p
1 q32	120620/50	Complement receptors	c
1 q43	131390	Nidogen (entactin)	p
1 q	278700	Xeroderma pigmentosum group A	p
1		Epidermolysis bullosa simplex	t
1	133200	Erythrokeratoderma variabilis	p
1	152445	Loricrin	p
1		Trichohyaline	p
2 p12	147200	Immunoglobulin κ constant region	c
2 p	101850	Focal acral hyperkeratosis of Costa	p
2 q13–q21	176860	Protein C (coumarin skin necrosis)	c
2 q21	133510	ERCC-3 (xeroderma pigmentosum group B)	c
2 q31–q37		HOX gene cluster	p
2 q31–q32.3	120180	Collagen III α_1 (Ehlers–Danlos syndrome IV)	c
2 q32–q33	120190	Collagen V α_2	c
2 q34–q36	135600	Fibronectin (Ehlers–Danlos syndrome X)	c
2 q35	125660	Desmin	c
2 q35–37	120070	Collagen IV α_3	p
2 q37	120250	Collagen VI α_3	p
2 q37	193500	PAX-3 (Waardenburg syndrome)	c
2		Integrin α_6	p
3 p24	180220	Retinoic acid receptor beta	c
3 p	193300	Von Hippel–Lindau disease	c
3 q28–q29	155750	Melanoma-associated antigen p97	c
3 q26.3	122470	Cornelia de Lange syndrome	p
3	120120	Collagen VII (dystrophic epidermolysis bullosa)	p

179

Continued on p. 180

Chromosome region	MIM	Locus name (deficiency disease)	Status
4 p16.3	134934	Fibroblast growth factor receptor 3	p
4 p16–p16.1	142983	*HOX-7*	c
4 p16	194190	Wolf–Hirschhorn syndrome	c
4 q12–q21	172800	Piebald trait	c
4 q21	165190	Fibroblast growth factor 5	p
4 q21	155730	Melanoma growth stimulating activity	c
4 q25	131530	Epidermal growth factor	c
4 q25–q27	134920	Fibroblast growth factor (basic)	c
4 q28	134820, 30, 50	Fibrinogen polypeptides	c
4 q28–q31	181600	Sclerotylosis of Huriez	p
4 q	266300	Hair colour (red)	t
5 p14–p12	120940, 217050/70	Complement components	c
5 p14–p12	262500	Growth-hormone receptor	c
5 q21.22	175100	Adenomatosis polyposis coli/Gardner syndrome	c
5 q23.31	153455	Lysyl oxidase	c
5 q23.3–q31.2	121050	Fibrillin (congenital contractural arachnodactyly)	p
5 q31–q32	138040	Glucocorticoid receptor	c
5 q31.3–q33.2	134910	Fibroblast (endothelial) growth factor (acidic)	c
5 q31–q34	222600	Diastrophic dysplasia	p
5 q33–qter		Fibroblast growth factor receptor	p
5	278720	Xeroderma pigmentosum group C	
6 pter–p21	125647	Desmoplakin I and II	p
6 p21.3	217000, 120810	Complement components 2,4 (lupus erythematosus)	c
6 p21.3		Class I and II major histocompatibility complexes	c
6 p12–11	113810	Bullous pemphigoid antigen 1	c
6 q24–q27	133430	Estrogen receptor	c
7 p15–p14	186970	T-cell receptor γ cluster	c
7 p15–p14	142950	*HOX-1*	c
7 p13–p12	131550	Epidermal growth factor receptor	c
7 q11.2	130160	Elastin	p
7 q11.23	233700	Neutrophil cytosolic factor 1 (chronic granulomatous disease autosomal 1)	p
7 q21.3–q22.1	120160	Collagen I α_2	c
7 q21.3–q22.1	166220	Osteogenesis imperfecta IV	c
7 q22–q31	150240	Laminin B_1 polypeptide (cutis laxa with marfanoid phenotype)	c
7 q35	186930	T-cell receptor β cluster	c
7	173325	Desmoplakin III/plakoglobin	p
8 q24.12	190350	Trichorhinophalangeal syndrome type I	c
8 q24.11–q13	150230	Trichorhinophalangeal syndrome type II	c
8	131950	Epidermolysis bullosa simplex (Ogna)	p
9 pter–p22	115501	Tyrosinase related protein	c
9 p13–p22	155600	Familial melanoma	p
9 p	125645	Desmocollin 1	p
9 q22.3–q31	109400	Gorlin syndrome	c
9 q22–q31	132800	Self-healing epitheliomas	p
9 q34.1	278700	Xeroderma pigmentosum group A	c
9 q33	120900	Complement 5	c
9 q34.1–q34.2	191100	Tuberous sclerosis 1	c
9 q34.2–q34.3	120215	Collagen V α_1	p
9 q34	161200	Nail–patella syndrome 1	c

Continued

Chromosome region	MIM	Locus name (deficiency disease)	Status
9	121300	Coproporphyrinogen oxidase (coproporphyria)	c
9	187380	Tenascin	p
10p13	193060	Vimentin	c
10p11.2	135631	Fibronectin receptor β polypeptide	c
10q11	133540	ERCC-6 (Cockayne syndrome group B)	p
10q11.2	171400, 162300	Multiple endocrine neoplasias IIA and B	c
10q22–q23	193065	Vinculin	c
10q25.2	263700	Uroporphyrinogen III synthase (congenital erythropoietic porphyria)	p
11pter–p15.4	130650	Beckwith–Wiedemann syndrome	c
11p15.4	114130	Calcitonin/calcitonin-related peptide α	c
11p15	148022	Cuticle keratin	p
11p14.2–p12	114160	Calcitonin-related peptide β	c
11q12–q13.1	106100	Complement component 1 esterase inhibitor (hereditary angioedema)	c
11q12–q13	147050	Atopy (allergic asthma and rhinitis)	c
11q13	148021	Cuticle keratin	c
11q14–q21	203100	Tyrosinase (oculocutaneous albinism)	c
11q22–q23	191090	Tuberous sclerosis 2	p
11q21–q22	226600	Collagenase	c
11q22–q23	208900	Ataxia telangiectasia groups A,C,D	c
11q22–q23	264080	Progesterone receptor	c
11q23–qter	176000	Porphobilinogen deaminase (acute intermittent porphyria)	c
12p13	134921	Fibroblast growth factor 6	p
12q11–q13		Keratin type II gene cluster (epidermolytic hyperkeratosis, epidermolysis bullosa simplex)	c
12q11–q13	135620	Fibronectin receptor alpha polypeptide	p
12q12–q13	155740	Melanoma antigen 1	p
12q12–q13	142970	*HOX* 3 region	c
12q13	180190	Retinoic acid receptor gamma	c
12q22–q24.1	191091	Tuberous sclerosis 3	t
12q23–q24	124200	Darier's disease	c
12q24.1	261600	Phenylalanine hydroxylase (phenylketonuria)	c
13q33	133530	Excision repair cross-complementing (*ERCC-5*)	c
13q34	120130, 120090	Collagen IV α_1 and α_2	c
14q11.2	186880, 186810	T-cell receptor α and δ	c
14q11.2	164050	Nucleoside phosphorylase (severe combined immunodeficiency)	c
14q32.1	107400	α_1-antitrypsin	c
14q32.33		Immunoglobulin heavy-chain gene cluster	c
14q32–q33	158000	Monilethrix	
14q	176200	Protoporphyrinogen oxidase (variegate porhyria)	p
15q11–q13	203200	P gene (oculocutaneous albinism type II)	c
15q13–q15	109710	β_2 microglobulin regulator	c
15q21.1	134797	Fibrillin 1 (Marfan syndrome)	c
15q21–q22.2	109700	β_2 microglobulin	
c15q25–qter	120340	Collagen 1 α receptor	p
15	278760	Xeroderma pigmentosum group F	p
15	180230	Retinoic acid binding protein 5	p
16p13.3	180849	Rubinstein–Taybi syndrome	p
16p13	191100	Tuberous sclerosis	p
16q21	120360	Collagenase IVA (basement membrane)	c

Continued on p. 182

Chromosome region	MIM	Locus name (deficiency disease)	Status
16q22.1	276600	Tyrosine amino-transferase (Richner–Hanhart syndrome)	c
16q24	233690	Cytochrome b-245 α polypeptide (chronic granulomatous disease)	p
17p12–p11		Keratin type 1 gene cluster	c
17q11.2	162200	Von Recklinghausen neurofibromatosis (NF-1)	c
17q11–qter		Integrin β_4	p
17q12–q23		Keratin type 1 gene cluster (epidermolytic hyperkeratosis, epidermolysis bullosa simplex, pachyonychia congenita)	p
17q21.1	180240	Retinoic acid receptor α	c
17q21.3–q22	120150	Collagen 1 α_1 (Ehlers–Danlos VIIB)	c
17q21–q22		HOX-2	c
17q22–q24	139250/40	Growth hormone 1 and 2	c
17q23–q25	146630	Intercellular adhesion molecule 2	p
17q		Fibrillin	
18p11.32–p11.2	150320	Laminin A polypeptide	p
18q21.3	177000	Ferrochelatase (erythropoietic protoporphyria)	p
18	125670	Desmoglein I	p
19p13.3	151445	Receptor for Fc fragment of IgE	c
19p13.3–p13.2	120700	Complement component 3	c
19p13.3–p13.2	147840	Intercellular adhesion molecule 1	c
19p13.3–p13.2	147670	Insulin receptor (acanthosis nigricans)	c
19p	135631	Fibronectin receptor β polypeptide-like	c
19cen–q13.11	170100	Peptidase D (prolidase deficiency)	c
19q13.3	126380	ERCC-1	c
19q13.3	126340	ERCC-2 (xeroderma pigmentosum group D)	p
19	147840	Intercellular adhesion molecule 1 (CD54)	p
19	227240	Green/blue eye colour	p
19	113750	Brown hair colour	p
20q12–q13.11	102700	Adenosine deaminase (subacute combined immunodeficiency)	c
20q13.2	139320	Stimulatory guanine nucleotide binding protein (McCune–Albright syndrome)	c
20q	227650	Fanconi anaemia	c
21q22.3	120220	Collagen VI α_1	c
21q22.3	120240	Collagen VI α_2	c
21q22.3		Down syndrome chromosome region	c
22q11–q13.1	101000	Bilateral acoustic neuromas (NF-2)	c
22q11.1–11.2	147220	Immunoglobulin light-chain λ gene cluster	c
X p22.32	302950	Chondrodysplasia punctata, X-linked recessive	c
X p22.32	308100	Steroid sulphatase (X-linked ichthyosis)	c
X p22.31	305600	Goltz focal dermal hypoplasia	c
X p22.2–p22.1	303600	Coffin–Lowry syndrome	c
X p22.2–p21.2	308800	Keratosis follicularis spinulosa decalvans	p
X p21.1	306400	Cytochrome b-254 β polypeptide (chronic granulomatous disease)	c
X p11.3–p11.21	301000	Wiskott–Aldrich syndrome	c
X p11.21–cen	308300	Incontinentia pigmenti (sporadic)	c
X q12	313700	Androgen receptor (testicular feminization)	c
X q12–q13.1	305100	Hypohidrotic ectodermal dysplasia	c
X q13.1–q21.1	300400	Severe combined immunodeficiency	c
X q13.2	314670	X-chromosome inactivation centre	c
X q13.2–q13.3	309400	Menkes syndrome	c

Continued

Chromosomes region	MIM	Locus name (deficiency disease)	Status
X q21.3–q22	300300	X-linked agammaglobulinaemia	c
X q21.3–q22	301500	α-galactosidase (Fabry disease)	c
X q25–q27	300700	Albinism–deafness	c
X q27–q28	305000	Dyskeratosis congenita	c
X q26–q28	308310	Incontinentia pigmenti (familial)	c
X q28	308840	L1 cell-adhesion molecule	c
X	302000	Epidermolysis bullosa, macular type	p
X	302960	Chondrodysplasia punctata, X-linked dominant	p
Yq11		Steroid sulphatase pseudogene	

Further reading

Moss C. Dermatology and the human gene map. *Br. J. Dermatol.* 1991; 124: 3–9.

Human Gene Mapping 11 (1991) Eleventh International Workshop on human gene mapping. *Cytogenet. Cell Genet.* 1991; 58: 1–2197.

B: SUPPORT GROUPS FOR FAMILIES OF PATIENTS WITH GENETIC SKIN DISORDERS

Albino Fellowship
Mr Henry McDermott, 16 Neward Crescent, Prestwick,
Ayrshire, Scotland KA9 2JB, Tel. 0292-70336

Ataxia Telangiectasia Society
Mrs Glynis Watkins, 42 Parkside Gardens, Wollaton,
Nottingham NG8 2PQ, Tel. 0602-287025

Rare Unspecified Chromosome Disorder Support Group
Mrs Edna Knight, 160 Lockett Road, Harrow Weald,
Middlesex HA3 7NZ, Tel. 081-863-3557

Chronic Granulomatous Disease Support Group/ Research Trust
Rene and Paul Numan, Seafields, Shootersway
Lane, Berkhamstead, Hertfordshire HP4 3NP,
Tel. 0442-863116

Cockayne Syndrome Contact Group
Mrs A Khan, 18 Eden Way, Brickhill, Bedford MK41 7EP,
Tel. 0234-270417

Cornelia de Lange Syndrome Foundation
29 Victoria Avenue, Grays, Essex RM16 2RL,
Tel. 0375-376439

Down's Syndrome Association
Information Officer, 155 Mitcham Rd, London SW17 9PG,
Tel. 081-682-4001, Fax. 081-682-4012

Dystrophic Epidermolysis Bullosa Research Association (DEBRA)
Mr John Dart, Suite 4, 1 Kings Rd, Crowthorne, Berkshire
RG11 7BG, Tel. 0344-771961, Fax. 0344-762-777

Ectodermal Dysplasia Contact/Support Group
c/o Contact a Family, 16 Strutton Ground, London SWIP
2HP, Tel. 071-222-2695

National Eczema Society
Mrs Tina Funnell, 4 Tavistock Place, London WCIH 9RA,
Tel. 071-713-0377, Fax. 071-713-0733

Ehlers–Danlos Support Group
Mrs Valerie Burrows, 2 High Garth, Richmond, North
Yorks DL10 4DG, Tel. 0748-823867

Fabry's Disease Research Group
Mrs Carol Lummon, PO Stores, Leake Commonside,
Boston, Lincolnshire PE22 9QQ, Tel. 0205-870223

Facial Disfigurement: Changing Faces
Mr James Partridge, 27 Cowper Street, London EC2A 4AP,
Tel. 071-251-4232, Fax. 071-251-1610

Disfigurement Guidance Centre
Mrs Doreen Trust, PO Box 7, Cupar, Fife KY15 4PF,
Tel. 0334-839-084, Fax. 0334-839-105

Lets Face It
Mrs Christine Piff, 10 Wood End, Crowthorne, Berkshire
RG11 6DQ, Tel. 0344-774405

Junior Lets Face It
Mrs Pearl Fowler, Villa Fontana, Church Rd, Worth,
Crawley, W. Sussex RH10 7RS, Tel. 0293-885901

Fanconi's Anaemia; F.A.B. UK
4 Pateley Road, Woodthorpe, Nottingham NG3 5QF,
Tel. 0602-269634

Hereditary Haemorrhagic Telangiectasia: Telangiectasia Self Help Group
Mrs Diana Lawson, 39 Sunny Croft, Downley,
High Wycombe, Buckinghamshire HP13 5UQ,
Tel. 0494-528047

Hypomelanosis of Ito Support Group
Mrs Eileen Atkinson, 30 Grange Rd, Bury, Lancashire BL8
2PE, Tel. 061-797-5204

Lupus UK
Queens Court, 9–17 Eastern Rd, Romford, Essex RM1
3NG, Tel. 0708-731251

Marfan Association
Mrs Diane L Rust, 6 Queens Rd, Farnborough,
Hampshire GU14 6DH, Tel. 0252-547441/617320,
Fax. 0252-523-585

Research Trust for Metabolic Diseases in Children
Lesley Greene, Golden Gates Lodge, Weston Road,
Crewe, Cheshire CW1 1XN, Tel. 0270-250221,
Fax. 0270-250244

The Society for Mucopolysaccharide Diseases
Christine Lavery, 7 Chessfield Park, Little Chalfont,
   Buckinghamshire HP6 6RU, Tel. 0494-762789

Naevus Support Group
Ms Renata O'Neill, 58 Necton Rd, Wheathampstead,
   Hertfordshire AL4 8AU, Tel. 058-283-2853

The Neurofibromatosis Society (Link)
Colonel Jon Blackwell, 120 London Rd, Kingston-
   upon-Thames, Surrey KT2 6QJ, Tel. and
   Fax. 081-547-1636

Noonan Syndrome Society

12d Low Street, Cheslyn Hay, Walsall, Staffordshire WS6
   7HP, Tel. 0922-415500

The Primary Immune Deficiency Association
PO Box 1490, Halstead, Essex CO9 2SW, Tel. 0787-478299

The Psoriasis Association
Mrs Linda Henley, Milton House, 7 Milton Street,

Northampton NN2 7JG, Tel. 0604-711129,
   Fax. 0604-792-894

Sturge–Weber Foundation (UK)
Mrs Lynn Buchanan, 53 Brookland Road West, Old Swan,
   Liverpool L13 2BG, Tel. 051-220-5290

Tuberous Sclerosis Association of Great Britain
Mrs Janet Medcalfe, Little Barnsley Farm, Catshill,
   Bromsgrove, Worcester B61 0NQ, Tel. 0527-71898

The Vitiligo Society
Mrs Margaret Bown, 97 Avenue Rd, Beckenham, Kent
   BR3 4RX, Tel. 081-776-7022

Reference

*The CaF Directory of Specific Conditions and Rare
Syndromes in Children with their Family Support
Networks*, published by Contact a Family, 16 Strutton
Ground, London SW1P 2HP, Tel. 071-222-2695,
Fax. 071-222-3969.

GLOSSARY

Acrocentric a chromosome in which the short arm is a mere satellite, and the centromere is very close to one end (chromosomes 13,14,15,21,22 and Y). These chromosomes are susceptible to **Robertsonian translocation,** in which the short arms are lost and the long arms join up at the centromere.

Allele one of a pair of genes.

Aneuploidy deviation from disomy; for example, monosomy, trisomy, tetrasomy, etc., due to failure of a pair of chromosomes to separate during meiosis (**nondisjunction**).

Anticodon see **transfer RNA.**

Anticipation earlier onset of a genetic disorder in successive generations, particularly shown by myotonic dystrophy where it is due to increasing numbers of **trinucleotide repeats.**

Antisense DNA the strand of DNA that acts as the template for mRNA. The other DNA strand of the double helix is considered 'sense' because its sequence is identical (not complementary) to the mRNA product. Exogenous antisense DNA introduced into cells mops up the mRNA: a technique useful experimentally and therapeutically.

Antisense RNA RNA formed by transcription of sense DNA. This can hybridize with and inactivate the normal mRNA, providing an internal regulatory mechanism.

Autosome any chromosome other than X and Y.

Barr Body nuclear inclusion seen in any individual with more than one X chromosome. It represents the inactive X chromosome. See **X-inactivation.**

Blotting the transfer of molecular material from an agarose gel to a nitrocellulose filter, which can be baked to immobilize the material. This process links two important techniques, **restriction enzyme digestion** and **hybridization.**

Southern blot single-stranded DNA fragments are blotted, then hybridized with labelled DNA probes.

Northern blot mRNA is blotted then hybridized with labelled DNA probes.

Western blot protein is blotted then stained, or 'hybridized' with specific antibodies (immunoblot).

Dot or Slot blot not strictly a blot, as material (usually genomic single-stranded DNA) is applied directly to the filter for hybridization. Used to detect presence or absence of a particular DNA sequence but gives no information on size or position of the sequence.

CCAAT box see **promoter sequence.**

Centimorgan the distance separating two loci that show recombination in 1 out of 100 gametes (i.e. $\theta = 0.01$). It represents about 1 million base pairs, but cannot be converted exactly to a physical distance because recombination events are not uniformly distributed (e.g. hotspots at the telomeres).

Chimaera an individual composed of two genetically different cell lines resulting from fusion of two zygotes, or fertilization of an ovum by two sperms (cf. **mosaicism**).

Chromosome painting the use of multiple fluorochromes for **FISH** (see below).

Chorion villus biopsy a technique whereby fetal DNA can be sampled during the first trimester via the cervix or through the abdominal wall.

Clonality the presence of the same genetic constitution in every cell, implying origin in a single cell.

Codominance the terms dominant and recessive apply to gross phenotypes: if, at a molecular level, the products of the two alleles can be distinguished, the genes themselves are codominant.

Codon a three-base sequence or triplet coding for a particular amino acid (See also **stop-codon**).

c(complementary)DNA the expressed segments (exons) of a gene, complementary to the corresponding mRNA (unlike genomic DNA, which contains the introns as well).

Compound heterozygote an individual with a recessive disorder who is homozygous in the sense of having two abnormal alleles, but is heterozygous at the molecular level because there is a different mutation on each allele.

Constitutive not subject to normal control mechanisms.

Contiguous gene syndrome a condition in which overlapping deletions of different sizes give different clinical pictures, due to the loss of different numbers of closely linked genes.

Cosmid an artificial vector for large DNA fragments, composed of plasmid DNA packaged into a phage particle.

Crossing over the normal process of exchange (**recombination**) between the maternal and paternal chromatids during the first stage of meiosis. On average about 52 crossovers occur; one to six per chromosome.

Cytogenetics the microscopic study of chromosomes.

Diploidy the normal complement of 46 chromosomes (two sets of 23), as opposed to **triploidy** (69 chromosomes), **tetraploidy** (92) and **polyploidy** ($23 \times n$). In **myxoploidy** n is variable. these abnormalities are usually lethal antenatally, except **myxoploidy** with a significant number of diploid cells.

Disomy the normal presence of two copies of each chromosome as opposed to **monosomy** and **trisomy** (cf. **aneuploidy**). Normally one is derived from each parent: occasionally both are derived from the same parent (**uniparental isodisomy**) increasing the risk of recessive disorder because of homozygosity of the whole chromosome.

DNA a double-stranded helical molecule composed of deoxyribonucleotide building blocks, i.e. base (adenine, guanine, cytosine and thymine), deoxyribose and phosphate. The sequence of bases along the sugar phosphate backbone is infinitely variable. The two strands are joined by hydrogen bonds between A and T and between C and G, and they separate at these points for synthesis of new complementary daughter strands.

DNA fingerprint Southern blot in which lengths of DNA (**VNTRs**) are hybridized with labelled **minisatellite probes**, generating a pattern unique to each individual, but the same in identical twins.

DNA polymerase enzyme responsible for the synthesis of a new complementary strand of DNA, using uncoiled, single-stranded DNA as template.

Dominant negative effect the phenomenon whereby heterozygosity for a mutation reduces functional gene product by more than 50%, even though a normal allele is present. This may be due to the production of a **nonfunctional heterodimer** as in the case of piebaldism and the **p53** gene.

Dosage analysis a procedure used in gene mapping, whereby involvement of a particular gene in a deletion or duplication is deduced by comparing the level of the gene product with normal.

Exon the expressed DNA sequences of a gene.

Expression (i) biological activity resulting from a gene. All tissues contain the same DNA but express different genes at different times. See **regulation**.

Expression (ii) variation in the penetrant phenotype (see **penetrance**).

FACS (fluorescence-activated chromosome sorter) used to separate individual chromosomes for purposes of mapping or preparation of libraries.

FIGE (field inversion gel electrophoresis) see **pulsed field gel electrophoresis**

FISH (fluorescent *in situ* hybridization) a mapping technique using *in situ* hybridization, where the DNA probe is labelled with fluorochrome and its chromosomal position visualized under the fluorescence microscope. Probes labelled with fluorochromes of different colours can be used simultaneously to establish the relative positions of different sequences (**chromosome painting**).

Fragile site a chromosome locus with a heritable susceptibility to deletion in the presence of nutritional (usually folate) deficiency in culture. The best known is responsible for **fragile X syndrome**, but at least 10 others have been identified.

Fragile X syndrome the most common cause of inherited mental retardation, in which a fragile site is present at the end of the long arm of the X chromosome. In the most common type there is a **trinucleotide repeat** (CGG).

Frameshift loss of the normal divisions between triplet codons (reading frame), so that although the sequence of bases is unchanged it can no longer be transcribed into amino acids. This is well illustrated by a sentence (= sequence) composed of three letter words (= triplets), when one letter (= base) is omitted (= point mutation) the sentence becomes unreadable; for example, TOM DID NOT SEE THE FOX might become OMD IDN OTS EET HEF OX. (Readers may like to compose a sentence in which the frameshift, like that responsible for haemoglobin Wayne, produces a novel, readable sentence.)

Gamete germ cell (ovum or sperm).

Gene the unit of heredity; a DNA sequence coding for one or more proteins.

Gene cloning amplification of DNA by inserting the required sequence into a vector (usually a plasmid) which will replicate autonomously in a host bacterial cell, providing multiple identical copies of the original sequence. The starting point is a **library.**

Gene tracking see **linkage analysis**.

Genetic code the universal language whereby a specific sequence of three bases in DNA (or corresponding RNA) specifies a particular amino acid. There are four different bases and 64 possible triplets (4^3), but only 20 amino acids, so (like all languages) the genetic code is degenerate having more than one code word for each 'meaning'.

Genotype the unique genetic constitution of an individual.

Giemsa banding in use since 1968, this technique of staining chromosomes in a metaphase spread reveals a pattern of dark and light bands in all the chromosomes (**karyotype**), which is constant in normal individuals. Regions have been divided into bands, sub-bands and sometimes sub-band divisions, all numbered outwards from the centromeres along the long (q) and short (p) arms. Conventional mapping terminology numbers the 22 autosomes in decreasing order of size, and names the divisions as follows: chromosome/arm/region/band/./sub-band/sub-band subdivision, for example, 7q11.22.

Gonadal mosaicism presence of a mutation affecting some but not all gametes. The carrier may be phenotypically normal but can pass on a full-blown disorder. This phenomenon can cause recurrence of an apparently sporadic dominant disorder.

Half chromatid mutation a mistake in DNA polymerization during the first meiotic division of gametogenesis, whereby the wrong base is synthesized at one point, resulting in a mismatched double strand. If this mismatched chromosome is passed on to the next generation, the first time it separates in mitosis it will provide two templates that are not exactly complementary, giving rise to two different lines of daughter cells (**mosaicism**).

Haploid: having only one set of 23 chromosomes (the normal situation in gametes).

Haploid insufficiency a condition in which homozygosity for a **dominant** disorder gives a more severe phenotype than heterozygosity, for example, familial hypercholesterolaemia. In most dominant disorders the clinical expression is the same in homozygous and heterozygous individuals.

Haplotype a group of closely linked alleles inherited as a unit.

Hardy–Weinberg law the frequency of carrier state for a recessive disorder (q) can be deduced from the frequency of affected homozygotes (q^2), for example, cystic fibrosis, $q^2 = 1/2500$ or 0.0004, $q = 0.02$ or $1/50$.

Hemizygous having only one of a pair of alleles, for example, due to deletion of the other allele, or an X-linked gene in a male.

Heterozygous having two different alleles of a gene.

Homozygous having an identical pair of alleles.

Homozygosity mapping a strategy for localizing recessive disorders in affected offspring of consanguineous parents, by mapping homozygous regions and comparing them with those of inbred patients from unrelated families.

Hotspot a locus particularly susceptible to mutation or recombination.

HOX gene homeobox gene involved in organization of embryogenesis.

Hybridization (i) a fundamental concept in **recombinant technology**—the principle that a single strand of DNA will bind only DNA or RNA with the complementary base sequence.

Hybridization (ii) fusion of the nuclei of two species generating a hybrid organism (see **somatic hybridization**).

Imprinting the influence of parental origin on the behaviour of genes, a concept not considered by Mendel. Examples include Huntingdon disease, where inheritance from the father is associated with rigidity rather than chorea, and 15q deletions where mutation of the maternal chromosome 15 produces Angelman syndrome while the same deletion on the paternal 15 gives rise to Prader–Willi syndrome. The mechanism may involve **methylation**.

Initiation codon the triplet ATG near the 5′ end of a gene, indicating the start of the region to be translated. 5′ and 3′ refer to the numbering of carbon atoms in the deoxyribose phosphate backbone.

***In situ* hybridization** a direct method of mapping a DNA segment to a specific chromosomal locus. A labelled cloned DNA sequence (probe), rendered single stranded by heating, applied to a similarly denatured metaphase spread will anneal to its complementary sequence. Excess labelled probe is removed, then the position of the signal is determined by cytogenetic inspection. Tritium has now been superseded as a label by fluorochromes, which give a faster, more precise and easily visualized result (see **FISH**).

Intron the non-translated DNA sequences of a gene.

Karyotype the chromosomal constitution of an individual. The normal male and female karyotypes are 46XY and 46XX. Chromosomal abnormalities detected on **Giemsa banding** are denoted according to established conventions; for example, a balanced translocation in a female, between the short arm of chromosome 1 and the long arm of chromosome 17, with breakpoints at 1p34.3 and 17q11.2 is written 46XX,t(1;17) (p34.3;q11.2).

Library a 'clone bank' containing fragments of DNA, which serves as a source of material for the preparation of various probes. Libraries can be prepared from genomic DNA, DNA from a particular chromosome (obtained by **FACS**) or mRNA from a particular tissue, according to the subject of the study. The DNA is broken down into relatively large fragments and stored in **cosmid** or **YAC** vectors.

Linkage the principle that genes close together on the same chromosome are likely to be transmitted together to future generations because they are unlikely to be separated by **recombination** at meiosis.

Linkage analysis study of the segregation of an inherited disease and other inherited traits within families. It is used (a) to map genes in families where affected individuals and various marker traits can be recognized and (b) in counselling, to predict whether an undiagnosed (e.g. unborn) individual is affected, knowing the segregation of the disease with a linked marker in the rest of the family (**gene tracking**).

Linkage disequilibrium the preferential linkage of particular polymorphisms (not to be confused with ordinary linkage between genetic loci, which is independent of the form of the allele). An example useful in counselling is the mutant cystic fibrosis gene which is preferentially associated with haplotype B of an RFLP tightly linked to the cystic fibrosis locus.

Locus position on a chromosome.

Lod score a term derived from 'logarithm of the odds'. It is a measure of whether two genetic markers are linked or segregating independently within a particular family (see **linkage**). The lod score is calculated for different values of θ the **recombination fraction**. The question that the lod score answers is 'supposing these two markers are closely linked (e.g. θ = 0.1), what is the logarithm of the odds (lod score) of finding by chance the number of recombinations seen in this family?' An answer of more than 3 means that the observed values would occur only once in 10^3 times, i.e. there is close linkage. This is repeated for other values of θ from 0 (inseparable) to 0.5 (no linkage at all). The value of θ giving the highest lod score greater than 3 indicates the distance between the two loci. Results from more than one family can be combined simply by adding the lod scores, increasing the significance of the study.

Loss of heterozygosity somatic mutation involving a previously normal allele, conferring homozygosity for a recessive trait. This is found in some tumours in individuals heterozygous for a cancer-prone mutation; for example, patients with the dominant disorder familial polyposis coli are heterozygous for a mutation at the FAP locus on chromosome 5, and their tumours show homozygosity for this mutation.

Lyonization random **X inactivation**. Mary Lyon proposed the idea that in each female cell only one X chromosome is active, the other having been inactivated early in embryogenesis (see **Barr body**). Whether the paternal or maternal X chromosome is inactivated is random, but once the choice has been made it is the same in all daughter cells.

Marker see **polymorphism**.

Meiosis the particular form of cell division that occurs in the gonads and produces gametes. In the first stage, crossing over occurs between paternal and maternal chromosomes, and in the second the chromosome number is reduced from diploid to haploid.

Methylation a mechanism of gene suppression involving the covalent linkage of ($-CH^3$) to carbon 5 in cytosine in DNA, at sites where cytosine is followed by guanine. Degree and distribution of methylation within the genome are inherited. Methylation is implicated in: (1) X inactivation, the inactive X chromosome being hypermethylated; (2) differentiation, demethylation being a way of switching on a gene; (3) imprinting, as maternal genes are more methylated than paternal genes.

Minisatellite probe a DNA probe that hybridizes with the repeating unit of a **VNTR** (variable number tandem repeat), used in **DNA fingerprinting**.

Missense mutation a base substitution leading to generation of a different amino acid.

Mitochondria cytoplasmic bodies which may have originated from bacteria captured early in evolution. Each contains a circular chromosome of which there may be thousands of copies within a cell. The mitochondrial DNA codes for enzymes involved in the respiratory chain and oxidative phosphorylation.

Mitochondrial inheritance all the cytoplasm of the zygote comes from the ovum and none from the sperm, so inheritance of mitochondrial DNA and its disorders (e.g. Leber's optic atrophy) is matrilineal.

Mosaicism the coexistence of genetically different cell lines within an individual or organ, the abnormal clone or clones having arisen by mutation (cf. **chimaerism**).

Multifactorial disorder a condition for which there appears to be a genetic predisposition interacting with environmental factors (e.g. psoriasis and eczema).

Multiplexing amplification of different DNA sequences by simultaneous **PCRs**.

Mutation a change in genetic constitution that can involve a large part of the genome (e.g. **aneuploidy**), a large part of a chromosome, a whole gene, or a single nucleotide (point mutation). Gene mutations can affect the coding sequences (exons), or the removal of introns (RNA splice mutations), or other regulatory functions; for example, promoter sequence mutations. Different forms of mutation include **missense**, **nonsense**, **stop-codon** and **frameshift**. The same mechanisms that produce pathogenetic mutations are responsible for the variability in DNA used in linkage studies; for example, RFLPs and VNTRs.

Naevoid (i) linear, presumably due to a mutant clone of epidermal cells that migrated embryologically along Blaschko's lines.

Naevoid (ii) round and dome-shaped like a naevocytic (melanocytic) naevus; for example, naevoid basal-cell carcinoma syndrome.

Non-disjunction the failure of chromosomes to separate during either meiosis or mitosis, resulting in daughter cells with too many or too few chromosomes.

Non-functional heterodimer some gene products dimerize in order to function, in which case a mutation on one allele may produce a product that can still dimerize but the dimeric product is non-functional, thus mopping up the normal monomer, reducing function to less than 50% (**dominant negative effect**).

Nonsense mutation a point mutation that converts an amino acid specifying codon to a stop-codon. The opposite is a **stop-codon mutation**.

Oligonucleotide probe synthetic DNA fragments corresponding to part of a gene, capable of recognizing point mutations.

Oncogene a gene that can undergo a mutation rendering it capable of inducing tumours. Oncogenes were first discovered in retroviruses (v-*onc*); homologues of viral oncogenes were then found to be part of the vertebrate cell's normal genetic machinery (cellular oncogenes, or c-*onc*). Because v-*onc*s are thought to derive originally from vertebrate c-*onc*s, the latter are sometimes called proto-oncogenes.

Oncogenesis activated (i.e. mutant) oncogenes cause cancer by encoding any of the following: (a) growth factor; (b) growth factor receptor; (c) factors conveying messages from cell surface to nucleus; (d) mediators of DNA transcription.

P53 a tumour suppressor gene on 17p whose 53 000 molecular weight product binds DNA thus regulating growth. *P53* mutations, particularly homozygous deletion, are the most common mutations found in tumours. Even heterozygosity for a *P53* mutation can cause cancer as the mutant product forms non-functional heterodimers with the product of the normal allele (a **dominant negative effect**).

PCR (polymerase chain reaction) a rapid *in vitro* technique for producing millions of copies of a selected region of the genome. PCR can amplify DNA of known or unknown sequence provided the flanking sequences are known. First, genomic double-stranded DNA is denatured by heat. Next it is cooled to allow two oligonucleotide probes, one complementary to one end of the sense strand and the other complementary to the other end of the antisense strand, to anneal to the native DNA. These primers are extended on to the unknown region using a thermostable DNA polymerase, yielding two complete complementary strands. The primers are present in excess, so this process can be repeated 20 or 30 times by alternately heating and cooling, the amount of the required sequence doubling every time.

Penetrance whether or not a gene is detectable phenotypically. It is 'all-or-nothing' for an individual, unlike **expressivity** which refers to variation in the penetrant phenotype.

Phage a virus that inserts itself into the bacterial genome.

Phenotype biological appearance resulting from a particular **genotype.**

Plasmid a simple organism that normally lives in the cytoplasm of bacteria.

Polymorphism a variable genetic trait used in linkage studies. Examples include: the presence or absence of a disease; sex; a biochemical or immunological variable such as glucose-6-phosphate dehydrogenase (G6PD) type or blood group; the sequence of a particular DNA segment (DNA polymorphism); the length of a DNA fragment between cutting sites for a particular restriction enzyme (RFLP).

Positional cloning cloning of a gene of unknown sequence (usually a disease gene) by mapping it to a particular chromosome region by linkage studies, then using more closely linked markers to define the candidate region to be cloned. This technique is used in **reverse genetics.**

Primer an oligonucleotide probe complementary to a short segment of DNA on to which DNA polymerase can synthesize the adjacent segment of DNA.

Promoter sequence a sequence at the 5′ end (upstream) of a gene indicating to RNA polymerase the start of a region to be transcribed; for example, CCAT and TATA boxes.

Pulsed Field gel electrophoresis (PFGE) a method of separating segments of DNA larger than 50 kb that all electromigrate through agarose gels at the same rate because they move end-on. Switching between two perpendicular electric fields realigns the molecules and slows down the larger ones. A variation on this is **field inversion gel electrophoresis** in which the two fields are at 180°.

Recombinant a cell or individual in which crossing over has occurred so that two genes previously on the same chromosome are now on different chromosomes.

Recombinant technology see **hybridization**

Regulation control of gene transcription in different cells and at different times is mediated by a variety of mechanisms including alteration of chromatin structure, **methylation, promoter sequences** and DNA binding proteins (**regulatory sequences**).

Regulatory sequences a large family of genes coding for binding proteins that regulate gene expression, such as zinc fingers.

Restriction enzyme a bacterial endonuclease that cuts DNA at a specific site, usually a sequence of four to six bases, which recurs several times in the genome. Over 1000 are now available. An example is *Hinf*I (named after its source, *Haemophilus influenzae* strain f).

Restriction fragment length polymorphism (RFLP) variation between individuals in the length of a DNA sequence between two cleavage sites for a particular **restriction enzyme.**

Retrovirus a virus that enters a host cell, transcribes its RNA into double-stranded DNA using a reverse transcriptase, then integrates this DNA into the host's genome.

Reverse genetics establishing the molecular basis of a disorder by: (a) linkage analysis to map the gene; (b) cloning the candidate region (**positional cloning**); (c) inferring the amino acid sequence of the gene product in normal and affected individuals.

Ribosome a cytoplasmic organelle that mediates **translation** by moving along mRNA allowing anticodons of a **tRNA** to recognize appropriate codons in mRNA.

RNA a molecule similar to **DNA** except that the sugar is ribose not deoxyribose and RNA contains uracil in place of thymine. Antisense DNA is transcribed into RNA, from which the introns are then removed leaving mRNA. mRNA is then stabilized at the 5′ end by a 5′5′ pyrophosphate link (CAP) and at the 3′ end by the attachment of a polyadenylate tail, before moving out of the nucleus.

RNA splice mutation mutations in genomic DNA at intron–exon boundaries preventing normal RNA **splicing**. The regions concerned in splicing are donor and acceptor sites, and consensus sequences.

Robertsonian translocation the long arms of two **acrocentric** chromosomes joined together at the centromere.

Splicing the removal of introns and joining together of exons to form mRNA.

Single-strand conformation polymorphism (SSCP) a method for detecting point mutations.

Somatic mutation a mutation occurring after conception (i.e., postzygotic) rather than in gametogenesis.

Somatic cell hybridization an important mapping technique whereby human cells are fused with rodent cells. The resultant hybrids are passaged and preferentially lose human chromosomes. Eventually the line stabilizes with a predominantly rodent karyotype containing one or more fragments of human chromosome, which can be identified cytogenetically. Several lines are isolated and their functional properties *in vitro* (indicating the presence of particular genes) can be correlated with the presence of particular chromosome fragments.

Stop-codon a triplet indicating the end of the translated region of a gene.

Supergene family a large number of specialized genes of common ancestry; for example, the immunoglobulin genes.

TATA box a **promoter sequence**.

Telomeres the stabilized, non-sticky ends of chromosomes.

Theta (θ) the recombination fraction, i.e. the frequency of crossovers between two genes, ranging from 0 (if they are inseparable) to 0.5 if they are unlinked (e.g. on different chromosomes).

Topoisomerase nuclear enzymes involved in packaging of chromatin. They are targets for a variety of antibiotic and antimitotic agents.

Transcription the production of mRNA from DNA.

Transfection the transfer of functional DNA from one organism to another.

Transfer RNA (tRNA) a short segment of RNA carrying an amino acid and an anticodon (recognition site for the appropriate triplet codon).

Transgenic mouse animal containing a foreign gene inserted into the male pronucleus at conception.

Translation the production of protein from mRNA.

Translocation a form of mutation in which chromosomes are broken and the sticky, broken ends join together incorrectly.

Trinucleotide repeats three nucleotide bases that are repeated serially; for example, CGGCGGCGG etc. These occur at various loci in normal individuals, the number of repeats being increased in certain disorders, and sometimes correlating with severity; for example, at the myotonic dystrophy locus CTG repeats 5–27 times in normals, 50–100 times in mildly affected patients, up to 1000 in severe adult-onset disease and more than 1000 in affected babies. Progressive increase in successive generations may explain **anticipation**.

Triplet see **codon**.

Tumour suppressor gene a gene, deletion of which allows a tumour to develop.

Two-hit hypothesis the idea that tumours occurring sporadically and in dominant cancer syndromes (e.g. Wilm's tumour) are due to mutation in both alleles of a tumour suppressor gene; either both alleles undergo sporadic mutation, or one mutation is inherited and the other occurs by chance.

Variable number tandem repeat (VNTR) a block of DNA in which a short sequence (nine to 70 base pairs) is repeated, the number of repeats differing between individuals. Restriction enzymes that cut outside the repeat region thus generate different-sized fragments in different individuals, which can be detected on a Southern blot using a **minisatellite probe**. This is the basis of **DNA fingerprinting**.

Wild type the form of an allele found in the normal population.

X inactivation a mechanism for 'dosage compensation', which avoids females having a double dose of X-linked genes (see **lyonization**). However, two X chromosomes are required early on in embryogenesis, otherwise XO individuals would be normal. The mechanism is unknown but probably involves an inactivation centre near the centromere, which sends a signal along both arms. The steroid sulphatase gene at the end of the short arm is not completely inactivated. In patients with X-autosome translocations the translocated X is preferentially active, presumably to avoid spread of the inactivation signal to the autosome, with serious loss of genes more vital than those on the X chromosome.

Yeast artificial chromosome (YAC) a vehicle for large fragments of DNA used in cloning. The target DNA is introduced into a plasmid containing a centromere and two telomeres from a yeast, generating a synthetic chromosome.

Zinc finger a type of DNA-binding domain found on some regulatory proteins. It contains zinc, with amino acids jutting out like fingers.

INDEX